# THE SOCIOECONOMIC DIMENSIONS

## OF

## HIV/AIDS IN AFRICA

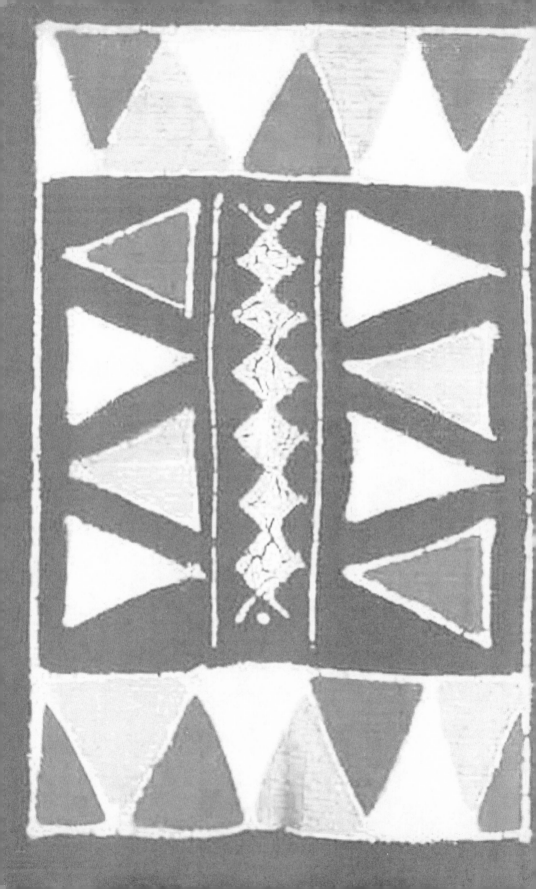

# THE SOCIOECONOMIC DIMENSIONS

## OF

## HIV/AIDS IN AFRICA

*Challenges, Opportunities, and Misconceptions*

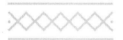

*edited by*

DAVID E. SAHN

PUBLISHED IN COOPERATION

WITH THE

UNITED NATIONS UNIVERSITY

CORNELL UNIVERSITY PRESS    ITHACA AND LONDON

Copyright © 2010 by Cornell University

First published 2010 by Cornell University Press in cooperation with the United Nations University

Printed in the United States of America

Library of Congress Cataloging-in-Publication Data

The socioeconomic dimensions of HIV/AIDS in Africa : challenges, opportunities, and misconceptions / edited by David E. Sahn.
    p.   cm.
    "Published in cooperation with the United Nations University."
    Includes bibliographical references.
    ISBN 978-0-8014-7693-8 (pbk. : alk. paper)
  1. AIDS (Disease)—Social aspects—Africa, Sub-Saharan.
  2. AIDS (Disease)—Economic aspects—Africa, Sub-Saharan.
  3. HIV infections—Economic aspects—Africa, Sub-Saharan.
  4. HIV infections—Social aspects—Africa, Sub-Saharan.
  I. Sahn, David E. II. United Nations University. III. Title.
    RA643.86.A357S63 2010
    362.196′97920096—dc22

2010033351

# CONTENTS

# FIGURES

# TABLES

# FOREWORD

This is the second volume of the Africa Series, a collaborative initiative involving leading scholars from around the globe that addresses some of the most intractable societal challenges that impede efforts to reduce poverty and sustain development on the African continent. The primary goal of the series is to generate new insights and knowledge that will inform the establishment of policies that facilitate progress towards achieving the Millennium Development Goals for sub-Saharan Africa, and to provide a platform for sharing best practices in the unique African context. The project brings together two academic institutions, the United Nations University and Cornell University, which share a common commitment to original scholarship that enhances the capacity of people, governments, and institutions to improve human health and well-being.

HIV/AIDS remains one of the greatest threats to the people of sub-Saharan Africa and is certainly amongst the greatest contemporary threats to global public health. The pandemic has revealed the hubris and stark limitations of modern western medicine, and fundamentally questions our understanding of human behavior and our ability to affect individual and societal change, even when human life at its prime is at risk on a massive scale. In this volume, the authors offer unique perspectives and collectively provide an evidence base that questions conventional wisdom which continues to inform current public policies focused on controlling the spread of HIV/AIDS, including the wide dissemination of antiretroviral drugs. The tension between the seemingly complementary approaches of treatment and prevention is highlighted from multiple perspectives, including their comparative effectiveness and sustainability. The authors indicate new directions for future resource allocations and offer a roadmap for new research in the social and behavioral sciences that will be essential to ensure Africa's future.

There are many individuals responsible for the success of this volume and the related symposia held at the United Nations in New York City. Foremost, the authors and symposium speakers, each internationally renowned in his or her area of expertise, provided the intellectual contributions that are the foundation of this initiative. The organization and content areas of the volume directly reflect the inspiration and vision of David Sahn, and I am grateful for his steadfast commitment to this project. The Africa Series was conceived by Jean-Marc Coicaud of the United Nations University, New York, who has played an essential role in developing this project. The funding for this volume and the symposia was generously provided by the Turkish Mission to the United Nations, UNAIDS, the World Food Programme, the World Health Organization, the United Nations University, and Cornell University through the Division of Nutritional Sciences. I would also like to extend my appreciation to the devoted staff of the United Nations University including Sara Shapiro of the Food and Nutrition Programme, and Luna Abu-Khadra and Jin Zhang from the United Nations University's New York City office.

Patrick J. Stover
*Director, Division of Nutritional Sciences, Cornell University*
*Director, United Nations University Food and Nutrition Programme for*
*Human and Social Development*

# ACKNOWLEDGMENTS

XXXXXXX

I am grateful to several individuals and institutions that contributed in a variety of ways to the publication of this book. First, I would like to acknowledge the support of the United Nations University. Patrick Stover, the chair of the United Nations University (UNU) Food and Nutrition Program and director of the Division of Nutritional Sciences at Cornell University, and Jean-Marc Coicaud, the director of the UNU office in New York City, provided the vision and resources that enabled me to organize the symposium held at the United Nations headquarters in New York City that was the source of many of the papers included in this volume. Additionally, they have been instrumental in bringing this volume to fruition and guiding the publication process.

I would also like to express my appreciation to the contributors to this volume. It has been my privilege to work with such a committed and extraordinary group of scholars, all of whom were patient and responsive throughout the process of organizing the symposium and preparing the manuscript for publication. A large number of anonymous reviewers also contributed greatly to the quality of the book. I also am deeply grateful to Patricia Mason. Her tireless work editing the manuscript, communicating with authors, and preparing the book for publication was truly an extraordinary effort. I am humbled by her professionalism and enduring friendship.

# ABBREVIATIONS

×××××××

| | |
|---|---|
| ACASI | Audio computer-assisted self-interview |
| AFASS | Acceptable, feasible, affordable, sustainable, and safe |
| AIDS | Acquired Immune Deficiency Syndrome |
| AMPATH | Academic Model Providing Access to Healthcare |
| ANC | Antenatal clinic |
| ANRS | French National Agency for Research on AIDS |
| ART | Antiretroviral Therapy |
| ARV | Antiretroviral drug |
| ASCI | AIDS, Security and Conflict Initiative |
| CGE | Computable General Equilibrium |
| CHAP | Children with HIV Antibiotic Prophylaxis (randomized trial) |
| CHGA | Commission on HIV/AIDS and Governance in Africa |
| CHS | Community and Household Survey |
| CPOL | Community popular opinion leader |
| DALYs | Disability-Adjusted Life Years |
| DFID | United Kingdom Department for International Development |
| DHS | Demographic Health Surveys |
| FAO | United Nations Food and Agriculture Organization |
| GAVI | Global Alliance for Vaccines and Immunisation |
| GDP | Gross Domestic Product |
| GFATM | Global Fund to Fight AIDS, Tuberculosis and Malaria |
| GHP | Global Health Partnership |
| GUD | Genital ulcer disease |
| HAART | Highly Active Antiretroviral Therapy |
| Hb | Hemoglobin |
| HIV | Human Immunodeficiency Virus |
| HMIS | Health Management Information System |
| HSV-2 | Herpes Simplex Virus Type 2 |
| IAS | International AIDS Society |
| IDU | Injecting drug user |
| IFPRI | International Food Policy Research Institute |
| IHP+ | International Health Partnership and Related Initiatives |
| IMAGE | Intervention with Microfinance for AIDS and Gender Equity Project, South Africa |

| | |
|---|---|
| IOM | Institute of Medicine |
| IPV | Intimate partner violence |
| JFFLS | Junior Farmer Field and Life Schools |
| KHDS | Kagera Health and Development Survey |
| KIDS | KwaZulu-Natal Income Dynamics Study |
| LMICs | Lower and middle income countries |
| M&E | Monitoring and evaluation |
| MAP | Multi-country AIDS Program of the World Bank |
| MaSoSHA | The Malawi Social Science and HIV/AIDS Research |
| MC | Male circumcision |
| MCH | Maternal and child health |
| MDG | Millennium Development Goals |
| MDICP | Malawi Diffusion and Ideational Change Project |
| MLSFH | Malawi Longitudinal Study of Families and Households |
| MOH | Ministry of Health |
| MOS-HIV | Medical Outcomes Study HIV Health Survey |
| MSM | Men who have sex with other men |
| MTCT | Mother-to-Child Transmission |
| NAC | National AIDS Commission |
| NIC | U.S. National Intelligence Council |
| NIH | National Institutes of Health |
| ODA | Offical development assistance |
| OECD | Organisation for Economic Co-operation and Development |
| OGAC | Office of the Global AIDS Coordinator |
| PEPFAR | U.S. President's Emergency Plan for AIDS Relief |
| PMTCT | Preventing mother-to-child transmission |
| PMU | Project Management Unit |
| PYO | Person-years of observation |
| RCT | Randomized controlled trial |
| RENEWAL | Regional Network on AIDS, Livelihoods and Food Security |
| SACU | South African Customs Union |
| SADC | Southern African Development Community |
| SFTF | U.S. State Failure Task Force |
| SGBVE | Sexual and gender-based violence and exploitation |
| SHAZ! | Shaping the Health of Adolescents in Zimbabwe Program |
| STD | Sexually transmitted disease |
| STI | Sexually transmitted infection |
| SW | Sex worker |
| SWAp | Sector-wide approach |
| TASO | The AIDS Support Organization |
| TRIPS | Trade-Related Aspects of Intellectual Property Rights |

| | |
|---|---|
| UNAIDS | Joint United Nations Programme on HIV/AIDS |
| USAID | United States Agency for International Development |
| VCT | Voluntary counseling and testing |
| VL | Viral load |
| WFP | World Food Programme |
| WHO | World Health Organization |
| WTO | World Trade Organization |

# INTRODUCTION

Since HIV/AIDS came into the public spotlight in the 1980s, it has occupied a singular position because of the rapidly emergent threat and devastation the disease has caused, particularly in sub-Saharan Africa. The grim statistics are readily available and speak for themselves: the latest estimates, for 2008, suggest that 33.4 million people presently are infected, and their numbers continue to grow, beyond the 2 million people who died of the disease in the previous year. New infections continue to create a formidable challenge to households, communities, and health systems: last year alone, 2.7 million new infections occurred globally. Sub-Saharan Africa remains the epicenter of the suffering with around two-thirds of infected individuals worldwide found there, and correspondingly, with a disproportionate number of deaths and new infections.

Across the continent, the ravaging effects of HIV/AIDS are quite unequally distributed along numerous dimensions, including, in particular, geography—with Southern Africa by far hit the hardest, and West Africa the least afflicted. Within countries, there are important differences by demographic characteristics and socioeconomic status as well. In Southern African countries, the toll of the disease has taken on enormous proportions. In Swaziland, life expectancy has fallen by half, and in South Africa and Zimbabwe, prevalence rates hover between 15 and 20 percent. Within countries, there is also wide geographic variability. For example, there is a 15-fold greater probability of being infected with HIV in Nyanza province than the North Eastern province of Kenya (UNAIDS 2009a). Women, aged 15 to 25, are particularly vulnerable, as are women of all ages who are divorced or separated. Their heightened risk indicates the role gender and gender inequality in power within relationships are likely to play. It is also well known that individuals engaged in certain occupations or living situations are especially vulnerable, including commercial sex workers, migrants, and truck drivers. While across regions of the globe and across countries within Africa, HIV/AIDS prevalence is positively associated with poverty, within countries in Africa, it is the better off and better educated who are more likely to be infected, reflecting urban residence of the better off but also the greater access to sexual partners that comes with higher income. This clearly differentiates HIV/AIDS from other leading causes of death in Africa, such as malaria, tuberculosis, and upper-respiratory infections, which disproportionately affect the poor.

For years there have been widespread and concerted efforts to prevent the spread of HIV/AIDS, identify a cure, and understand and mitigate the deleterious social and economic ramifications of the disease. Guarded scope for optimism is found in some recent statistics, even for hard-hit sub-Saharan Africa. Deaths are being delayed by the rollout of, and rapidly increasing access to, antiretroviral drugs (ARVs). Among those fortunate enough to receive the drugs, their impact, measured by declines in mortality, has been dramatic. Similar strides are being made to increase access to voluntary counseling and testing (VCT) services, although the benefits of such services are far less clear. In most countries, awareness of the causes of HIV/AIDS is now high. Further, and most importantly, there have been declines in risk behaviors (as self-reported in surveys) as well as prevalence in a number of countries, beginning early on with Uganda but now recorded in other countries such as Kenya and Zimbabwe. Despite these efforts and some apparent successes, there is still a long way to go in terms of altering behaviors in order to realize the objective of dramatic reductions in the spread of HIV/AIDS in Africa (Glick and Sahn 2007, 2008).

The context of a persistent HIV/AIDS crisis in Africa, despite major strides in averting deaths due to antiretroviral therapy (ART), motivates this volume. The objective is to tell an important story of the distinct nature of the disease, its socioeconomic implications, as well as to assess the misconceptions and evidence on the results of efforts at controlling its spread and impact. The various chapters focus on the most salient socioeconomic dimensions of HIV/AIDS in the region. The perspectives captured in this book are unique in several ways. Most important, the chapters examine the new realities of HIV/AIDS, in an era of growing availability of antiretroviral drugs that are now providing a realistic hope for significantly extending life while offering an opportunity for a vast improvement in quality of life and ability to function. Unlike in upper income countries, the prospects of treatment for those who are infected are relatively new to Africa. Only a few years ago, coverage was less than 5 percent of the infected population; at present, ART is reaching nearly 50 percent of those with AIDS. It is in this context of rapidly expanding access to antiretroviral therapy that the implications of HIV/AIDS across a multiplicity of dimensions need to be revisited. This includes considerations ranging from how access to treatment might affect the spread of the disease, efforts at prevention, the livelihoods of families and the future prospects of children, gender relations, and the economic vitality of countries and communities. There is a need to consider the potentially harsh fiscal realities of paying for costly treatment programs, and the implications of such efforts for a broad range of institutions, ranging from international organizations to local health delivery systems, in countries now on the front lines of the battle against HIV/AIDS.

In exploring these issues, this book also takes a step back to examine, and in many respects, to challenge some of the conventional wisdom about the spread, consequences, and potential control of the disease. It thus looks at the response and implications of a late twentieth-century pandemic that challenged governments and the public health establishment in new ways, as the disease itself invoked fears and provoked misconceptions in a public that remains confused by its origins, consequences, and control. How governments, international institutions, communities, households, and individuals confronted this new and unexpected pandemic is thus one theme of this book. While the global burden of other more traditional communicable diseases such as malaria, diarrheal disease, and respiratory infection have proven relentless and formidable health challenges in Africa, the rapid emergence of HIV/AIDS and the heightened attention that it has commanded often overshadows these other killers, and even contributes to the neglect of other public health needs in Africa. Several contributors to this book argue that the emotional and reflexive reaction to this new threat contributed to the obfuscation of some fundamental truths about who gets AIDS, why, its implications, and what can be done to combat the social and economic consequences and causes of the epidemic. One objective of this book, therefore, is to reflect upon what has made HIV/AIDS appear exceptional, examining this question from a range of disciplinary perspectives, including anthropology, economics, epidemiology, political science, and sociology. In doing so, the authors discuss lessons learned and their implications as we move forward to combat HIV/AIDS and mitigate its consequences. This evaluation is especially important as the perceptions of the disease are rapidly evolving from being a death sentence to a chronic disease. Still, like other life-threatening and untreated ailments that affect the poor in Africa, access to antiretroviral drugs remains uneven and unpredictable.

While this collection is not intended to be contentious, distilling some of the lessons learned about the efforts to combat HIV/AIDS in Africa and ameliorate its consequences forces us to take a hard look at the expectations and prospects for controlling the disease, as well as to objectively assess prior experience in addressing this tragedy. The careful analytic work in this book is directed at helping us to better understand and circumscribe the socioeconomic dimensions of HIV/AIDS in Africa, about which there remains a great deal of conjecture and anecdote, despite the growing body of evidence and knowledge that has emerged in recent years, some of which is compiled in this volume.

The first few chapters of this volume focus on the causes and consequences of HIV/AIDS. This includes an examination of the macro level implications, as well as those that look at the more microeconomic implications of HIV/AIDS. In the case of the former, Markus Haacker points out that while HIV/AIDS is often thought of as the most prominent health threat to emerge in recent history, causing dramatic reductions in health outcomes such as life expectancy in many countries, the macroeconomic implications have been modest. Likewise, Haacker notes that the macroeconomic evidence seems, at first glance, to be inconsistent with the microeconomic picture, including that discussed in later chapters in this volume. Several reasons may explain this seeming contradiction. Enterprises with high value added per employee may be able to cushion the shocks from high rates of HIV/AIDS in the population, unlike those at the bottom end of the income distribution or in the informal sector, who contribute little to GDP. Also, average incomes mask distributional effects across households, with losses to households affected by HIV/AIDS offset by improved employment opportunities to other households. Thus, even when impacts on GDP are not substantial, HIV/AIDS may contribute to increases in poverty and inequality, an outcome that is also conditioned by the shape of the income distribution and the socioeconomic characteristics of those afflicted. Of course, the rollout of ART reverses some of the economic impacts of HIV/AIDS, mitigating losses in output and productivity. But once again, distributional impacts may arise, especially to the extent that those at the lower end of the income distribution are less likely to get access to therapy. Indeed, there is some evidence that the more educated, urban, and better-off households are the first to receive treatment, the same groups that are more able to absorb the economic shocks associated with the disease.

The concern of the potentially deleterious macro level impacts of HIV/AIDS goes beyond economics and includes the prospect of the pandemic contributing to political destabilization and social fragmentation. This was a concern that was shared by local political elite, foreign powers, and international institutions worried about potential security threats, such as the prospect of increased terrorism. These concerns are the subject of the contribution to this volume by Alex de Waal. As HIV/AIDS began to inflict a devastating toll on the population, many voiced concern that this would in turn contribute to state crisis. Manifestations such as the collapse of and disarray among armies and police forces, (which in many countries are high-prevalence groups), in turn could contribute to an even broader violent conflict. While de Waal tells the story of social and political collapse averted, he also notes that at the local level, state institutions have not been immune from disruption related to the AIDS crisis in Africa. And, at the national level, while the epidemic has generally not become a major political and electoral issue, even in South Africa where the former president denied the link between HIV and AIDS, it has had important implications internationally. These range from the case of Uganda, where the president's aggressive prevention policies were in part used to burnish his image abroad, to the international health diplomacy of both developed countries and international organizations. Likewise, the HIV/AIDS crisis has given rise to a new importance for activism of civil society and grassroots organizations that have played key roles as partners of the state and international efforts to combat the disease.

In the case of the micro perspectives, Kathleen Beegle, Markus Goldstein, and Harsha Thirumurthy explore both the direct economic impacts of HIV/AIDS in terms of declines in productivity and loss of income, as well as impacts on future-oriented socioeconomic behaviors. The latter may result in a range of adverse outcomes, as an array of decisions are impacted in dimensions such as investment choices that affect asset accumulation and decisions regarding investment in the education and health of children and other household members. They make an important distinction between the behavioral response and socioeconomic consequences of those changes during the initial period in which an individual is initially diagnosed but is not yet suffering the physical ravages of disease; the subsequent period of illness when an individual's productivity and income are directly affected; and the period after the individual's death when the legacy of the disease may affect the well-being of surviving family members. The authors thus focus not just on the affected individual, but also on how his or her behavior and those of others have consequences for non-infected members of the family and extended community. Perhaps the most dramatically distinguishing characteristic of HIV/AIDS is that the prime-age disabling morbidity and premature mortality due to HIV/AIDS contributes to hardships for children, regardless of whether they are infected themselves. But again, important caveats exist to the likelihood and consequences of being orphaned, such as the differential effects by socioeconomic groups and the nature of social networks and relationships.

In keeping with the general theme of this book, this chapter highlights how the provision of ART has altered the landscape in terms of thinking about the economic impact of HIV/AIDS. There is conclusive evidence that treatment reduces mortality and has strong positive impacts on labor supply and productivity as well as the nutrition and schooling outcomes of children in treated adults' households. Likewise, there are many variables that will affect the size of the microeconomic impacts of ART, such as when treatment begins. For example, Beegle, Goldstein, and Thirumurthy point out that if treatment occurs earlier in the disease cycle, the effects on labor supply will be lower, as will the losses associated with pretreatment morbidity. Such considerations have important policy implications, such as how aggressively testing strategies should be pursued.

Despite the successful nature of treatment, access to lifesaving pharmaceuticals remains limited and the challenges of expanding coverage daunting—thus, the importance of also according priority to policies and programs that mitigate the long-term negative impact of HIV/AIDS on family members, and especially, on orphans that are left behind. This same reasoning applies to prevention programs. To date, however, there is a paucity of empirical evidence on the effectiveness of such efforts, including various forms of cash transfers and programs targeting orphans, as well as prevention efforts such as information campaigns and male circumcision. Likewise, the potential role of other types of interventions, such as nutrition programs and microfinance, to both reduce the probability of infection and mitigate its consequences must be considered as competing options in combating the spread and consequences of the disease. Beegle, Goldstein, and Thirumurthy thus emphasize the need for more rigorous evaluations of these efforts. In the final analysis, they come back to one of the main themes of this book—that we need to concentrate on reducing the numbers of new infections and mitigating the consequences of illness, and not let those priorities be over-shadowed by the successful treatments now available.

Suneetha Kadiyala and Antony Chapoto focus on the relationship between HIV/AIDS and food security and nutrition, and how this has changed in recent years with the introduction of ART. They briefly address the deleterious synergism between HIV/AIDS and malnutrition, noting that both afflictions compromise the immune system and reduce the ability to fight infection and ward off disease. Thus, there is in essence a vicious nutrition-HIV cycle which, until recently, could only be partially addressed through nutrition-related interventions that mitigated to a modest extent the harsh consequences of this downward spiral.

As with other aspects of the pandemic, the nature of the interactions between HIV/AIDS and nutrition and food security has changed dramatically in the era of ART. Notably, nutrition has an important impact on the success of ART, and at the same time, ARVs can contribute to substantial improvements in nutritional status. But from a socioeconomic perspective, the deleterious impact of HIV/AIDS on rural livelihoods, agriculture, and non-farm income and assets are emphasized by Kadiyala and Chapoto. Of particular concern is the prospect for irreversible and adverse outcomes across generations that result from the AIDS epidemic. The emerging, albeit still very limited, evidence, however, suggests that the availability of ART will have positive impacts on labor market outcomes, rural livelihoods, and so forth, as the drug therapy becomes more available in rural areas. Perhaps no impact is more important than the pervasive poverty that has been in part caused by the AIDS epidemic in rural Africa.

While ART is clearly a crucial element in improving productivity and employ-ment, numerous challenges remain. These include reducing constraints that have limited the rollout of, and access to, the ARVs. Indeed, while ART improves pro-ductivity, there remain numerous barriers to re-entry into the work force and to redressing the loss of assets and earnings that result from having AIDS, even as an individual's health improves. But even when labor market outcomes are less than what would be desired, ART improves household welfare by other mecha-nisms, such as enabling labor reallocation away from caregiving to the sick to pro-ductive activities and enabling investments in children's schooling and nutrition. Despite the emerging evidence on the bi-directional relationship between nutri-tion and food security and the AIDS epidemic, a far greater understanding is required of the extent to which nutrition and agricultural interventions will mit-igate the harsh socioeconomic consequences of HIV, and how efforts to control HIV/AIDS will contribute to improved livelihoods, especially in rural areas.

In considering the appropriate response to the spread of HIV/AIDS, the role of education is highlighted in the chapter by Damien de Walque and Rachel Kline. Based on an empirical study of several countries in sub-Saharan Africa as well as review of prior research in this area, they note that the impact of education on the probability of contracting AIDS is ambiguous. Education, for example, may reduce risky sexual practices as it increases understanding of the connection between behavior and outcomes. On the other hand, the more educated have wider social and sexual networks, which may be a risk factor, as will the greater income associated with higher educational attainment, particularly for men. In considering why the association between HIV and education is so weak in the six countries' data they analyze, they point out that there are likely countervailing behaviors operating: that the more educated are more likely to use condoms, but also more likely to have sexual partners outside of marriage. Additionally, the results reported by the authors are suggestive of an evolving epidemic, where education is a factor in responding earlier and faster to the dissemination of knowledge. Perhaps more important is that the relationship between education and HIV status is not static, and in fact, amenable to change through programs and policies. For example, interventions aimed at teenagers have successfully altered sexual behaviors, as have school-based programs designed to raise incentives for students to remain in school longer. Thus, it seems likely that there is a shift from a positive to negative gradient between education and HIV, as more educated individuals who initially had more resources, traveled more, and thus engaged in more risky behaviors have more rapidly incorporated information about risks into their behavior.

While these previous papers take a hard look at empirical evidence derived largely from survey data, they are complemented by Susan Watkins's examination of the of the conventional wisdom that women are particularly vulnerable to the ravages of HIV/AIDS in Africa, as well as the role that gender relations is assumed to play in the spread of the disease. More specifically, Watkins takes a close look at the evidence on the widely held notion that women and, even more so, young women, are of greater vulnerability to HIV/AIDS than are males. Statistics from various sources do indeed suggest that *younger* women have higher rates of infection than younger men. Watkins, however, points to a number of reasons why the reported sex ratios in infection at younger ages, which are calculated from surveys, may be misleading. These range from bias arising from differences in refusal to get tested to a simple demographic explanation: in a growing population (where fertility is higher than mortality), each birth cohort is larger than the one that preceded it. Since women are infected with HIV at younger ages than men, it would be expected that at ages 15–24, more women would be infected than men even in the absence of norms or any physiological differences that made women particularly vulnerable. She concludes that, in some high-HIV prevalence countries, the gender ratio of new infections changes across age cohorts, from higher incidence among young women than young men to higher incidence among older men than older women. Indeed, there is compelling evidence that over the entire spectrum of ages, men are as likely to contract HIV as women.

But more central to Watkins's chapter is her effort to gain a better understanding of the explanation for the widespread misconception that women are particularly vulnerable to HIV because of gender inequality and women's lack of empowerment, especially with respect to control over sexual relationships. The nearly universal perspective of international organizations and AIDS researchers has been focused on the ideas that dominant males refuse to wear condoms, perpetrate sexual violence, and subordinate women in their sexual relationships; this is nowhere more acute than in the case of cross-generational sex where young girls suffer in silence. Here again, the careful work of Watkins and colleagues in rural Malawi challenges this view, as she finds little evidence that intergenerational sex and sexual violence contribute to the epidemic in this high-prevalence country. Extensive reviews of existing programs and studies that attempt to protect women from HIV/AIDS, through various empowerment and related programs designed to alter sociocultural norms in gender relations, provide virtually no evidence that such programs achieve this goal. And even more troubling is the evidence that rural women in Malawi, even those who are HIV positive, disagree with the "AIDS exceptionalism" of the donor community: they would prefer that more resources go to everyday problems such as clean water and agricultural development than to AIDS programs.

It is not only in terms of the micro pictures where there is a great deal of contentious debate in terms of how governments and international institutions have responded to the disease. Chapter 7 by Roger England presents a provocative discussion of the "exceptionality" of the nature and institutional response to HIV/AIDS. His argument is quite straightforward: that the response of the international community to HIV/AIDS has been out of proportion to the threat that the disease has, and continues to pose to the public health. This imbalance has led to a range of distortions in terms of health priorities and has contributed to substantial inefficiencies in the health sectors of countries in the region. Thus, HIV/AIDS has cut with a double-edged sword: being a devastating disease, but one that has contributed to the neglect of health challenges out of all reasonable proportion. The policy implications that England draws from his analysis are profound and suggest the need for a major rethinking of the role of international aid in not just the fight against HIV/AIDS in Africa, but in terms of overall priority setting and resource allocation. In that context, he raises a rather controversial issue of whether too many scarce resources, both financially and institutionally, are being committed to ART that has proven so effective in improving longevity and the ability of affected individuals to lead fuller and more productive lives.

Mead Over's chapter on the costs associated with antiretroviral therapies picks up on that point and expands on the future implications of meeting the needs of the population infected with HIV/AIDS in Africa. Indeed, the evidence about the life-prolonging benefits of treatments now available to an increasing number of Africans is overwhelming. Well over a million lives have been saved through the highly successful President's Emergency Plan for AIDS Relief (PEPFAR), whereby the United States continues to provide medicine to millions of Africans who would otherwise be facing certain and painful deaths that would leave their children without parents, their families without a vital source of income, and their communities facing even more economic stress from the loss of otherwise productive members of society. These irrefutable benefits, however, come into conflict with some stark realities: the escalating treatment costs are financially unsustainable; they have partly come at the expense of failed efforts to promote measured focus on prevention; and there is the emerging prospect that funding PEPFAR will not only be at the expense of other health priorities but runs the risk of crowding out the entire foreign assistance budget. Indeed, the prospect of what Over refers to as a grand global "entitlement" program was not the original intent of PEPFAR. But in light of the constellation of factors that led to this reality, he argues for strong and urgent actions to forestall what is likely to be an unsustainable global welfare program whose success in the present will likely breed future failure. To begin, there is a need to better manage the treatment entitlement, including reducing unit costs and limiting the share of antiretroviral treatment that is supported by the United States Treasury. Likewise, far greater effort is required to find and fund innovative treatment options.

The opportunities and prospects for prevention of new infections in adults, and how prevention efforts may be impacted by the emergence of effective treatment for HIV-positive individuals are taken up in a number of contributions to this volume. Peter Glick points out that resources for prevention have grown far more slowly than for treatment in recent years and remain grossly inadequate. While this reflects a number of factors, the lack of clear success or understanding about what works in prevention remains a major challenge. In his chapter, Glick thus explores the evidence for three classes of interventions: biomedical, that focus on blocking infection or decreasing infectiousness; behavioral, that seek to reduce risk; and structural, that attempt to alter the underlying social and economic contexts of HIV risk. The overall conclusions of Glick's review are sobering. With the exceptions of partner reduction campaigns and male circumcision, few interventions—including control of other STIs, HIV testing and counseling, condom promotion, programs targeting students or youth, microbicides, and microcredit programs for women—have proven consistently effective. While structural interventions (including microcredit to empower women) are generating considerable enthusiasm, evidence for these interventions remains slim. Finally, the impacts of ARV provision on prevention—and in particular, the possibility of "treatment optimism" leading to greater risk behaviors—have not been adequately explored. Glick notes, however, that despite the lack of compelling evidence for the effectiveness of many prevention initiatives, at least as stand-alone interventions, there remains an important role for efforts such as condom promotion to prevent transmission within serodiscordant couples or sexually active single people, or school-based programs that target messages of risk reduction to youth. In the final analysis, achieving sustained behavioral change and avoiding unintended effects, such as compensation in risk behaviors that may result from the widespread availability of lifesaving pharmaceuticals or perceived effectiveness of circumcision, remains a very formidable challenge. It will require multi-pronged national strategies that are context specific as well as greater commitment of leaders, both at the national and community levels. Further, in order to provide a better evidence base for policy, there is a need for a renewed commitment to rigorous research on prevention programs discussed in Glick's chapter. This includes using a range of modern evaluation techniques, as well as focusing greater attention on the impacts of combinations of strategies.

Elizabeth Pisani further elucidates the complexity of the nexus between treatment and prevention with her probing examination of the epidemiology of the disease. She reaches a disturbing conclusion that the expansion of treatment will contribute to more new infections in the absence of invigorated and more successful efforts at prevention. Pisani reaches her conclusion after examining issues of infectiousness related to virology, co-infection, and health service access, as well as various behavioral considerations. The evidence suggests that, on the one hand, rapid and widespread treatment programs will reduce viral loads, and thus the transmission of the disease from an infected person to another during unprotected sex or through sharing of needles. However, these benefits are likely to be outweighed by the fact that there will be a large increase in the number of people living with HIV/AIDS, coupled with the fact that those infected often view the disease as both chronic and inconvenient but not a deterrent to engaging in risky behaviors. While the evidence that Pisani draws upon to reach this conclusion is largely from outside of Africa, she makes a compelling argument that, if anything, this pessimistic scenario is more likely in Africa than elsewhere. For example, the high prevalence of untreated sexually transmitted diseases in Africa increases the likelihood of transmission; and similarly, to the extent that the compliance with drug regimes is lower in Africa, this will also increase the risks associated with the interrupted use of ARVs.

The intended audience for this book is wide and diverse. It includes academic audiences from a range of disciplines, including public health, economics, epidemiology, political science, sociology, and anthropology. In addition, the book is written in a way that will be accessible to those professionals from a wide range of occupations and from internationally focused institutions working on and interested in the broader questions of economic and social development in Africa. This includes health care professionals, as well as economists, program planners, and so forth. But perhaps the most important audience will be non-professional readers who have a general interest in understanding and improving the living standards and well-being of the poor, particularly those in developing countries. Here are lessons and insights that we gain from examining the saga of HIV/AIDS in Africa, in and of itself a compelling story of human tragedy and suffering, and the strenuous efforts being made to understand and control its consequences.

# CHAPTER 1

## HIV/AIDS, Economic Growth, Inequality[1]

*Markus Haacker*

## I. Introduction

The evolving HIV epidemic can be considered as the most significant adverse health development in modern history. In many countries, it has reversed gains in life expectancy and related health indicators that had been achieved over many decades. However, the impacts of HIV/AIDS on key macroeconomic indicators, such as economic growth and income per capita, have been modest so far. This chapter reviews the available evidence on the macroeconomic impacts, discussing the interactions between the economic impact of HIV/AIDS and the structure of the economy. In particular, we will argue that a high degree of inequality mitigates the impacts of HIV/AIDS on economic growth and income per capita, while (and because) HIV/AIDS tends to exacerbate inequality.

As a point of reference for our analysis, Section II provides a brief review of the impact of HIV/AIDS on demographic and health indicators, as well as a discussion of the contribution of HIV/AIDS to the burden of disease.

Section III reviews the available evidence on the impacts of HIV/AIDS on economic growth, and contrasts it with the literature on health and growth, as well as the more specific studies analyzing the impacts of HIV/AIDS on growth. Empirical studies typically find a small impact of HIV/AIDS on growth, and this finding is matched by growth analyses in a neoclassical mold in which some adverse impacts of HIV/AIDS (productivity, population growth) are offset by an increase in the capital-labor ratio. We relate these outcomes to the broader growth literature, in which health (usually measured by life expectancy) is frequently used as a proxy for human capital and a determinant of productivity.

Section IV discusses the interactions between the macroeconomic impact of HIV/AIDS and the structure of the economy. Specifically, we will argue that the structure of many economies with high HIV prevalence (which is associated with high degrees of income inequality) mitigates the macroeconomic impacts of HIV/ AIDS, owing to their dual character and—in some countries—the prominent role of resource extraction in the formal sector. We will argue that the increased availability of antiretroviral therapy (ART) has strengthened this link between the structure of the economy and macroeconomic impacts of HIV/AIDS.

Some (but not all) of the mechanisms described in Section IV imply that, while (and because) inequality mitigates the impacts of HIV/AIDS on growth, HIV/AIDS exacerbates inequality through its asymmetric impacts across sectors and households. This issue is developed further in Section V.

Section VI discusses the findings from our analysis. Most generally, our analysis underlines that the impact of HIV/AIDS on growth is not a good measure of its development impacts. This has been observed by other analysts—it does not require rocket science (or growth analysis) to see that the declines in life expectancy associated with HIV/AIDS signify a development catastrophe. Our analysis, however, goes a step further, suggesting that the apparent small impacts of HIV/ AIDS on economic growth so far mask distributional effects which are problematic in their own right.

## II. Demographic and Health Impact of HIV/AIDS

A full discussion of the demographic and health impact of HIV/AIDS is beyond the scope of this chapter. However, a brief review of some demographic and health aspects of the impact of HIV/AIDS is useful to provide some context for our economic analysis, and because economic studies build on these direct impacts of HIV/AIDS. Specifically, we review the impact of HIV/AIDS on life expectancy in a global context, discuss the impacts of HIV/AIDS on the rate of population growth, illustrate the age profile of HIV/AIDS-related mortality, and address the contribution of HIV/AIDS (and other diseases) to the burden of disease.

Figure 1.1A illustrates the impact of HIV/AIDS on life expectancy, based on estimates by the United Nations Population Division (2009a, 2009b). After life expectancy in sub-Saharan Africa had grown roughly in line with the global average between 1965 and 1985, the growth rate of life expectancy essentially dropped to zero between 1985 and 2005, with an increase of only 0.8 years between the 1985–90 period and the 2000–05 period. Evidently, this decline can be attributed to HIV/AIDS, as the declines are highly correlated with HIV prevalence on the country level (as illustrated by Figure 1.1B, showing developments in life expectancy in countries with high HIV prevalence).[2]

To understand the magnitude of this slowdown, it is important to bear in mind that it took place in the context of otherwise positive trends on the global level; consequently, the gap in life expectancy between sub-Saharan Africa and the global

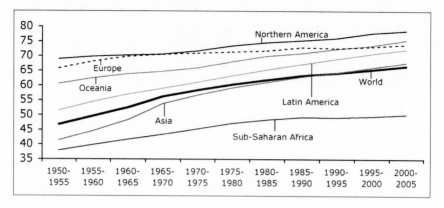

*Figure 1.1a*    Life Expectancy at Birth, by Period and Major World Region (Years)
SOURCE: United Nations Population Division (2009b).

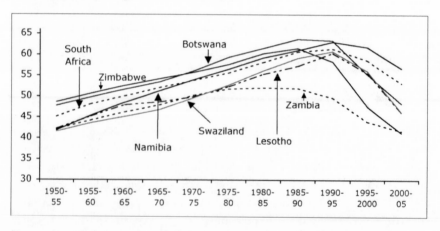

*Figure 1.1b.*    Life Expectancy at Birth, in Seven Countries with High HIV Prevalence
(Years)
SOURCE: United Nations Population Division (2009b).

average increased from 13.4 years in 1980–85 to 16.4 years in 2000–05. [3] Another useful point of reference is the estimation of changes in life expectancy that would have occurred in the absence of HIV/AIDS, produced by United Nations Population Division (2009b). These estimates suggest that life expectancy in sub-Saharan Africa would have improved by 5.7 years between 1985–90 and 2000–05 in the absence of HIV/AIDS. This means that the estimated small increase in actual life expectancy of 0.8 years masks an average decline of about five years across sub-Saharan Africa owing to HIV/AIDS, more than offsetting the positive health developments in other areas over this period.

One well-known aspect of HIV/AIDS is the fact that HIV prevalence and mortality are concentrated among the economically most active age groups. This is illustrated in Figure 1.2 for Zambia, a country with an estimated HIV prevalence

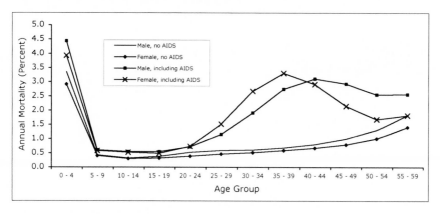

*Figure 1.2*    Zambia: Mortality by Age and Sex, 2000–05
SOURCE: Author's calculations based on United Nations Population Division (2009b).

of about 15 percent among the population of ages 15–49, which compares to an average of 5 percent for sub-Saharan Africa (UNAIDS 2008a,b).

The estimates by United Nations Population Division (2009b), summarized in Figure 1.2, imply that overall mortality (population weighted) almost doubles from 1.1 percent to 1.9 percent for females, and that it increases from 1.2 percent to 2.0 percent for males. The increase is most pronounced between ages 15 and 49, where annual mortality increases from 0.5 percent to 1.6 percent for females, and from 0.6 percent to 1.4 percent for males. HIV/AIDS-related mortality for women peaks at an earlier age (30–34) and at a higher level than for males, reflecting an earlier average age of infection and somewhat higher HIV prevalence among women.

An immediate consequence of increased mortality is a decrease in the rate of population growth. Additionally, increased morbidity and mortality among women result in a decline in reproduction rates, reinforcing the slowdown in population growth.[4] According to the estimates of the United Nations Population Division (2009b), the slowdown in population growth has been dominated by increased mortality so far. For Malawi, for example, the estimates suggest that population growth in 2000–05 is 0.8 percent lower (3.4 percent rather than 2.6 percent) as a consequence of HIV/AIDS, reflecting an increase in mortality of similar magnitude (from 1.0 percent to 1.8 percent).

One useful point of reference regarding the mortality and health impact of HIV/AIDS are the Global Burden of Disease estimates produced by the WHO (2008b), because they can be used to place HIV/AIDS in the context of other diseases, and as they also include estimates of "disability-adjusted life years" (DALYs) lost owing to various diseases or other reasons. Overall, WHO (2008b) estimates that the contribution of HIV/AIDS to mortality in sub-Saharan Africa amounted to about 14 percent of the total burden of disease, accounting for 1.7 million

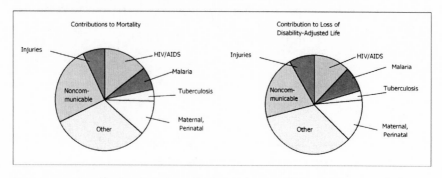

*Figure 1.3*   Sub-Saharan Africa: Contributions to Burden of Disease, 2004
[a] Contributions to Mortality
[b] Contribution to Loss of Disability-Adjusted Life Years
SOURCE: Data from WHO (2008b).

out of a total of 11.7 million deaths.[5] In terms of the loss in DALYs, the contribution of HIV/AIDS is less pronounced, at about 12 percent of the total. The less than proportionate role of HIV/AIDS in terms of lost DALYs primarily reflects that infant mortality accounted for only about 14 percent of HIV/AIDS-related deaths, whereas it accounted for 41 percent of deaths overall.

Regarding the age profile of HIV/AIDS-related deaths, the estimates produced by WHO (2008b) broadly match those included in United Nations Population Division (2009b). The role of HIV/AIDS-related mortality is most pronounced in the 30–44 age bracket, where HIV/AIDS-related mortality accounted for 40 percent of mortality among men and 56 percent of mortality among women.

Another important aspect of the health impact of HIV/AIDS regards the distinction between mortality and morbidity (or death and disability, in WHO diction). For HIV/AIDS, the years lost to disability play a subordinate role (9 percent of DALYs lost), similar to malaria and tuberculosis where years lost to disability account for 11 percent and 10 percent, respectively, of the loss in DALYs. These rates are markedly different from those for maternal conditions or non-communicable diseases where years lost to disability account for about half of the loss in DALYs.

## III. Health, HIV/AIDS, and Growth

Our discussion now turns to the available literature on the impact of HIV/AIDS on growth. We proceed in three steps. First, we look at recent trends in economic growth in countries with high HIV prevalence, and check if we can—literally— see the growth impact of HIV/AIDS. This discussion is complemented by some empirical analysis. Second, we discuss some of the literature on health and growth, which might be directly relevant, but also motivates research focusing on the economic impacts of HIV/AIDS. Finally, we review the literature specifically addressing the impacts of HIV/AIDS on growth.

## HIV/AIDS and growth—some data

Figure 1.4 illustrates trends in the growth rates of real GDP (Figure 1.4A) and real GDP per capita (Figure 1.4B) from 1990–2007 for the 10 countries with the highest HIV prevalence rates at the end of 2005 (all in sub-Saharan Africa).[6] We do not

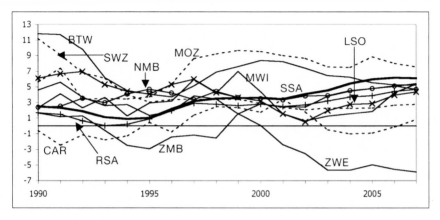

*Figure 1.4*    Growth Trends in 10 Countries with High HIV Prevalence, 1990–2007. BTW–Bowswana, CAR–Central African Republic, LSO–Lesotho, MWI–Malawi, MOZ–Mozambique, NMB–Namibia, RSA–South Africa, SWZ–Swaziland, ZMB–Zambia, ZWE–Zimbabwe, SSA–Sub-Saharan Africa (Includes 10 countries shown).

*Figure 1.4a*    Growth of Real GDP (Average annual growth in 5-year period ending in year indicated)

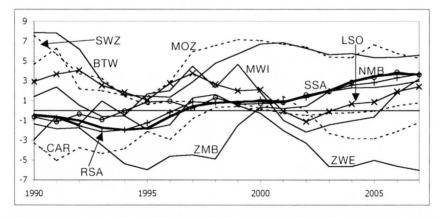

*Figure 1.4b*    Growth of Real GDP per Capita (Average annual growth in 5-year period ending in year indicated)

SOURCE: Data from IMF (2009).

see a dramatic decline in real GDP growth in countries with high HIV prevalence, although the data suggest that growth in these 10 countries may have decelerated somewhat relative to the average for sub-Saharan Africa, where growth has increased during the period shown. Regarding changes in GDP per capita, the picture is similar (Figure 1.4B). This seems counterintuitive at first sight, as HIV/AIDS results in a decline in population growth, so that the growth of GDP per capita in countries with high HIV prevalence should accelerate relative to GDP growth. However, many of the countries with high HIV prevalence are further advanced in the demographic transition, with higher life expectancies (before the arrival of HIV/AIDS) and lower fertility rates than the average for sub-Saharan Africa. For this reason, the rate of population growth, over the 1990–2007 period, declines less in the countries with high HIV prevalence than in the rest of sub-Saharan Africa.

Taking a closer look at the data presented in Figure 1.4, it appears that some of the largest swings in GDP growth shown are arguably not related to HIV/AIDS. Growth in Swaziland is high in the early years shown because it benefited from foreign direct investment serving the South African market until the end of apartheid, but the country has lost this competitive advantage. GDP growth in Botswana is dominated by the diamond sector, the production of which has plateaued for geological reasons (and preceding the escalation of the HIV epidemic in that country); and the collapse in economic growth in Zimbabwe in the later years shown is attributed by most observers to the adverse impact of economic policies.

### Health and growth

The study of the impact of health on growth is complicated by an apparent interdependency between health and income.[7] Additionally, the correlation between health and growth (or income) may reflect underlying factors that affect both health and growth (Deaton 2006). While this issue is rarely acknowledged explicitly in the broader growth literature, it is an important issue in some of the recent literature addressing specifically the impacts of health on productivity and growth.

A useful workhorse for conceptualizing the impact of health on growth (and one frequently referred to in the relevant literature) is the framework developed by Mankiw, Romer, and Weil (1992) which augments the classical Solow growth model by allowing for accumulation of *human* as well as physical capital, with an aggregate production function of the form

$$Y_t = K_t^{\alpha} H_t^{\beta} (A_t E L_t)^{1-\alpha-\beta}, \tag{1}$$

where $Y$, $K$, $H$, and $L$ stand for aggregate output, the stock of physical capital, the stock of human capital, and the size of the labor force.[8] One addition to the

Mankiw-Romer-Weil (MRW) framework that we introduce is an efficiency parameter $E$, which stands for the effectiveness of labor inputs, in addition to a productivity parameter $A$ capturing technological progress (assumed to grow at rate $g$).
Dividing through by effective units of labor $AEL$, the production function becomes

$$y_t = k_t^\alpha h_t^\beta , \tag{2}$$

where $y_t \equiv \dfrac{Y}{AEL}$, $k_t \equiv \dfrac{K}{AEL}$, and $h_t \equiv \dfrac{H}{AEL}$. The accumulation of $k$ and $h$ is
described by

$$\dot{k}_t = s_k y - (n + g + \delta_k)k , \text{ and} \tag{3}$$

$$\dot{h}_t = s_h y - (n + g + \delta_h)h . \tag{4}$$

This means that the accumulation of physical capital (relative to effective units
of labor) depends on investments (= savings, $s_k$) in physical capital and a term
that captures the depreciation of physical capital $\delta_k$ and the dilution that occurs
through growth $n$ in the size of the labor force $L$ and technological progress (with
$A$ growing at rate $g$). The terms in the equation describing the accumulation of
human capital are defined correspondingly.

One further extension to the MRW framework is embodied in Eqs. (3) and (4),
as we allow the depreciation rates of physical capital ($\delta_k$) and human capital ($\delta_h$)
to differ. Specifically, we think of $\delta_h$ as the mortality rate among the population,
with the following reasoning (abstracting, for a moment, from technological
progress $g$): To maintain some capital-labor ratio, it is necessary to make investments to increase the capital stock by the same rate as the population growth rate
$n$. However, *human* capital is embodied in people. To retain a constant level in $h$,
it is therefore necessary to make investments $s_h y$ to bring new entrants to the
labor force "up to speed" with their peers. The rate at which new workers enter
the labor force is equal to the (net) growth rate of the labor force $n$, plus the rate
at which new entrants replace workers who died, $\delta_h$, which motivates our interpretation of the depreciation rate for human capital.

To link key parameters of the growth model to health indicators, it makes
sense to operate in terms of birth rates and mortality rates, rather than the rate
of population growth (affected by births and deaths) and mortality. We therefore
define the birth rate $\mu$ and the mortality rate $\omega$. The parameters of the growth
model are linked to these demographic/health variables as $n = \mu - \omega$, and $\delta_h = \omega$.
Substituting for $n$ and $\delta_h$, in Eqs. (3) and (4) yields

$$\dot{k}_t = s_k y - (\mu - \omega + g + \delta_k)k , \text{ and} \tag{5}$$

$$\dot{h}_t = s_h y - (\mu + g)h. \tag{6}$$

Solving Eqs. (2), (3), and (4) for the steady state level of output per efficiency unit yields

$$y_t^* = \left( \frac{s_k}{\mu - \omega + g + \delta_k} \right)^{\frac{\alpha}{1-\alpha-\beta}} \left( \frac{s_h}{\mu + g} \right)^{\frac{\beta}{1-\alpha-\beta}}. \tag{7}$$

Additionally, one could be interested in output per capita (Y/L), which—along the steady-state growth path—follows

$$\left( \frac{Y}{L} \right)^* = AEy_t^* = AE \left( \frac{s_k}{\mu - \omega + g + \delta_k} \right)^{\frac{\alpha}{1-\alpha-\beta}} \left( \frac{s_h}{\mu + g} \right)^{\frac{\beta}{1-\alpha-\beta}}. \tag{8}$$

In the framework described by Eqs. (1) – (6), changes in health can affect the steady-state level of output along numerous channels:

1) An increase in mortality rates would increase GDP per capita through its impact on the accumulation of physical capital (Eq. (5)). As more people depart from the labor force, the capital/labor ratio increases.
2) A decline in birth rates would raise GDP per capita through its impact on physical capital accumulation, as the existing capital stock is less diluted by new arrivals (Eq. (5)). At the same time, it would become less expensive to sustain a given level of human capital; alternatively, for given investment rates in human capital, the steady state level of $h$ would rise (Eq. (6)).[9]
3) A decrease in the (average) efficiency of labor $E$, as a result of a deteriorating health state among the population, would decrease $Y/L$.
4) A decline in the investment rate in physical capital, to accommodate higher health expenditures or reflecting a deteriorating economic outlook, would result in a decline in the steady-state capital stock and output per capita.[10]
5) A decline in the investment rate in human capital would result in a decline in $h$. In addition to the factors noted for physical capital, the decline in human capital could also reflect a more pessimistic outlook regarding the expected returns to human capital (which decline as expected mortality increases).
6) Additionally, a decline in the health outlook may reduce the steady-state growth rate $g$, for example, if there is a feedback effect from human capital to the rate of technological progress.

In the literature on determinants of growth, health is typically discussed in the context of human capital. Barro and Sala-i-Martin (1995) adopt "an empirical framework that relates the real per capita growth rate to . . . the stock of human capital in the forms of educational attainment and health," proxied by life expectancy at birth (421). Bosworth and Collins (2003) largely equate human capital with educational attainment, but also include life expectancy "as a measure of health." Weil (2004) discusses health as one of the forms of human capital (the other being education), and provides some discussion of the interactions of health and income (with higher income also "buying" better health), and of the links between climate, disease, and productivity.

More recently, Durlauf, Johnson, and Temple (2005) find that life expectancy appears as the most common "health indicator" used in the literature; others include the prevalence of malaria and survival rates (i.e., the probability of reaching some age $y$, starting at age $x$). Caselli (2005, 709), in his discussion of "accounting for cross-country income differences," finds that, "a correction for differences in health status is a first-order requirement in the measurement of human capital," when the adult mortality rate is used as a health proxy. Another health-related variable discussed by Caselli (2005) is "experience," i.e., the average level of work experience among the population, a variable that is influenced by demographic and health variables.

The analysis by Bloom, Canning, and Sevilla (2004) is based on a similar framework as the one outlined above, using a measure of human capital that includes educational attainment (years of schooling, $s$); health (life expectancy, $h$); and "experience" of the workforce. They suggest that "a one-year improvement in a population's life expectancy contributes to an increase of 4 percent in output" (11).[11]

Bhargava and others (2001) focus on the link between growth and the adult survival rate (i.e., the probability of surviving to age 60 after reaching age 15), which arguably is a better measure of health as it relates to productivity since it excludes child mortality. They find a positive effect of adult survival rates on GDP growth only for low-income countries. Lorentzen, McMillan, and Wacziarg (2005) suggest that mortality is an important determinant in explaining growth (the coefficients cannot easily be interpreted, as three different measures of mortality are included in the regressions), and that adult mortality may affect fertility rates, physical capital investment rates, and school enrolment.[12]

Weil (2007) is among the more recent studies adopting approaches that take into account the endogeneity of health outcomes. His approach involves transforming available estimates from microeconomic and historical studies on the link between height and labor productivity into estimates of more commonly used health indicators like adult survival rates.[13] Weil finds that health differences account for about 10 percent of the cross-country variation in income. Acemoglu and Johnson (2006) address the issue of interdependency of health outcomes and income by focusing on declines in mortality that can be attributed to the international epidemiological transition that began in the 1940s (i.e., changes in mortality that can be arguably attributed to medical innovations rather than economic factors). They find no evidence suggesting that the large exogenous increase in life expectancy led to a significant increase in per capita economic growth in the longer run.

A number of papers have developed a more explicit analytical framework focusing on the impact of changes in mortality on human capital accumulation and growth. Kalemli-Ozcan, Ryder, and Weil (2000) develop a model in which an agent's decisions to invest in human capital depend on the anticipated mortality. They suggest that the negative impact of increased mortality on schooling would double the elasticity of steady-state output with respect to changes in the mortality rate. Kalemli-Ozcan (2002) proposes that an increase in mortality also results in an increase in demand for children and a decline in investment in each child. Another study linking mortality, educational attainment, and fertility, along similar lines, is Soares (2005), although his paper is not primarily geared toward the growth implications.

## Health and growth

The adverse health impacts of HIV/AIDS have motivated a body of literature dealing specifically with the growth impacts of HIV/AIDS. The discussion of the links between health and growth already provides many pointers regarding the economic impacts of HIV/AIDS, and indeed motivates much of the applied literature in this area. However, the findings of that literature do not necessarily translate directly to the study of the impacts of HIV/AIDS, as the health consequences of HIV/AIDS are different from health developments underlying the literature on health and growth.

The empirical evidence regarding the effects of HIV/AIDS on economic growth is weak. One early study, Bloom and Mahal (1997), does not find any impact of HIV/AIDS on growth,[14] while Mahal (2004), updating this earlier work, finds a negative (but insignificant) impact. McDonald and Roberts (2006) specify a model in which child mortality enters growth regressions as an explanatory variable, and in turn depends on HIV prevalence. Their estimates imply that an HIV prevalence of 10 percent initially reduces growth by 1.2 percent, and that this effect is highly persistent. Similarly, Dixon, McDonald, and Roberts (2001, 2002) and Bonnel (2000), specify models in which HIV/AIDS negatively affect economic growth through declining life expectancy. Among recent studies, Papageorgiou and Stoytcheva (2009) find a negative (but very small) impact of reported AIDS cases on growth. Lovász and Schipp (2009) report a negative link between HIV/AIDS and HIV prevalence, but caution that it is not robust.

One striking aspect of the empirical literature on the growth impacts of HIV/AIDS is the fact that the most "successful" approaches adopt indirect approaches (from HIV/AIDS, to life expectancy or mortality, to growth), while the evidence from direct approaches (adding HIV prevalence or mortality to growth regressions) is much weaker. This suggests that misspecification may play a role in the "indirect" approaches, merging one well-established correlation between growth and life expectancy (or mortality) from the cross-country literature with the apparent health impact of HIV/AIDS. Alternatively, the general growth literature may reflect longer-term trends; the discrepancy between the findings from the direct and indirect approaches may, therefore, reflect that the impact of HIV/AIDS has not fully materialized yet.

A number of studies of the impact of HIV/AIDS on the microeconomic level are also relevant for a macroeconomic analysis. Fox and others (2004), and Morris, Burdge, and Cheevers (2001) find evidence regarding the impacts of HIV/AIDS on workers' productivity, although these findings cannot easily be generalized. Regarding access to education, Fortson (2010) finds that areas with a higher level of HIV prevalence experienced a decline in schooling.

The increasing recognition of HIV/AIDS as a serious development issue in the early 1990s has motivated a "first wave" of studies modeling the macroeconomic effects of HIV/AIDS. Two early studies apply a one-sector neoclassical growth model similar to the one outlined above to assess the potential growth impacts of HIV/AIDS in Tanzania (Cuddington 1993a) and Malawi (Cuddington and Hancock 1994). Cuddington (1993b) and Cuddington and Hancock (1995) extend the analysis to a dual economy model; Over (1992) also uses a dual-economy framework and allows for different categories of labor inputs (according to skill level). One common feature of these studies is that the size of the impact of HIV/AIDS on GDP per capita is small, as negative impacts on human capital, savings, or productivity are offset by an increase in the capital-labor ratio brought about by increased mortality and the corresponding fall in the rate of population growth.

Most recent work expands the analysis either by introducing a more differentiated sectoral structure, or by including behavioral relationships with important (and sometimes large) implications for the long-run impact of HIV/AIDS.

Kambou, Devarajan, and Over (1992) apply a "computable general equilibrium" (CGE) model to studying the macroeconomic impacts of HIV/AIDS, distinguishing 11 sectors which differ with respect to the intensity of inputs of rural labor, urban unskilled labor, and skilled labor, with a share of skilled labor that ranges from 0 percent (food crops) to 28 percent (public services). They find that the economy appears most vulnerable to shocks to the supply of skilled labor, as this factor is disproportionally used in sectors accounting for a relatively large share of GDP. Arndt and Lewis (2001) and Arndt (2006) follow similar approaches, also including more detailed assumptions regarding the impact of HIV/AIDS on spending patterns (Arndt and Lewis 2001) or discussing policy interventions to offset an adverse impact of HIV/AIDS on access to education. The studies by

Arndt and Lewis (2001, on South Africa) and Arndt (2006, on Mozambique) find a large impact of HIV/AIDS on GDP growth, reflecting strong assumptions on the impact of AIDS incidence on productivity growth.[15] Thurlow, Gow, and George (2009, focusing on KwaZulu-Natal) complement the analysis with a discussion of the impact of HIV/AIDS across households.

A number of studies (Ellis, Laubscher, and Smit 2006; ING Barings South African Research 2000; and Laubscher, Visagie, and Smit 2001) have adapted large macroeconomic models designed for economic policy analysis to the study of the economic impacts of HIV/AIDS. While the sectoral structure of these models compares to the CGE models described above, they are also designed to capture demand-side effects of HIV/AIDS on GDP (for example, owing to increased demand for health expenditures), but return similar impacts of HIV/AIDS on growth as the CGE models.[16] Ellis, Laubscher, and Smit (2006) is also noteworthy, because it is one of the few studies available that explicitly addresses the economic implications of increasing access to ART.

Several recent studies have explored more complex and indirect effects of HIV/AIDS which arise when economic agents adjust their behavior in response to the macroeconomic and disease environment. Understanding these factors is important especially in order to project the long-term economic consequences of HIV/AIDS. Robalino, Voetberg, and Picazo (2002) argue that increased mortality will result in a decline in the savings rate and investment that exceeds any direct effects arising from higher health expenditures. In Corrigan, Glomm, and Mendez (2005), HIV/AIDS also reduces investments in children's education, as higher mortality risk means that parents are less likely to benefit in old age from investments in their children.[17] Bell, Devarajan, and Gersbach (2006) cover similar ground but provide a more elaborate model of the growth of human capital. In this study, the most significant impacts of HIV/AIDS arise as early mortality disrupts the transmission of knowledge between generations.

A related group of studies focuses on the potential impact of HIV/AIDS on fertility. Young (2005, 2007) focuses on two effects of HIV/AIDS, namely the adverse impact on the human capital accumulation of children, and the reduction in fertility that arises through a reduction in unprotected sex and because HIV/AIDS results in an increase in the of scarcity of labor (as the capital/labor ratio rises) and thus in the value of women's time. Young (2005) argues that the fertility effect, primarily through reduced population growth, translates into increased GDP per capita; Young (2007) provides some empirical analysis in support of this argument. However, these findings run contrary to earlier work on the links between mortality and fertility (e.g., Soares (2005); Juhn, Kalemli-Ozcan, and Turan (2008a); and Fortson (2009)).

In summary, the available evidence suggests that the impact of HIV/AIDS on economic growth (both of real GDP and real GDP per capita) has been small so far. The literature applying a neoclassical growth framework (and the related CGE and large-scale macroeconomic models) provide some pointers as to why this is the case for GDP per capita, identifying adverse impacts of HIV/AIDS (e.g., reduced savings and productivity), but also an increase in the capital-labor ratio brought about by reduced population growth. If this is true, and the impact of HIV/AIDS on GDP per capita is small, this would mean that the rate of GDP growth, in the long run, would decline roughly in line with reduced population growth.[18] Looking ahead, there is considerable uncertainty regarding the long-term impacts of HIV/AIDS, and concern in particular regarding the large numbers of orphans in countries with high HIV prevalence and the implications for the accumulation and transmission of human capital.

A puzzling aspect of the evidence on the impacts of HIV/AIDS on growth is the fact that the impact appears much lower than predicted by the literature on growth and health (as far as it uses life expectancy or mortality as a meter for health). Within the confines of this chapter, we can only point to some possible explanations. First, HIV/AIDS, unlike other diseases, is a very lethal disease, following a largely asymptomatic period. Its contribution to sickness (as measured by WHO (2008b)) is therefore much smaller than its contribution to mortality, which could mean that the impact of HIV/AIDS on productivity could be smaller than suggested by cross-country evidence conditioning economic variables on mortality or life expectancy.[19] Second, the positive correlation between health outcomes (such as life expectancy) and economic outcomes could reflect factors (such as the quality of institutions) which have an impact on both health and income (as suggested by Deaton (2006)), and which are not directly affected by HIV/AIDS. Relatedly, much of the empirical literature does not adequately capture the endogeneity of health outcomes and may therefore produce biased results. Third, some of the correlation between health indicators and economic variables could reflect longer-term effects (e.g., working through the impacts of impaired health or orphanhood on education) which, in the case of HIV/AIDS, have not fully materialized yet.

## IV. HIV/AIDS, Economic Growth, and the Structure of the Economy

In our discussion of the impacts of HIV/AIDS on economic growth, we found that the evidence suggests that HIV/AIDS did not have a large impact on the growth or level of GDP or GDP per capita so far. In this section, we discuss some factors that may contribute to this finding but have played a subordinate role in the literature so far—notably the dual structure of economies and high degrees of inequality found in many economies with high HIV prevalence, and the role of resource extraction in some of these economies.

## Data

The extent of inequality in many economies with high HIV prevalence is very high. This is illustrated in Table 1.1, providing summary indicators for the distribution of income for the nine countries with the highest HIV prevalence (at the end of 2007). These data should be interpreted with caution, as some of the data are more than a little outdated.[20] However, more recent country-level data (applying somewhat different methodologies) for Namibia, Lesotho, and Botswana are broadly consistent with the data presented in Table 1.1, suggesting that income inequality has declined moderately in Namibia and Lesotho, although the extent of inequality remains among the highest in sub-Saharan Africa (and globally).

The apparent correlation between high degrees of inequality and high HIV prevalence is sometimes interpreted causally. For example, Piot, Greener, and Russell (2007) discuss links between poor governance, inequality, and HIV prevalence, pointing at the "clear pattern of association between income inequality . . . and HIV prevalence across countries in sub-Saharan Africa" (1571). They find that "inequality is a stronger predictor of HIV prevalence than poor governance," and suggest "that economic growth that is not pro-poor and that leads to greater income inequality may even fuel the HIV epidemic" (1572).

We find that the data do not support these findings regarding the role of inequality. Economic transformation in the context of development can be associated with high degrees of inequality, and it is apparent that the economies with high degrees of inequality in Table 1.1 include some of the most advanced economies in sub-Saharan Africa. Table 1.2 summarizes some regressions exploring the

*Table 1.1.* Income Distribution in Nine Countries with High HIV Prevalence

| | | Share in Income or Expenditure (Percent) | | | | |
|---|---|---|---|---|---|---|
| | Survey year | Poorest 10% | Poorest 20% | Richest 20% | Richest 10% | Gini index |
| Namibia | 1993 | 0.5 | 1.4 | 78.7 | 64.5 | 74.3 |
| Lesotho | 1995 | 0.5 | 1.5 | 66.5 | 48.3 | 63.2 |
| Botswana | 1993 | 1.2 | 3.2 | 65.1 | 51 | 60.5 |
| South Africa | 2000 | 1.4 | 3.5 | 62.2 | 44.7 | 57.8 |
| Zambia | 2004 | 1.2 | 3.6 | 55.1 | 38.8 | 50.8 |
| Swaziland | 2000–01 | 1.6 | 4.3 | 56.3 | 40.7 | 50.4 |
| Zimbabwe | 1995–96 | 1.8 | 4.6 | 55.7 | 40.3 | 50.1 |
| Mozambique | 2002–03 | 2.1 | 5.4 | 53.6 | 39.4 | 47.3 |
| Malawi | 2004–05 | 2.9 | 7.0 | 46.6 | 31.8 | 39.0 |
| Average, 30 countries[a] | | 2.0 | 5.0 | 53 | 37 | 47.5 |

SOURCE: UNDP (2008)

[a] Unweighted average, thirty sub-Saharan countries for which data were available from UNDP (2008).

*Table 1.2* HIV Prevalence, GDP per Capita, and Inequality

|  | Dependent variable: HIV prevalence (2007) | | | |
|---|---|---|---|---|
| Constant | −12.9** | 3.5** | −5.8 | 4.4 |
|  | (2.1) | (2.6) | (−1.0) | (0.8) |
| Gini coefficient | 0.43*** |  | 0.21 | 0.007 |
|  | (3.3) |  | (1.66) | (0.06) |
| GDP per capita (1995) |  | 0.006*** | 0.005*** | −0.001 |
|  |  | (4.6) | (3.2) | (−0.35) |
| SACU[a] dummy |  |  |  | 17.9 |
|  |  |  |  | (3.8) |
| Number of observations | 30 | 30 | 30 | 30 |
| $R^2$ | 0.28 | 0.43 | 0.48 | 0.67 |

SOURCE: Author's estimates based on data from IMF (2009), UNDP (2008), and UNAIDS (2008a).
NOTE: One, two, and three stars indicate estimated coefficients significant on a 10-, 5-, and 1-percent level of confidence, respectively.
[a] SACU (South African Customs Union) includes South Africa, Botswana, Lesotho, Namibia, and Swaziland.

correlation between HIV prevalence, the Gini coefficient, and GDP per capita. Clearly, GDP per capita is much more closely correlated with HIV prevalence than the Gini coefficient (which turns—just—insignificant at the 10 percent level if GDP per capita is included in the regression). More problematic for hypotheses regarding economic determinants of HIV is the fact that the coefficients for both the Gini coefficient and GDP per capita are not robust and essentially fall to zero when a dummy for the five South African Customs Union (SACU) countries is included. Thus, apart from the fact that HIV prevalence is high in the five SACU countries (which also happen to feature relatively high levels of GDP per capita and income inequality), the cross-country evidence does not support the hypothesis that HIV prevalence is related to inequality or GDP per capita.

However, inequality is nevertheless relevant for our analysis of the economic impacts of HIV/AIDS. Below, we will argue that economic activity, in terms of value added or incomes, is concentrated in a fairly narrow segment of the economy in many countries facing a severe HIV epidemic. This is captured by the notion of a dual economy which plays a role in some of the studies of the macroeconomic impact of HIV/AIDS discussed above. Alternatively, one may distinguish between manufacturing and services on one hand, and agriculture (characterized by a lower level of value added per head) on the other hand.

From Table 1.3, we see that value added per employee can differ substantially across major sectors, notably between industry and agriculture, where value added per employee differs between the sectors by a factor of up to 20 (for Botswana); the second highest gap (14) occurs for Zambia. It is not a coincidence that these

*Table 1.3* Employment and Value Added Across Sectors, Six Countries

| Country | Year | Share of Employment (Percent) | | | Value Added per Employee (2000 US$) | | |
|---|---|---|---|---|---|---|---|
| | | Agriculture | Industry | Services | Agriculture | Industry | Services |
| Botswana | 2003 | 21.2 | 22.6 | 56.1 | 409 | 8,231 | 2,909 |
| Lesotho | 1997 | 56.5 | 15.2 | 28.2 | 432 | 4,452 | 2,331 |
| Namibia | 2000 | 31.1 | 12.2 | 56.0 | 1,075 | 7,088 | 3,305 |
| South Africa | 2003 | 10.3 | 24.5 | 65.1 | 2,356 | 8,750 | 6,761 |
| Zambia | 1998 | 70.0 | 7.0 | 23.0 | 188 | 2,603 | 1,346 |
| Zimbabwe | 1999 | 60.0 | 11.8 | 24.3 | 311 | 1,952 | 2,238 |

SOURCE: Data from World Bank (2008b), and author's calculations.

are economies which feature a large mining sector. In Botswana (IMF 2008a, 2007), exports of diamonds accounted for about 30 percent of GDP in 2005–07 (and exports of copper nickel for around 4 percent of GDP); in Zambia, exports of metals accounted for 28 percent of GDP in 2006 (IMF 2008b); and in Namibia (also showing high value added in the industrial sector in Table 1.4 below), exports of diamonds and other minerals accounted for 21 percent of GDP in 2006 (IMF 2008c).

The fact that resource extraction is associated with a high degree of concentration in terms of the distribution of value added across the economy is illustrated by data on the value added per employee from Namibia, which specifically account for the mining sector (Table 1.4). We see that employment in the mining sector is miniscule as a percentage of the total labor force. As value added per employee is very high (US$71,500—25 times the level of value added per employee observed in agriculture), the share of mining in GDP is much higher (8.6 percent).[21]

*Table 1.4* Namibia: Employment and Value Added Across Sectors, 2004

| Labor Force Status | No. of People (Thousands) | No. of People (Percent of Total) | Value Added per Employee |
|---|---|---|---|
| Total employment | 385 | 78.1 | $13,300 |
| Mining | 8 | 1.6 | $71,500 |
| Agriculture | 103 | 20.9 | $2,800 |
| Other employment | 275 | 55.8 | $15,500 |
| Public sector | 83 | 16.8 | n.a. |
| Private sector | 192 | 38.9 | n.a. |
| Unemployment | 108 | 21.9 | n.a. |
| Labor force | 493 | 100.0 | n.a. |

SOURCE: Data from Namibian Labor Force Surveys, as quoted in IMF (2008d).

## The Structure of the economy and the macroeconomic impact of HIV/AIDS

The uneven structure of many economies facing severe HIV epidemics does have some implications for the macroeconomic impacts of HIV/AIDS. Very generally, the macroeconomic impact of HIV/AIDS is dominated by its impact in the formal sector. Correspondingly, the impacts in the informal or the agricultural sector carry little weight, even though they account for the livelihoods of a large share of the population. Additionally, considering the relatively low levels of value added for the agricultural sector reported in Table 1.3, the impact of HIV/AIDS in that sector could exacerbate poverty even though aggregate indicators like GDP per capita show a small impact of HIV/AIDS. (We will discuss this issue in some more detail in the next section.)

One of the impacts through which HIV/AIDS may affect growth is the impact on the productivity of sick workers. The most compelling evidence comes from the agricultural or agro-processing sector. For example, Morris, Burdge, and Cheevers (2001) document productivity losses among workers in a sugar mill, while Fox and others (2004) estimate that tea pickers on an estate in Kenya who retired or died from AIDS-related causes earned 16 percent less in their penultimate year at work and 17.7 percent less in their final year. These estimates, however, cannot be transformed into estimates of losses in labor productivity on an aggregate level, as the estimates regard demanding physical labor which is not typical for the economy overall. Indeed, Fox and others provide some indirect evidence suggesting that average productivity losses on the plant level are lower than these direct effects, as workers who cannot do hard physical labor may get shifted to physically less demanding jobs.

Additionally, companies can incur certain expenditures to mitigate the losses associated with increased mortality and morbidity among staff. In addition to just hiring more people,[22] they can invest more in training to compensate for higher turnover or increase the flexibility of staff across tasks. Additionally, they can provide or finance medical services that would mitigate the impacts of HIV/AIDS. (In this context, one of the most significant developments is the expansion in access to ART, which we will return to below.) Additionally, it is important to bear in mind that, according to WHO burden of disease estimates, the extent of morbidity, relative to mortality, is relatively low for HIV/AIDS. Compared to other health conditions, times lost to sickness for HIV/AIDS are relatively small until the last stages of the disease preceding death. Thus, the primary costs associated with HIV/AIDS may be related to increased turnover rather than declining productivity on the job.

These conjectures are consistent with perceptions of the impact of HIV/AIDS in the business community, where companies would typically note an impact of HIV/AIDS on their employees but not regard it as one of the most critical issues facing the company. For example, according to Ellis and Terwin (2005), only between 0 percent (motor sector) and 16 percent (transport sector) reported a significant impact of HIV/AIDS on businesses, although a much larger proportion of the same businesses—between 22 percent (motor sector) and 52 percent (transport sector)—anticipated a significant impact over a five-year period. In a study focusing on small- and medium-sized enterprises, Connelly and Rosen (2005) report that that HIV/AIDS ranked 9th of 10 major business concerns (although some higher-ranking concerns, such as worker productivity, are related to HIV/AIDS).

One consistent feature of studies of the business response to HIV/AIDS is that the response differs across companies (and sectors) depending on the size of the companies. Ellis and Terwin (2005) report that almost all large companies have implemented an HIV awareness program, while only about one-third of small companies have done so. In this regard, Connelly and Rosen (2005) point at the role of HIV awareness among managers of small and medium enterprises, and at barriers (essentially arising from scale economies) to extending HIV services to small companies.

The points we have made about dual economies and asymmetries in the impact of and the response to HIV/AIDS across companies or sectors applies in particular to resource extraction, which is dominated by large companies. Historically, large mining companies were among the first to address the impact of HIV/AIDS and implement policies to address (and mitigate) the impact of the epidemic.[23] However, there is one aspect that is unique to resource-extracting industries—rents from resource extraction may account for a large proportion of value added.[24] Among other macroeconomic implications (such as the disproportionate role in government revenues), the presence from large rents from resource extraction implies that wages are not a good indicator for the marginal contribution of an employee to a company's output. This is apparent, for example, from the labor market data from Namibia quoted in Table 1.4, estimating the value added per employee at $71,500. In this setting, it is likely that stakeholders in the mining operations find it cost-effective to incur substantial outlays to prevent disruptions to production processes associated with increased morbidity or mortality among employees, and mining output may well remain unchanged, even in the context of a serious epidemic.

Another consequence of the presence of large rents from resource extraction is that the models commonly applied to studying the macroeconomic impacts of HIV/AIDS are misleading.[25] Two studies addressing the macroeconomic impacts of HIV/AIDS in Botswana—a textbook example for an economy built on resource extraction—implicitly acknowledge that the models commonly applied to the study of the macroeconomic impacts of HIV/AIDS are ill-suited to analyze an economy where rents from resource extraction play a dominant role. BIDPA

(2000) assume that mineral rents are unaffected by HIV/AIDS (which would be consistent with our reasoning), while MacFarlan and Sgherri (2001) restrict their analysis to the non-mining sector.

## Role of increased access to antiretroviral treatment

The increase in access to access to ART over the last year has also transformed the economic impact of HIV/AIDS, by reducing mortality among people living with HIV/AIDS and extending their life expectancy.[26] To the extent that ART reduces mortality and morbidity among the working-age population, we would also expect to see reduced macroeconomic impacts.[27] However, access to ART is far from universal; the distribution of access to treatment across the population has implications for the economic impacts of HIV/AIDS.

Globally, access to ART in low- and middle-income countries has increased from about 400,000 people at the end of 2003 to about 4 million people at the end of 2008, corresponding to a treatment coverage rate of 42 percent (WHO, UNAIDS, and UNICEF 2009). For sub-Saharan Africa, the increase is much more pronounced, from 100,000 people at the end of 2003 (coverage: about 2 percent) to 2,925,000, i.e., a treatment coverage rate of 43 percent. In spite of this large increase, the majority of the population who would require treatment does not receive it, which means that—through explicit or implicit mechanisms—rationing of access to ART does occur. In this regard, Rosen et al. (2005) distinguish between explicit mechanisms (such as programs prioritizing access to treatment for pregnant women) and implicit mechanisms. Below, we argue that implicit rationing contributes to mitigating the macroeconomic impacts of HIV/AIDS.

One implicit rationing mechanism is the cost of accessing treatment. Even where treatment is provided for free, patients have to incur the costs of accessing health facilities, which can be substantial for poor households. Rosen et al. (2007d) find that the average cost of a visit to a health clinic for patients receiving ART is R120 (about $20), in addition to travel and waiting time, and that it is incurred at least six times in the year in which patients start ART. Together with other costs such as non-prescription medicines, special foods, other medical expenses, etc., these are high costs for a substantial portion of the population. As a key aspect of the costs of accessing treatment is transportation, this example understates obstacles to access to treatment in rural areas where the density of health facilities is lower. Another dimension of rationing is inequity in the quality of services provided across sites. In this regard, Scott et al. (2005) analyze the quality of HIV/AIDS-related services and find large differences between an urban and two rural sites.

The other element of implicit rationing that is particularly relevant for our discussion regards the link between access to health services and the employment status of a person seeking health services. Many large companies provide access to health services to their employees, either directly or through some financial arrangement with health providers. These facilities were instrumental in providing access to ART before the large increase in access through public health services experienced since 2003. Additionally, large employers are more likely to provide medical insurance for employees in lieu of, or in addition to, company-controlled health facilities.

In addition to the availability of health services through employment relations (an important factor in a context where access to health services is uneven across the population), there are studies suggesting that provision of ART does yield immediate financial benefits to companies extending it to their employees. Based on an assumed treatment cost of US$360 per year, Rosen et al. (2006) find that providing ART saves money for all categories of employees (managers, skilled workers, and unskilled workers) for a number of companies, although this may not hold for labor-intensive, low-technology industries where the costs of labor attrition are relatively low.

Thus, there is substantial circumstantial evidence suggesting that access to ART is higher among employees in the formal sector, especially those working for large companies. This adds another dimension to our argument that key sectors of the economy, in terms of the contribution to GDP, but not necessarily in terms of the number of people depending on them, have certain tools at their disposal to mitigate the adverse impacts of HIV/AIDS. This may help explain the small magnitude of the macroeconomic impacts of HIV/AIDS observed so far.

## V. Impact of HIV/AIDS on Inequality

Some of the factors described in the previous section—such as privileged access to health services for people employed in or associated with the formal sector—while mitigating the magnitude of macroeconomic impacts of HIV/AIDS, have distri-butional implications. Uneven access to health services and other interventions, which—as we argue—mitigates the impacts of HIV/AIDS on GDP, exacerbates existing inequities across the population. Another reason why an analysis of the dis-tributional impacts of HIV/AIDS is crucial for understanding and evaluating the economic impacts of the epidemic flows from the uneven impact of the epidemic across households (primarily depending on whether a household is directly affected by the epidemic or not). Thus, small impacts of HIV/AIDS on the macro-economic level may mask impacts of HIV/AIDS on the household level which are relevant from a welfare perspective, in terms of poverty- or development-related policy objectives, and may have macroeconomic consequences in the longer run.[28]

Against this background, our discussion of the impacts of HIV/AIDS on pov-erty and inequality proceeds in three steps. First, we review the macroeconomic impact of HIV/AIDS in the context of the dual economy and explain why GDP per capita is not a reliable indicator of living standards in this context. Second, we review the available literature on the impacts of HIV/AIDS on the household level. Third, we discuss the implications of the evidence on the impacts of HIV/AIDS on the household level for risks of poverty and income distribution. This also includes a discussion of the available evidence on equity aspects of access to treatment.

### GDP per capita and HIV/AIDS in the dual economy

One implication of the dual structure of many economies facing high rates of HIV prevalence and the high degrees of inequality in the region, is that GDP per capita is an unreliable indicator for changes in material living standards associated with HIV/AIDS. This point is illustrated in Figure 1.5, which presents a very stylized description of the impact of HIV/AIDS.

For our illustration, we assume that the economy consists of two sectors, and that output per capita is much higher in the formal sector than in the informal sector, but that it is even within sectors. As a consequence of HIV/AIDS, value added per capita in both sectors declines, and the population shrinks owing to increased mortality. Since the impact of increased mortality is somewhat larger in the informal sector,[29] its share in the working population increases. This means that GDP per capita increases, although survivors in each sector are worse off.[30]

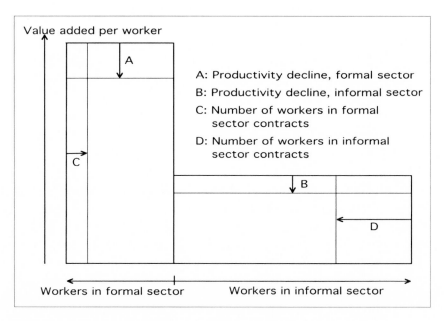

*Figure 1.5*   HIV/AIDS: Productivity Losses, Sectoral Shifts, and GDP per Capita

More generally, the macroeconomic perspective misses out on one crucial aspect of the economic impact of HIV/AIDS: the impacts differ significantly across households, ranging from households that may become impoverished owing to loss of income or health-related costs, to households experiencing only indirect effects, to households who may financially benefit, e.g., through additional employment (filling jobs vacated by people who have died or are too ill to work). We explore these points in more detail in the two sections below, focusing first on the direct impacts of HIV/AIDS for the affected households, and then discussing the implications of HIV/AIDS for poverty and inequality from a bird's eye perspective.

## The impact of HIV/AIDS on the household level

There are two principal sources of information on the impact of HIV/AIDS on the household level—studies analyzing features of or trends among households affected by HIV/AIDS, and studies analyzing the implications of mortality on households. Additionally, for a macroeconomic assessment, it is also necessary to understand the "socioeconomic gradient" of the epidemic, i.e. the extent to which HIV incidence differs across population groups. Among studies of the first type, Steinberg and others (2002) find that households affected by HIV/AIDS spend about one-third of their income on health care, compared with a national average of 4 percent, and that funeral expenses are, on average, equivalent to four months of salary. They also find that the cost of the disease relative to household income is twice as large in rural as in urban areas, which means that the lowest deciles are bearing disproportionately large expenses. Over two-thirds of caregivers are women, and 22 percent of caregivers have to take time off from work and other income-generating activities.

Bachmann and Booysen (2003) find that incomes and expenditures for households affected by illness are substantially lower than for households not affected, and that expenditures and incomes for households affected by HIV/AIDS are lower than for households facing other forms of illness. While this could point to higher HIV incidence among households in the sample, or a stronger impact of HIV/AIDS compared to other health conditions, both would be consistent with an asymmetric impact of HIV/AIDS on poor households. Booysen (2005) provides a more dynamic analysis, showing that the income ranking of households affected by HIV/AIDS is more likely to deteriorate and less likely to improve than that of other households.

As HIV/AIDS accounts for a significant share of adult deaths in sub-Saharan Africa (especially among the working-age population), and deaths and their aftermath represent an important aspect of the impact of HIV/AIDS, the other useful branch of literature regards the impacts of adult mortality more generally. Mather and others (2004) synthesize studies of the impact of adult mortality on rural households from five countries (Kenya, Malawi, Mozambique, Rwanda, and Zambia), finding households affected by adult deaths do not uniformly have less available prime-age labor than non-affected households (a finding that may reflect the ability of those households to attract new members); and that the death of a male household head is associated with a larger decline in crop production and non-farm income than the death of any other type of household member. Yamano and Jayne (2004), whose study is one of those covered by Mather and others (2004), suggest that the impact of adult mortality on households in Kenya is related to household wealth. They "find negative impacts on the net value of crop production, assets, and off-farm income only in the case of male head-of-household mortality among relatively poor households" (115).

In addition to understanding the impacts of HIV/AIDS for the affected households, an assessment of the economic impacts of HIV/AIDS also requires an understanding of who becomes infected. The early literature (e.g., Over and Piot (1993)) suggested that the epidemic primarily affected individuals who are better educated and belong to higher occupational classes. Similarly, Hargreaves and Glynn (2002), in a systematic review of the literature, noted that HIV prevalence across four African regions was higher among the well-educated (primarily for the older cohorts). However, de Walque (2006), using recent Demographic and Health Surveys that include HIV testing for a representative sample of the adult population, arrives at more differentiated results—education is associated with a higher level of infidelity and a lower level of abstinence, but also with preventive behavior and knowledge, and overall there is no clear correlation between HIV prevalence and education. HIV prevalence also tends to be positively correlated with wealth (although findings differ across countries). Mishra et al. (2007b) and others, using a similar but more comprehensive dataset as de Walque (2006), emphasize the positive correlation of HIV prevalence with wealth. Most recently, Fortson (2008a) finds a robust link between HIV/AIDS and the level of education, but uneven results for wealth variables. The primary limitation of this literature regarding the impact of HIV/AIDS is the fact that the analysis is based on HIV prevalence rather than incidence. As survival rates are arguably correlated with socioeconomic factors like education and wealth, the available studies suffer from selection bias and do not adequately assess the impact of HIV/AIDS across population groups.

## Implications of HIV/AIDS for poverty and inequality

Our discussion of the impacts of HIV/AIDS on the household level suggested that HIV/AIDS resulted in an impoverishment of the affected households, and that poor households were less able to cope with the disease. However, finding an adverse impact of HIV/AIDS or increased mortality in household studies is not sufficient to establish a link between HIV/AIDS, poverty, and inequality, or to quantify its impact, for two reasons: First, to assess the significance of HIV/AIDS as a contributor to poverty, it is necessary to relate data on the household impact of HIV/AIDS to estimates on HIV prevalence across the population or across types of households (as HIV prevalence may be correlated with household characteristics, including income). Second, it is necessary to take into account indirect effects arising in households not directly affected by HIV/AIDS, which could include financial support to households directly affected by HIV/AIDS, but also financial gains through economic opportunities associated with HIV/AIDS-related vacancies.[31]

The most significant efforts so far discussing the implications of the microeconomic evidence on household impacts of HIV/AIDS for poverty and inequality are the studies by Greener, Jefferis, and Siphambe (2000); Greener (2004); and Salinas and Haacker (2006). Their approach involves combining data on the household impacts of HIV/AIDS with economy-wide data on household characteristics, treating the costs and income losses associated with HIV/AIDS as shocks to the existing income and expenditure patterns.

Salinas and Haacker (2006) extend the earlier studies by adding a labor market, allowing for vacancies associated with HIV/AIDS-related attrition to be filled again. Their analysis is based on data from Demographic and Health Surveys or sentinel reports (as well as data and estimates on the household impacts of HIV/AIDS), and add a cross-country perspective, covering Ghana, Kenya, Swaziland, and Zambia. They find that in three of the sample countries, poverty incidence and the poverty gap increase more than would be expected from the decline in income per capita. Key determinants of the impact of HIV/AIDS on poverty are the size of the population at risk of falling into poverty and the HIV prevalence among this population group. Their findings also provide some additional insights on informal insurance mechanisms whereby households affected by HIV benefit from financial and others forms of support, suggesting that these would have some impact in terms of avoiding extreme poverty, but that they may not have an impact on common poverty indicators, once the households providing support (i.e., experiencing a deterioration in living standards) are included in the analysis.

The principal shortcomings of the studies described are the simplistic assumptions regarding the structure of households in treating HIV/AIDS as a shock to otherwise static households. This excludes important mechanisms of coping with and mitigating the impacts of HIV/AIDS, such as remarriage, joining a different household, and children growing up and leaving the household. While the studies described go some way toward a macroeconomic analysis of the impacts of HIV/AIDS on poverty and the distribution of income, our understanding of this issue remains limited.

One area not well researched thus far is that of the implications of the increased availability of ART for the economic impacts of HIV/AIDS, including poverty and inequality. Medical data, as well as the few available economic studies, suggest that ART reverses or mitigates the adverse impacts of HIV/AIDS on productivity. For example, Larson and others (2008), in a study focusing on the productivity of tea pluckers, find that workers on ART quickly returned to their primary work assignment, and that men quickly returned to nearly similar work patterns as the general workforce during the initial 12 months on ART, while women spent fewer days on plucking tea and more days on other tasks.

Meanwhile, ART adds a dimension to the distributional impacts of HIV/AIDS, as access to treatment is not necessarily even across population groups. This was obvious when access to ART was still very expensive, and access was de facto restricted to the most wealthy segments of the population and parts of the population depending on the formal sector. With the large increase in access to treatment, economic determinants of access have become less pervasive, but with coverage rates in sub-Saharan Africa estimated at about 30 percent at the end of 2007, uneven access to treatment could conceivably exacerbate the distributional impacts of HIV/AIDS.[32]

Available studies point to some disparities in access to treatment according to socioeconomic status. Rosen and others (2008a, 200) find that "relative to the HIV-positive population as a whole, ART patients are older, more likely to be female and have 1 long-term partner, live in informal housing, have reached secondary school, and earn an income from formal or informal employment." Scott et al. (2005) emphasize the difference in the quality of services between urban and rural sites. Tsai and others (2009) suggest that persons seen in clinic were more likely to have completed secondary or tertiary education, less likely to be unemployed, and more likely to live in households with access to a private tap water supply, compared to a community sample. Overall, these studies suggest some correlation between social status and access to ART. However, the point of reference for comparison with the sample of people receiving treatment is not fully satisfactory in each of these studies (a point discussed in Rosen et al. (2008a)), and our understanding of the equity implications of access to treatment is far from satisfactory at this stage.

## VI. Conclusions

In light of the magnitude of the demographic and health disruptions caused by HIV/AIDS in many countries, it is important to understand the economic and development impacts of the disease, as these may have implications beyond the immediate health impacts of the epidemic, complicating the attainment of development objectives or material living standards. Against this background, the chapter contrasts the large health impacts of HIV/AIDS with the moderate (if any) impacts on GDP or GDP per capita that can be observed thus far. A key hypothesis we pursue is that the dual structure of many economies affected by HIV/AIDS, where much value added is concentrated in fairly narrow segments of the economy, plays a role in mitigating the adverse impacts of HIV/AIDS on GDP. However, this argument implies that a disproportionate share of the impact of HIV/AIDS is borne by the low-income informal sector, suggesting that the small macroeconomic impact of HIV/AIDS masks adverse developments regarding inequality or poverty.

More specifically, our findings include the following: Econometric inference is complicated by the fact that the countries featuring the highest HIV prevalence rates in sub-Saharan Africa differ very substantially from other countries in the region in terms of their economic structure. Econometric findings are generally not robust to the exclusion of such outliers. The impact of HIV/AIDS on GDP or GDP per capita appears to be small so far, and countries with the highest prevalence rates do not show a marked slowdown in GDP growth, relative to the rest of sub-Saharan Africa.

We do not find compelling evidence for a link between inequality (Gini coefficient) and HIV prevalence. GDP per capita is more closely correlated with HIV prevalence than inequality and when—in light of the previous points—a dummy for SACU countries is included in the regression, any correlation between HIV prevalence, GDP per capita, and inequality disappears.

We also find the contributions to GDP across sectors are very uneven in countries with high HIV prevalence. This applies, in particular, to countries featuring a large mining sector.

Responses to HIV/AIDS also differ by company size. Most large companies have HIV policies in place, and many of them have been leading in extending access to treatment to employees (consistent with findings that, in companies with high value added per employee, providing access to ART tends to save money). On the other hand, in surveys HIV/AIDS does not feature among the most pressing concerns in small- and medium-sized businesses (let alone the informal sector), and establishing or accessing HIV-related services appears relatively difficult for small establishments. In the context of HIV/AIDS and a dual economy, GDP per capita is not a good indicator for material living standards across the population. Further, the (weak) evidence on macroeconomic impacts of HIV/AIDS contrasts with microeconomic evidence showing adverse impacts among households affected by HIV/AIDS. However, other households apparently gain from additional employment.

Studies integrating the microeconomic evidence on HIV/AIDS in a macro framework, including a simple model of the labor market, suggest that a small impact of HIV/AIDS on the macroeconomic level can coincide with increases in poverty and inequality. These findings are primarily driven by the large size of the shocks to households affected by HIV/AIDS. The shape of the income distribution and the socioeconomic profile of HIV/AIDS are important factors in determining the size of the impacts of HIV/AIDS on poverty.

Overall, regarding our hypothesis that the small size of the macroeconomic impact of HIV/AIDS is related to the uneven structure of many economies facing large HIV epidemics, we do not obtain a confession from the (weak) data, and the trial proceeds on the basis of circumstantial evidence. Consistent with our hypothesis, we see asymmetries in the response to HIV/AIDS across sectors, and economic data illustrating the incentives and scope for making outlays to protect high value added businesses from adverse impacts of HIV/AIDS. Conversely, our hypothesis implies that the brunt of the impact of HIV/AIDS is borne by households at the lower end of the income distribution and the informal sector, contributing to poverty and inequality, and the limited data at our disposal are consistent with this aspect of our hypothesis, too.

## Notes

1. Based on symposium held by United Nations University, New York Office at United Nations, New York, September 9, 2008.

2. It is worth noting that the estimates offered by the United Nations Population Division (2009b) are model-generated, based on a set of data and assumptions on the impacts of HIV/AIDS, as well as broader demographic trends. As the understanding of the health and demographic implications of HIV/AIDS is still evolving, the estimates are subject to some uncertainty.

3. The other major world region experiencing a substantial decline in life expectancy over a sustained period was Eastern Europe where life expectancy declined by about 1.9 years between 1990–95 and 2000–05. We argue that the adverse developments in Africa are more significant as they occur from a much lower base, as the population of sub-Saharan Africa is much larger than that of Eastern Europe, and as the declines in life expectancy in some of the countries with high HIV prevalence (15 to 20 years) are much higher than any declines experienced in Eastern Europe (up to four years, in Russia between 1985–90 and 2000–05, of which more than one year reflected the impact of HIV/AIDS).

4. As the impact of HIV/AIDS is fully realized by the population, it could also result in changes in the number of desired children. Fortson (2009, 170) finds that, "HIV/ AIDS had very little impact on fertility, both overall" (which could reflect both behavioral effects but also the direct effects of HIV infections), "and in a sample of HIV-negative women." Juhn, Kalemli-Ozcan, and Turan (2008a, 1) find that, "HIV-infected women have significantly lower fertility," and that "local community HIV prevalence has no significant effect on non-infected women's fertility." See also Juhn, Kalemli-Ozcan, and Turan (2008b) for a more concise discussion.

5. It is important to note that these estimates are averages across sub-Saharan Africa. WHO (2008b) does not provide country-level estimates. However, the earlier estimates

included in WHO (2004a) suggest that HIV/AIDS accounted for one-third of all deaths in Malawi, and more than half of all deaths in South Africa and Swaziland in 2002.

6. The countries for which growth trajectories are shown are: Botswana (BTW), Central African Republic (CAR), Lesotho (LSO), Malawi (MWI), Mozambique (MOZ), Namibia (NMB), South Africa (RSA), Swaziland (SWZ), Zambia (ZMB), and Zimbabwe (ZWE). SSA stands for sub-Saharan Africa (including the 10 countries shown).

7. Many of the key issues regarding the link between health and economic outcomes are discussed in a comprehensive (but somewhat outdated) survey by Strauss and Thomas (1998).

8. Sala-i-Martin (2005) also provides a discussion of different impacts of health on income or growth.

9. It is important not to equate birth rates with fertility rates (i.e., the average number of children a women bears). As birth rates are defined as the ratio of births to population size, an increase in mortality can result in an increase in the birth rate if it primarily affects people after childbearing age. On the other hand, an epidemic would reduce birth rates if behavioral changes, increased mortality, or lower health states among women of childbearing age results in a drop in the number of pregnancies, or if increased morbidity results in fewer successful pregnancies.

10. We focus on the direct effects of health shocks. Additionally, cross-effects between $h$ and $k$ may occur.

11. Additionally, Bloom, Canning, and Sevilla (2004) provide a survey of 13 earlier growth accounting exercises. In that literature, an increase in life expectancy of five years was associated with a growth rate that is between 0.0 and 0.6 percentage points higher than otherwise.

12. Additionally, Lorentzen, McMillan, and Wacziarg (2005) suggest that there may be an effect of mortality on risk behavior, as measured by smoking rates or HIV prevalence.

13. A second set of studies covered by Weil (2007) considers the link between age at menarche (first menstrual period) and labor productivity.

14. In Bloom and Mahal (1997), the key explanatory variable regarding the impact of HIV/AIDS (the number of AIDS cases) was constructed by the authors from very preliminary (and, from our perspective in 2010, obsolete) data.

15. Arndt (2006) assumes that an AIDS incidence rate of 1 percent translates into a slowdown in productivity growth of 1 percentage point. Arndt and Lewis (2001) apply a non-linear specification, whereby an AIDS death rate of 1 percent slows down productivity growth by 23 percent (not percentage points).

16. As the impact of these demand-side effects on GDP dissipates in the longer run, as the increased demand for health services is met by a reallocation of productive resources to the health sector (at the expense of other sectors), and as increased expenditures on health imply reduced budgets for other expenditures.

17. Another study, frequently quoted but as yet unpublished, that highlights the impacts of HIV/AIDS on investments in physical capital and education, is Ferreira and Pessoa (2003).

18. As pointed out earlier, we cannot distinguish well, empirically, between the impact of HIV/AIDS on the growth of GDP and GDP per capita because of peculiarities in the demographic transition across countries in sub-Saharan Africa.

19. This argument is sometimes made comparing the impacts of HIV/AIDS to those of malaria, suggesting that malaria is characterized by stints of illness (and thus productivity losses) over a long period, which are not well captured by proxies like mortality. The estimates by WHO (2008b) suggest that these comparisons are misplaced, as the contributions of both HIV/AIDS and malaria to DALYs lost to disability is similarly small, relative to

their contribution to mortality. Disability associated with HIV/AIDS, however, is concentrated over a shorter time period.

20. The Central Bureau of Statistics (2006) of Namibia, based on 2003/04 data, reports a Gini coefficient of 0.6 (as decimal, rather than percentage as we use it), and provides data according to which the poorest 33.5 percent of the population command 6.4 percent of consumption, while the share of the richest 17.4 percent is 66.4 percent. For Botswana, the Central Statistics Office (2006), based on different methodologies, describes an increase in the Gini coefficient in terms of "disposable income," and a very small decline in terms of "disposable cash income." According to the Lesotho Bureau of Statistics (n.d.), the 2002/03 Household Budget Survey Report returns a decline in the Gini coefficient of 52 (down from 57 in the 1994/95 survey for which the United Nations Development Programme (UNDP), applying a different methodology, reports a Gini coefficient of 63).

21. As mining is intensive in capital and other inputs, e.g., energy, the share of mining-related activities in GDP exceeds the value added based figure.

22. Regarding the impact of health-related disruptions on productivity or GDP, it makes little difference whether the output of a given group of workers declines, or whether additional workers are hired to maintain output at the previous level. Both developments would signify a decline in productivity.

23. In line with this, the mining sector in South Africa is among the most active sectors in terms of the share of businesses implementing policies to address HIV/AIDS, according to Ellis and Terwin (2005).

24. Rents from resource extraction arise when the value of output substantially exceeds the costs of extracting the resources (e.g., in case of diamonds that can be extracted at low costs). Typically, these rents are taxed through royalties or profit-sharing arrangements between a company obtaining an extraction license and the government.

25. In the commonly applied macroeconomic models, there is no role for rents from resource extraction, as the marginal product of labor (and, similarly, capital) is equal to the wage rate, whereas the marginal product exceeds the wage rate in an economy where rents from resource extraction play a role.

26. United Nations Population Division (2009b), summarizing the available evidence, assume that antiretroviral treatment extends the life span by about eight years.

27. A more comprehensive discussion would also need to cover the macroeconomic implications of external and domestic resources being shifted to providing HIV-related services.

28. The latter point is most forcefully argued by Bell, Devarajan, and Gersbach (2006), who analyze the long-term impacts of HIV/AIDS, focusing on the impacts of premature mortality among parents on the accumulation of human capital.

29. For this exercise, we abstract from the role of population growth. The essential point is that in our example the share of the population depending on the formal sector increases.

30. Moreover, even though GDP per capita increases, it is not possible to construct any transfers which would offset the income losses across the population, so that all survivors are better off materially.

31. An additional element, not addressed in the literature in this context so far, is the increase in employment opportunities associated with the response to HIV/AIDS.

32. In view of the limited availability of ART in the region, a number of studies discuss the (implicit or explicit) rationing of treatment and its economic and ethical implications. Rosen et al. (2005) and Bennett and Chanfreau (2005) are good starting points to this literature.

# CHAPTER 2

## Governing a World with HIV and AIDS:
## An Unfinished Success Story

*Alex de Waal*

## Introduction

Contributing to a debate on why Africa's HIV/AIDS epidemic had not (yet) led
to political crisis, Peter Baldwin pointedly asked, "Why would one expect it to do
so in the first place?" (Baldwin 2007) His specific point was that illness ". . . has
never been the source of political action." His wider point was that the HIV/
AIDS pandemic is being successfully managed, so that it does not pose a political
threat. It was a rebuttal to alarming predictions made just a few years before that
the HIV/AIDS pandemic spelled political crisis for weak states in hard-hit regions
of the world. A seminal report by the U.S. National Intelligence Council (NIC)
concluded that "the persistent infectious disease burden is likely to aggravate and
in some cases, may even provoke economic decay, social fragmentation and political destabilization of the hardest hit countries in the developing world" (NIC
2000, 10).

The history of the last decade has resolved the debate between those who predicted the collapse of armies, state crises, and a vicious interaction between HIV/
AIDS and violent conflict, especially in Africa. These calamities did not come to
pass. In retrospect, the predictions appear to be an example of a misplaced apoc-
alyptic prediction made for the African continent that projected existing trends
into the future in an uncritical manner, assumed that worst-case interactions would
come to pass, and underestimated the resilience of African societies and states.
However, this conclusion obscures the ways in which militaries, conflicts, and
governance have actually influenced the course of HIV/AIDS epidemics, and vice
versa. First, it is necessary to chart the debates as they unfolded from the turn of
the millennium, and why such alarming predictions were made.

## Forecasting Doom

Epidemic disease has rarely been the cause of endogenous political crisis. Indeed if we examine the political histories of Europe in the fourteenth century, the demographic cataclysm of the Black Death warrants only passing mention (see Tuchman 1979)—and then because it led to events relevant to high politics such as the premature death of an English princess on her way to marry into the ruling lineage of Spain. We can trace the indirect consequences of syphilis and cholera on European armies and trade, but neither led directly to revolution or the collapse of regimes. The great influenza pandemic of 1918–19 passed off with minimal political impact (Barry 2004).

On the other hand, disease and hunger have been handmaidens to state collapse in the face of an aggressor. When the European conquistadores introduced new infections to immunologically naïve Native American populations, the epidemics that followed left the great pre-Columbian empires weak and vulnerable. The sequence of famines, epizootics, and epidemics that devastated much of China, India, and northeastern Africa in the 1880s was also a prelude to imperial conquest (Davis 2001). Disease has also been a challenge to sustaining and deploying armed forces, with armies historically losing several men to infection for every one killed or wounded in combat. Emperor Napoleon Bonaparte's stomach ailment that kept him away from personally commanding the French army at the Battle of Waterloo may have determined the result. Insofar as illness has altered the course of military history, it has also determined the fate of nations.

The collapse of the Soviet Union, and the failure of the American foreign policy and intelligence establishment to predict it, sparked a flurry of interest in the links between health crisis and state crisis. In the late 1970s, the rising infant mortality rate in the USSR sparked debate in America over whether this was real or an artifact of poor statistics. Some scholars argued that the rise was not only real but was an important signal marking the bankruptcy of the Soviet system (Davis and Feshbach 1980; Eberstadt 1988[1]). In contrast to silence from the CIA, demographers and public health specialists saw a crisis coming. Policy interest in health and life expectancy indicators was reinforced when the U.S. State Failure Task Force (SFTF) found that the best model for predicting state failure used three variables: openness to trade (lack of), democracy (lack of), and infant mortality (Esty et al. 1995).[2] The infant mortality factor was taken as a "broad measure of living standards and quality of life" (viii), but it is nonetheless striking that among 75 potential proxies for well-being that were tested, this was one of the three that stood out.

The SFTF sprang from the mainstream of American political science in its quantitative methods and liberal-democratic values. The four kinds of state failure of concern to the SFTF were revolutionary wars, ethnic wars, mass killings (genocides or politicides), and adverse or disruptive regime changes (involving extended periods of disorder and excluding "routine" *coups d'etat* or orderly government changes). A different political science tradition would have resisted placing episodes of revolutionary transformation in the same category with genocide, ethnic war, and anarchy. Moreover, the indicators used for defining state collapse, and subsequently state fragility, are all at a high level of aggregation, measuring only limited dimensions of state crisis.

More significant than the incipient collapse of weak states, was the impact of the prediction itself on the policies of major powers, and especially the U.S. The HIV/AIDS pandemic had already badly shaken the confidence of western governments and health establishments, which had assumed that epidemics of fatal infectious diseases had been consigned to history. Laurie Garrett's *The Coming Plague* (1994) popularized these fears. This built upon a deepening disorientation in Washington, DC, about what new security threats might be looming. In February, 1994, Robert Kaplan's article "The Coming Anarchy," subtitled "How scarcity, crime, overpopulation, tribalism, and disease are rapidly destroying the social fabric of our planet," reportedly so disturbed President Bill Clinton that he ordered it to be faxed to every American embassy around the world.

Two years later, as part of a broadening in the focus of national intelligence to cover topics such as humanitarian emergencies and the environmental crises as well as assessments of missile threats and the military capabilities of China, President Clinton requested that the NIC focus on the threats posed by emerging and resurgent infectious diseases. In January, 2000, the NIC reported on the subject (NIC 2000) and, in the same month, the historic UN Security Council debate on HIV/AIDS was held at the initiative of the U.S. The UN Security Council focused its attention on minimizing the threats to international peacekeeping operations, adopting Resolution 1308 in July, 2000 (UN Security Council 2000).

The NIC report contributed to a minor avalanche of publications on how disease in general and HIV/AIDS in particular might undermine militaries, states, democracies, and international peace and security (Schönteich 2000; Cheek 2001; Heinecken 2001; International Crisis Group 2001; Youde 2001; Price-Smith 2002). These publications shared two main features. First, little empirical evidence was presented, but rather deductions were made from anecdote and selective historical comparison. Second, they tended to make worst-case assumptions, arguing from "*may* happen" to "*will* happen" and rarely examined how factors might act in the opposite direction to mitigate impacts. The unfolding of the food crisis in southern Africa in 2002–03, unexpected in a subregion enjoying peace for the first time in a generation, also led to the fear that HIV/AIDS would contribute to "new variant famine" (de Waal and Whiteside 2003). The NIC itself then upped its predictions of disaster, forecasting a "second wave" of HIV/AIDS in Russia, India, and China, which would surpass in numbers (though not prevalence rates) the generalized epidemics in Africa (NIC 2002; Eberstadt 2002).

Very little social science literature was concerned with resilience or lack of impact. A rare example is Caldwell (1997), who noted that in hard-hit countries, "Life goes on in a surprisingly normal way. There has not even been any very marked change in sexual behaviour, and society is not dominated by government demands that there should be. There is no paranoia and little in the way of new religious or death cults. In some ways, it is very impressive" (180). A more influential contrary view came from some economic analyses that indicated modest impacts or even an increase in per capita GDP as the epidemic reduced unemployment (Bureau of Economic Research 2001). Concerned at the lack of political theory in the published literature, this author tried to examine how a major drop in adult life expectancy might impact governance (de Waal 2003), concluding (correctly) that "little is known about the governance impact of the epidemic" and (less correctly) that "HIV/AIDS and its impact are Africa's biggest problem" (23).

As this debate gathered momentum, the center of gravity of U.S. foreign policy abruptly switched to the "Global War on Terror." Concern with HIV/AIDS and state crisis was folded into this. Three weeks after the terrorist attack of September 11, 2001, British Prime Minister Tony Blair spoke at the Labour Party conference, linking social crisis to state failure to terrorism: "We are realizing how fragile are our frontiers in the face of the world's new challenges."[3] One principle of the war on terror was that no territory should be left ungoverned and hence prey to terrorist takeover or hideout, while the "one percent doctrine" (Suskind 2006) required the U.S. to deal with even the smallest contributory factors to the risks of terrorism. The logic was that U.S. security entailed confronting HIV/AIDS.

The responses of the countries considered at risk of HIV/AIDS-related crisis were diverse. Africans tended to see the epidemic as one misfortune and stress among many, not as a grave political threat. This is illustrated by the relatively low priority given to HIV/AIDS in public responses to opinion surveys (Afrobarometer 2004). Some governments simply denied the problem for as long as they could. Others' efforts were focused principally on designing programs that could attract international funding and policies that would win them international credit. President Yoweri Museveni in Uganda, following his early domestically-initiated HIV/AIDS efforts, became adept at using HIV/AIDS to polish his image abroad (de Waal 2006). A number of militaries, including South Africa's, took prompt and vigorous steps (see below). Botswana's President Festus Mogae was the most alarmist, repeatedly saying that his country's very existence was at stake (Mogae 2008).

Fears over the implications of the epidemic impelled the UN Economic Commission for Africa to set up the Commission on HIV/AIDS and Governance in Africa (CHGA) in 2003. It conducted a series of meetings, in which governments, civil society, and the private sector all expressed worries over the human security impacts and economic costs of HIV/AIDS (CHGA 2008). Over the course of its work, it stepped back towards a measured assessment of the impacts and risks: "The CHGA concluded, that African governments and societies could surmount the challenges of governance and development posed by HIV and AIDS" (31).[4] This writer also concluded that HIV/AIDS was not causing political crisis in Africa (de Waal 2006), and critiqued (among others) his own earlier writings as having been unduly pessimistic.

Two of the biggest countries of concern in the "second wave" of HIV/AIDS were Russia and China. In due course, each came to see the epidemic as a threat, in its own distinct way. The Russian government is concerned about the declining health of its adult male population, including both the population from which it recruits its soldiers and those soldiers themselves (Feshbach 2008). On this basis, President Vladimir Putin announced in April 2006 that HIV/AIDS was a national security issue, and he would increase HIV/AIDS spending twentyfold.

China, concerned with its standing in the world, sees HIV/AIDS as prominent among infectious diseases that pose a threat to its national image, and consequently a national security issue. China's belated response to the 2003 SARS epidemic was heavily criticized at home and abroad, while quarantine measures hit the country's exports. Less tangible but perhaps more serious was the Chinese leadership's fear that their country would be seen as a global source of disease. Taking a long view, the leadership resolved that secrecy was not an option, and that the effective management of the HIV/AIDS epidemic, including measures such as harm reduction for injecting drug users, was in its national interest. China has acted accordingly.

In 2008, the U.S. NIC revised its assessment of the security implications of infectious diseases (NIC 2008). Gone were the predictions of social crisis and state collapse in Africa and the predictions that hyperendemic HIV would become common in Asian populations. Rather, the focus shifted to a wider spectrum of diseases, including chronic diseases and accidents, and their economic impacts. For example, the report notes that poor health is costing Russia an estimated 1 percent of GDP annually, and this may rise to as much as 5 percent by 2020, and conversely notes that reduction in disease burden contributes to economic growth. The governance impacts of health, it suggests, are "less pervasive" and cites examples of how mishandling of health issues can undermine a government's credibility, citing Thabo Mbeki's stand on AIDS and China's dithering over SARS. It also refers to contrary cases in which organizations such as Hezbollah in Lebanon or Hamas in Palestine have provided basic health care, enabling them to build a political base. In terms of military readiness, the report points to the poor health status of army conscripts in Russia and North Korea but also revisits the NIC's earlier fears about how HIV/AIDS would undermine military capabilities in sub-Saharan Africa, suggesting both that the risks had been overstated and the responses effective.

Perhaps most significantly, the 2008 NIC report concludes with a section entitled "Health as Opportunity: A new look at a successful paradigm." Global health, it suggests, is a fruitful field for diplomacy, including effective engagement with rising powers, reconstruction and stabilization, smoothing relations with adversaries, easing tensions between the U.S. and the developing world, and advancing economic development. The earlier pessimism had given way to optimism that efforts such as the President's Emergency Plan for AIDS Relief (PEPFAR) and other initiatives on malaria and child survival could become one of the U.S.'s major sources of global influence.

Even though the HIV/AIDS pandemic, including its broader impacts, may not have materialized as feared, HIV/AIDS has had global social and governance consequences. Among them is PEPFAR itself, which surely would not have been established and placed under the authority of the Department of State, were it not for the fears outlined above.

The following sections of this chapter focus on the missing middle: the evidence and experience that contributed to the remarkable turnaround between the NIC's January 2000 and December 2008 reports, including attending to some of the impacts that did unfold and the responses to the perceived crisis. Some of the reassessment was driven by new and better data, some by observation of an unfolding reality, and some by a positive assessment of the actual and potential impacts of programs and policies, notably antiretroviral treatment.

The essential background to this reassessment is the downward revision of estimates for the global numbers of people living with HIV (UNAIDS 2005a, 2006b). New HIV infections, having accelerated at a faster rate than anyone expected in the 1980s and 1990s, had crested and begun to fall (slightly) earlier than had been anticipated. Models for global HIV incidence indicate a peak in new infections in the early 2000s (Shelton, Halperin, and Wilson 2006). This downward revision had several components. The most important was that the concentrated epidemics in Asia and Eastern Europe were not developing into generalized epidemics, so that even the lower-end estimates made by the NIC in 2002 were proving overstated. In Africa, only South Africa and some of its immediate neighbors were sustaining hyperendemic HIV, and most countries were registering declining HIV rates.

## Armies, Law Enforcement, and HIV/AIDS

The issue of HIV prevalence in armies has been the subject of a number of "factoids"—claims that are so regularly cited that their original provenance becomes obscure and their slender empirical basis becomes overlooked (Barnett and Prins 2005). Prominent among these is the claim that HIV rates among soldiers are typically two-to-five times higher than among civilians, and that this ratio can be many times higher still during conflict (UNAIDS 1998a[5]; Yeager, Hendrix, and Kingma 2000), a claim repeated in at least ten publications (Barnett and Prins 2005, 18)

The claim that soldiers had elevated rates of HIV stigmatized them, and in turn caused many armies to become secretive, both about their HIV/AIDS problems and also about the policies and practices they followed (Rupiya 2006). In fact, data indicate that this is rarely the case (Whiteside, de Waal, and Gebretensae 2006). One reason for this is that infantry armies commonly recruit from a population category with low HIV, namely young rural men. The biggest study of HIV prevalence among recruits was conducted using HIV screening data from the Ethiopian army which showed low HIV levels (Abebe et al. 2003). Comparable data were collected in Swaziland (Simelane, Kunene, and Magongo 2006). However, HIV prevalence among soldiers increases with time in service and appears to do so more rapidly than among civilian peers (ASCI 2009).

Sub-Saharan armies moved promptly to respond to the threat posed by higher-than-normal rates of incapacity and death. Armies are designed with an element of redundancy built in, especially at lower ranks, so they can withstand attrition during war. They are also ready to implement command measures that violate individual human rights, in this case mandatory testing and exclusion of those found to be HIV positive from enlistment, promotion, specialist training, or deployment—all measures that reduce HIV prevalence among the ranks, albeit by displacing the problem elsewhere. Because they are incompatible with human rights standards and contradict national (civilian) HIV policies, many militaries have kept quiet about these practices and implemented them without publicity. Court cases in Namibia and South Africa, both of which found military discrimination on the basis of HIV status to be unlawful, have exposed this gap. It presents military commanders with a dilemma, as their own medical analysis and interpretation of command responsibility often determines that they practice such discriminatory policies (ASCI 2009).

This poses a particular dilemma for UN peacekeeping operations, which are highly visible and expected to conform to international norms, but are also wholly dependent on the readiness of troop-contributing countries to provide the forces, often in short order. The UN's HIV-testing policy for uniformed peacekeepers is that the sole medical criterion for deployment and retention is "fitness for duty," based on clinical criteria rather than HIV serostatus (Office of Mission Support, 2004). While holding up the standard of exclusively voluntary confidential counseling and testing, the UN also recognizes that many countries, including most of its major troop contributors, have a mandatory HIV-testing policy and do not deploy HIV-positive personnel (Lowicki-Zucca, Karmin, and Dehne 2009), and the UN respects these national policies.

The story for police services is similar. Senior police officers also felt stigmatized by casual allegations of high levels of HIV in their ranks, an especially problematic claim because of the day-to-day interaction between police officers and the general public. This led to even greater opacity than among armies and more obstacles to researchers (Masuku 2007). As a result, even limited data are not available, and the issue of HIV/AIDS within law enforcement services remains neglected (ASCI 2009).

An emerging agenda concerns how law enforcement influences the trajectory of the epidemic itself. This is the most compelling, if little studied, example of how governance can determine HIV/AIDS. In many countries in the world, HIV transmission is concentrated among groups which are criminalized or stigmatized, or is associated with practices that infringe the law. Examples include injecting drug users (IDUs), sex workers (SWs) and their clients, gay men and individuals with variant sexual identities, and illegal immigrants. Those most vulnerable to HIV may be offenders, victims, or the socially excluded. Examples include survivors of rape and other forms of sexual and gender-based violence and exploitation (SGBVE), trafficked women, and street children. In one way or another, the principal point of contact with the authorities for most of these people is the police officer. It follows that law enforcement and policing practices can be a major influence on the course of the epidemic, either for good or ill.

Challenges for the police occur in situations in which the law and widely held social norms come into conflict with public health principles and human rights. The most acute examples concern harm reduction technologies and methods such as methadone substitution and needle exchange for IDUs. These are prohibited in many countries yet are an HIV prevention intervention of proven efficacy. In the best cases, the individual police officer has much discretion in whether and how to enforce the law. In some countries, police officers turn a blind eye to their obligations under the law, knowing that it would be counterproductive and wasteful to try to enforce impossible prohibitions. They prefer for their discreet tolerance of harm reduction to go unnoticed in the public realm, because they fear that populist politicians would demand zero tolerance of prohibited activities. In other instances, such as China, the authorities recognized the efficacy of harm reduction measures and implemented them rapidly at scale, with measurable success. Increasingly, international HIV/AIDS policymakers are taking seriously the challenge that HIV transmission through IDUs can be prevented entirely, and that this requires the universal adoption of harm reduction technologies and practices, which in turn demands the worldwide decriminalization of drug use.

Policing practices concerning SWs provide another example. In some countries, possession of a condom is taken as evidence for participation in illegal sex work, complicating HIV prevention efforts. In other countries, the police themselves regulate commercial sex work, including the sexual exploitation of underage girls and trafficked women, operating simultaneously on both sides of the law. This poses acute dilemmas for HIV/AIDS advocates and policymakers, who want instinctively to respond both to the abuse of women and girls and to the threat of HIV—priorities that might not always be fully aligned.

Rape and gender-based violence are risk factors for HIV as well as crimes in themselves. Policing practices are a major part of the social response to SGBVE. Policemen and police forces can be contributors to SGBVE, with survivors of sexual violence sometimes suffering additional abuse, including sexual abuse, from policemen, who may hold discriminatory attitudes and enjoy a culture of impunity.

## HIV/AIDS during Traumatic Social Transitions

The assertion that armed conflict contributes to inflating HIV levels was a standard assumption at the turn of the millennium. This derived in part from circumstantial evidence suggesting that the movement of Tanzanian military brigades through Uganda in 1979 had contributed to the first unfolding of the epidemic in east Africa (Hooper 2000), and military bases in Namibia and South Africa had been local epicenters for HIV (Shell 2000). A 2001 meeting of experts convened by the U.S. Institute of Peace reached a consensus that, "Although some might question the significance of AIDS as a contributor to conflict, no one denies the role of conflict in the spread of the virus" (Docking 2001).

This claim has since been convincingly challenged, using data that show that refugees do not have elevated HIV rates in comparison to host communities, and that conflict is often accompanied by a suppression of HIV rates (Spiegel 2004; Spiegel et al. 2007). Other researchers come to slightly varying conclusions (Davenport and Loyle 2009; Iqbal and Zorn 2010). The common ground among these studies is that the implications of conflict and displacement for the epidemiology of HIV vary greatly according to specific circumstances, and the effects are not as dramatic as was earlier anticipated. Increasingly, scholarly and policy attention now focuses on the post-conflict period, as one in which HIV risks may increase because of population mobility and mixing, while HIV/AIDS services may be neglected in the gap between humanitarian relief and reconstruction, and in disarmament, demobilization, and reintegration (ASCI 2009).

The shift in focus from war as such, to the specific forms of social disruption and change associated with war, or with the transition from war to peace, provides a more productive line of inquiry. At a macro level, Paxton (2009) has examined the impacts of transitions—changes in type of regime (principally, democratization), rapid economic growth, and the beginning and end of armed conflict—on

HIV. He used a dataset that included 162 countries over the period 1990–2006. He found that rapid economic growth had no significant impact on HIV prevalence, but that major political transitions from authoritarianism to democracy were associated with an increase of about 0.9 percent. Other forms of political transition had mixed or insignificant results (constrained by the low number of cases from which statistical analysis could be extracted). Paxton found that interstate war had no statistically significant effect on HIV prevalence, but that internal war was associated with a suppression of HIV prevalence by about 1.7 percent. (Note that this does not mean that war pushes HIV prevalence down, but rather that rates would have been higher were the country not at war.)

Ethnographic research, especially with a gender perspective, reveals the bluntness of the concepts used for macroanalyses and alerts us to how existing indices may completely miss the factors that matter. A fine exemplar is the study of Burundi during and after conflict by Seckinelgin, Bigirumwami, and Morris (2008).

The Burundi conflict is normally defined as lasting from 1993 to 2005, and as a low-intensity conflict, with occasional spikes of mass atrocity. However, the definition of the beginning and end of the conflict is political (from the formation of an insurgent movement to a peace agreement), and the calibration of intensity is based upon the conventional measure of violent fatalities, especially on the battlefield. Both are public/political and principally male-framed definitions and assume that "conflict" and "emergency" are deviation from an unproblematic norm, which resumes when the aberrant situation is over. In reality, the outbreak of organized political violence was preceded by widespread dislocation, while the "post-conflict" phase has also seen ongoing disruption and a failure to return to "normality." As Seckinelgin, Bigirumwami, and Morris (2008) show, Burundi is a patriarchal society with immense gender inequalities in "normal" times. Women's vulnerabilities were deepened and changed during the conflict. Pre-existing social relations were not restored after the peace agreement. Spatial patterns of human settlement, marriage and family arrangements, and the status of women were all changed during the twelve years. The conflict was sufficiently protracted and profound in its impacts that it changed the context in which women and men established and maintained sexual relationships and partnerships. Because of the difficulties in organizing marriages and paying bridewealth, fathers had less control over their adult daughters. This relative loosening of paternal control was accompanied by increasing physical insecurity. Young women responded by, among other things, seeking partners from among soldiers and guerrilla fighters. Women always faced disadvantages in negotiating these relationships, and often their best hope was to seek a liaison with an officer or commander, whose rank would protect them from the possibly violent attentions of junior soldiers or fighters. Young men, especially those who were members of armed groups, held the advantage over women in every encounter, but they too faced overwhelming

constraints in trying to find socially-sanctioned long-term partnerships, especially because, with their familial bonds also loosened and their families impoverished, they usually lacked the wealth needed for conventional marriage. Burundi
demonstrates how periods of "low intensity" conflict can also be periods of high
intensity ongoing traumatic social change.

The social implications of conflict do not end with a peace agreement. The
processes of disarmament and demobilization of former combatants, the return
of refugees and displaced people, the opening up of areas that were isolated during conflict, and the winding down of humanitarian assistance are all disruptions
in their own ways. There are numerous historical examples in which demobilizing
soldiers contribute to different forms of violence, including against their spouses,
as well as petty crime and organized crime. Post-conflict periods can witness dis-
possession of villagers' land, as well-connected entrepreneurs move in, and the
sudden creation of boom towns associated with new economic opportunities,
government centers, and aid efforts. In addition, the psychological effects of conflict and trauma, among combatants and civilians alike, can endure long into the
post-conflict period. Numerous studies show that war veterans can be vulnerable
to personal and social dysfunction, including intimate partner violence. All these
can reconfigure vulnerabilities to HIV.

One conclusion from these studies is that researchers and policymakers have
been asking the wrong questions and looking in the wrong place. Casting the
analysis at the level of "conflict" as such misses the significance of the different
kinds of conflict, the groups involved, and the varied forms of interaction among
them. Aggregation to the level of an entire conflict-affected population is less useful than looking at specific groups, times, and places. The concept of a "crisis" or
"emergency" may be useful for marshaling an immediate humanitarian response,
but it does not help shape an appropriate analysis for HIV/AIDS or a response to
the epidemic.

## HIV/AIDS and State Crisis

One of the most compelling claims in the January 2000 NIC report was that the
HIV/AIDS epidemic threatened state crisis and collapse. It has not happened.
Moreover, Barnett (2009) argues that, based on analysis across large datasets of
fragile states and case studies, the lack of any relationship between HIV/AIDS and
state failure is sufficiently robust to allow for a strong conclusion to be drawn,
which is that it is not going to happen.

There is a limiting case: Swaziland, a very small country, economically dependent with weak governance that is facing hyperendemic HIV. Swaziland has been
described as a long-wave social crisis, in which daily mortality rates now exceed

the levels conventionally used by humanitarian agencies as their thresholds for identifying an emergency—facts which require us to revisit how we define the concept "emergency" (Whiteside and Whalley 2007). Swazi citizens face a chronic reduction in living standards. Barnett (2009) points out, however, that a very small nation such as this cannot be taken as a model for larger states. His review includes studies of Manipur and Nagaland, northeast India (Jacob 2008) and the Papua region of Indonesia (Smith 2008), both of which have the highest HIV rates in their countries, and a comparative study of the South Pacific (O'Keeffe 2008). There is no possibility that localized HIV/AIDS crises in parts of India or Indonesia could destabilize the states in question or threaten their overall prosperity, and despite a debate in Australia about possible "Africanization" of the South Pacific epidemic, any similarities are superficial, and the prospects for these countries resembling Swaziland are remote.

Barnett (2009) also modifies his conclusion with respect to local government. Until very recently, the political impacts of HIV/AIDS had been studied only at national level, and there was very little interest in what it might mean for local institutions and their performance and accountability.[6] The largest study of this type to date is a study of twelve municipalities in South Africa (Chirambo and Steyn 2008), which finds measurable adverse impacts of the epidemic on various aspects of local government. They found a consistent pattern of elevated death rates among councilors aged 29–42, raising the prospect of some communities lacking any elected councillors and therefore being unrepresented. Although there are mechanisms to compensate for these losses, including alternate representation and by-elections, these place additional burdens on already overstretched institutions. Strains are intensified by increased AIDS-related absenteeism and lower productivity among staff. Chirambo and Steyn identified "cracks" in the system contributing to poor service delivery. They also noted high level of stigma around AIDS among councillors and found only one councillor openly living with HIV from among a sample of 3,895.

It is notable that HIV/AIDS has not become a major political issue that determines the outcome of elections, even in South Africa which has had the combination of hyperendemic HIV, a president who denies the link between HIV and AIDS, and a powerful activist movement. Public opinion surveys indicate that HIV/AIDS is rarely a priority for electorates (Afrobarometer 2004). In line with the observations by Baylies (2002) and Baldwin (2007), it appears that AIDS is regarded as personal misfortune rather than being the occasion for political outcry. There is a striking contrast with the way in which food crisis is commonly the focus of political mobilization and the relative political apathy over HIV/AIDS. While many nongovernmental organizations have formed around HIV/AIDS, most are service delivery focused and dependent on external money (Englund 2006) and only a few, such as South Africa's Treatment Action Campaign (TAC), are based on grassroots activism. It is striking that, in order to mobilize a broader constituency, the TAC leadership decided to embed the campaign for antiretrovirals within claims for better social services including electricity, water, and housing (Achmat 2004).

Although HIV/AIDS has not become an issue in adversarial politics, it has become an important element of governance in many sub-Saharan countries (de Waal 2006), especially with a proliferation of civil society organizations (Iliffe 2006). This is primarily because of the innovation of the international HIV/AIDS leadership in promoting a human rights-based approach to managing the disease (Piot 2008). The rights-based approach has its origins in the early leadership of the AIDS movement among gay men in America, many of them gay rights activists, and the human rights framework for health pioneered by Jonathan Mann at the World Health Organization. Not only has this led to an emphasis on the individual's right to privacy and the strictly voluntary nature of HIV testing, but it has also contributed to the high-level participation of civil society organizations and representatives of people living with HIV and AIDS in international organizations including UNAIDS and the Global Fund to Fight HIV/AIDS, TB, and Malaria. This approach has its critics, including De Cock and Johnson (1998), De Cock, Mbori-Ngacha, and Marum (2002), Chin (2007), Pisani (2008) and England (2008b), but none of these engage with the issue of the wider governance implications of the exceptionalist approach. The HIV/AIDS pandemic has marked a new era for the governance of international public health, characterized by epidemiological individualism (see Baldwin 2005) and pressures on African governments to conform to a liberal civil society-based framework for disease management (Iliffe 2006; Elbe 2009).

In modern history, the measures implemented to control infectious diseases have often had a greater governance impact than those diseases themselves. To give just one example, European colonial powers' efforts to prevent the spread of cholera and other communicable diseases along trade routes, including the sanitary management of the Muslim Haj, were instrumental in imperial penetration of the Middle East (Bashford 2007). We can see a similar pattern in the case of HIV/AIDS, from the health diplomacy of the U.S. to the ways in which national governments, from Africa to China, have adjusted their governance strategies in response to the unique place occupied by the pandemic in global perception and aid institutions.

Peter Piot, arguing in support of an "exceptional" strategy for HIV/AIDS policy and programming, notes that the international response has been an important factor preventing stigma and discrimination (Piot 2008). It has also contributed to the consolidation of liberal governance in aid-dependent countries in Africa. The 2008 NIC report, with its stress on the strategic benefits of "medical diplomacy" for the U.S., sees this as one of the major, if unanticipated, outcomes of the pandemic. Another consequence is the emergence of a new model for the consensual governance of global public goods, including other disease threats, food insecurity, and climate change. In looking at possible frameworks for its institutional response to the challenge of managing climate change, the UN has debated the merits of the "UNAIDS model" as a model for how to engage a wide range of nongovernmental stakeholders, in such a way that the technical policy demands of a response are made compatible with democratic values and human rights. The rise of public health diplomacy and participatory governance for global public goods may be one of the most significant impacts of the HIV/AIDS pandemic. The public health arguments in favor of promoting harm reduction technologies are now beyond dispute, and it is possible that the next historic contribution of HIV/AIDS to global governance will be in the field of decriminalizing drug use.

## The Long Wave of HIV/AIDS

The analysis above gives far less cause for pessimism than many imagined would be possible even half a decade ago. This is far short of claiming that the pandemic is out of the danger zone or that the instruments are at hand for overcoming it. At the Toronto conference of the International AIDS Society in 2006, Peter Piot insisted that "tragically, the end of AIDS is nowhere in sight."[7] The then Executive Director of UNAIDS felt obliged to make this statement because of the optimism implicit in some of the conference speeches, to the effect that the combination of pharmaceutical technology and huge increases in funds meant that 25 years after the human immunodeficiency virus was first isolated, the world had turned the corner on the HIV/AIDS pandemic. Shortly afterwards, Piot initiated the aids2031 project, intended to look ahead another quarter century to anticipate how the pandemic might unfold over this period, and what might be done to ensure that international commitment to tackling HIV/AIDS remained undiminished.

The combination of the scaling back of UNAIDS's estimates for global HIV infections, evidence for prevalence plateauing or declining in Africa, and the huge increases in resources available for HIV/AIDS since 2002, might make it appear that optimism should be the order of the day. However, Piot's caution is precisely in order. The demographer Roy Anderson has modeled it as an event lasting 130 years (Anderson 2003). Some of the most prominent scholars of HIV/AIDS insist, the pandemic is a "long wave event" (Barnett and Whiteside 2006). Projections for the demographic and socioeconomic impacts of HIV/AIDS epidemics typically cast themselves in terms of decades if not generations (Bell, Devarajan, and Gersbach 2003). While HIV/AIDS may not be leading to dramatic crises, long-wave suppression of life chances and development prospects is probable in hyperendemic countries.

The setbacks in the search for a vaccine are a salutary reminder that there may not be a "cure" for AIDS in the foreseeable future. While the "second wave" fears (Eberstadt 2002) have not materialized, dangers such as extremely drug-resistant strains of HIV, or secondary epidemics associated with the TB pandemic or the worldwide increase in injecting drug use, mean that constant epidemiological and virological vigilance will be required for the indefinite future.

In conclusion, the HIV/AIDS pandemic can no longer be considered an extraneous factor in social functioning or governance. The impacts of the epidemic have been absorbed into social and political systems, while the national and international institutions and initiatives set up in response to the disease have themselves become an integral part of governance. However, vital issues remain unresolved—for example, whether militaries can legitimately practice mandatory testing and selective exclusion of the HIV positive, and whether it will be possible to make harm reduction the guiding principle for law enforcement services towards injecting drug use. While the feared relationships between HIV/AIDS and conflict and state fragility have not transpired, in both cases the epidemic compels reconsideration, not only of specific policies, but of the basic frameworks on which policy is made.

## Notes

1. Eberstadt's 1988 book is a compilation of papers published from 1981 onward.

2. The SFTF was frustrated by the lack of good data on environmental indicators and could not therefore include them in its models.

3. Tony Blair, "Address at the Labour Party Conference," October 2, 2001, http://www.americanrhetoric.com/speeches/tblair10-02-01.htm.

4. The one-time director of CHGA took a different view, writing as late as 2007, "Amid the unrelenting catalogue of horrors . . . must be added the real possibility that with HIV/AIDS the very survival of the African state may well be at stake. . . . There is every reason to suppose that AIDS may well be the deciding factor in shaping the body politics [*sic*] in many societies on the continent" (Poku and Sandkjaer 2007, 1).

5. http://data.unaids.org/Publications/IRC-pub05/militarypv_en.pdf.

6. An exception is Manning (2003).

7. UN News Centre, "With end of AIDS 'nowhere in sight,' UN official urges Toronto meeting to look ahead," August 14, 2006.

# CHAPTER 3

XXXXXX

Microeconomic Perspectives on the Impacts of HIV/AIDS[1]

*Kathleen Beegle, Markus Goldstein, and Harsha Thirumurthy*

## I. Introduction

HIV/AIDS impacts individual, families, and communities across numerous dimensions. Beyond the serious consequences on the health and mortality of persons living with AIDS, the disease has implications for socioeconomic and psychosocial outcomes of families. At aggregate (macroeconomic) levels, the disease can affect the course of a country's economic development and fiscal policy. As financial resources allocated to fight AIDS increase—by seven-fold in the last decade (UNAIDS 2008a)—health spending overall is increasingly dominated by the disease (which van Dalen and Reuser (2008) characterize as an imbalance and a costly shift away from other health services). Much has been written in the last two decades on the theoretical impacts of HIV/AIDS, and numerous empirical studies have attempted to estimate the size of these impacts. Still, there remain important gaps in the empirical evidence and, as the nature of epidemic changes and treatment is scaled up, in topics for study. These gaps no doubt reflect the challenges of this topic, a point we return to in the discussion below.

This chapter presents several microeconomic perspectives on the impacts of HIV/AIDS. We begin by first considering the direct economic impacts of HIV/AIDS. Perhaps the most immediate economic impact of the disease is on household livelihoods—through lower productivity, loss of income, and costs of medical care and funerals. In addition to the consequences for income and livelihoods of households, HIV/AIDS may impact future livelihoods through lower human capital formation and reduction in other investments.[2] These microeconomic relations, in turn, are important for modeling the macroeconomic projections of the impact of AIDS on aggregate measures like gross national income. Knowledge about the microeconomic impacts of HIV/AIDS also provides valuable information to policymakers and consideration of the costs and benefits of various health interventions.

Secondly, this chapter emphasizes that in order to respond effectively to the AIDS pandemic there is a need to also understand how individuals' future-oriented behaviors respond to the morbidity and mortality risks posed by the disease. That is, we focus on social and economic behaviors induced by the disease and the economic consequences of these behaviors. Finally, we also consider what can be learned from recent studies of the economic impacts of providing people with AIDS antiretroviral therapy (ART), a combination of medications that slow the progression of HIV disease and prolong the lives of infected individuals. Provision of ART has been a major policy and medical intervention to combat the disease. We highlight what these studies can tell us about not just the costs and benefits of ART, but also about the economic impacts of HIV/AIDS.

Although HIV/AIDS is global in its reach, we focus this chapter on sub-Saharan Africa for two reasons. It is in this region that the epidemic has arguably had the largest impact, broadly defined. As a result, there are more empirical studies from the region, including in some cases longitudinal studies. Still, there are challenges in interpreting evidence due to the limitations from study design, and generalizability is difficult. The second reason to focus on Africa is that it would be difficult to adequately combine Africa with Asia and Western Europe, where the prevalence rates and socioeconomic patterns of the disease are starkly different (UNAIDS 2008a; World Bank 1999). Instead of providing a comprehensive review of the many existing studies of the microeconomic aspects of AIDS (there are several such reviews that we refer to below), we highlight the key economic channels of impact and highlight some of the salient studies.

When framing how and why HIV/AIDS may impact incomes and livelihoods, it is useful to consider the three distinct phases that HIV-infected individuals will experience after becoming infected. The first phase is when a person discovers that she/he is HIV-infected. The second phase is the morbidity associated with the virus. This can follow the first (i.e., if an individual is diagnosed when still asymptomatic), or it can precede it (an individual gets tested for HIV after becoming, or perhaps, because they become symptomatic). The third phase is the mortality associated with the virus.

The implications for economic behavior and the economic consequences vary significantly across these three phases. In the first phase, when diagnosed with HIV/AIDS, a critical question is how the individual then views the future. This view will be tempered by the person's knowledge about HIV/AIDS and the timeline of its progression, knowledge about the availability of medications that can combat the virus (treatment), and expectations on how others will react to revelation of his/her status. This revised perspective on the future, in turn, can affect a range of decisions in dimensions such as investment, how he or she engages with others, and health-seeking behavior. While these effects may largely be at the household level, as individuals change how much they spend on children's education and health, the cumulative effects in countries with high prevalence can be large. Unfortunately, this is also the hardest phase for researchers to study, since, among other reasons, we rarely have appropriate data to examine this.[3] As a result, there is very little evidence on this phase.

In the second phase, the individual is likely to become ill.[4] His/her ability to work and otherwise engage economically will decline. The illness impacts productivity, income, food security, and household economic welfare. In addition to inducing economic responses or costs in the person living with HIV/AIDS, the disease in these first two phases can also affect economic behaviors of non-infected persons, especially of household members and the extended family. As the individual becomes visibly affected by the disease, others may change how they interact with this individual in economic dimensions—providing assistance (in cash, labor, or kind), for example. In the third phase, the death of the person due to AIDS, his or her family, household, work partners (including firms), and community will be affected.

In the next section, we focus primarily on the economic consequences of HIV/AIDS during phase 2—the effects of morbidity. However, many of the studies discussed do not necessarily distinguish the separate effects of phase 1 and phase 2 and thus often represent some combination of the two effects. Section 3 examines the economic impacts of HIV/AIDS during phase 3—the period of AIDS-related mortality. This section also discusses how the changes in life expectancy due to AIDS mortality can influence economic behavior. Section 4 therefore explores the economic impacts of providing ART. A general discussion is presented in Section 5, with emphasis on gaps in the body of applied microeconomic studies.

## II. HIV Infection and Labor Productivity

We start our examination of the economic consequences of infection by exploring a growing literature which shows the impacts of HIV-related morbidity on labor supply and productivity. A significant body of evidence has documented physical declines among persons living with AIDS, most noted in the year of infection preceding death with some effects in the years preceding death (if untreated).

One of the most precise studies of the effects of HIV-related morbidity on labor productivity and worker income comes from the study by Fox et al. (2004) of a tea estate in Kenya.[5] Because workers work on picking a single crop and their output is measured daily by the management, this setting allows a clear insight into the path of the downward trajectory in productivity. Working backwards from deaths or medical retirements (which Fox et al. label AIDS-related termination), they are able to document effects in a number of dimensions. They find that the overall labor supply of workers starts to decline well before termination: sick leave and unpaid leave among HIV-positive workers is higher than for the reference population (those who do not terminate) up to 2–3 years before termination. When HIV-positive workers are at work, they are not doing as much for two reasons. First, managers tend to shift them to light duty as a result of morbidity, which represents a loss of income for the person with HIV. HIV-positive workers spent 19.2 days more on light duty in the second year before termination and 21.8 days more in the final year. Second, even when they are plucking tea, HIV-positive workers pick less. Productivity in tea plucking starts to decline about 1.5 years before termination, where the difference is 10 percent. Shortly before termination, this differential grows to 19 percent. Together these effects add up to a production loss of 30.5 percent in the second year (13–24 months) before termination and 35.1 percent in the last year before termination. Since workers are paid per kilogram of tea plucked (with a flat rate for light duty), Fox et al. are able to measure directly the workers' income loss as a result of HIV-related morbidity. In the second year before termination, this income loss amounts to 16 percent, rising to 18 percent in the final year. This study shows significant income losses associated with HIV-related morbidity, extending back at least two years before the individual stops work completely. The morbidity consequence manifests obviously through absence from work altogether, but also through an increasing shift to less strenuous tasks and lower levels of productivity when present.

From a household perspective, the picture is, however, more complicated since increases in labor supply by other household members can at least partially offset individual income losses due to illness. On the other hand, if HIV-infected individuals are ill and require caregiving, household members who are the main caregivers may be constrained in their ability to work more to offset income losses. Beegle (2005) finds little change in labor supply of other family members in the months preceding prime-age deaths in Tanzania, although increases in caregiving do not account for this.

Rosen et al. (2004) survey firms in Southern Africa to measure the productivity impact of AIDS illnesses. They also find an increase in absenteeism in advance of AIDS-related termination: firms report additional sick leave for HIV-infected workers in the second year prior to termination ranging up to 20.2 days. In the year preceding termination, this range is between 11.2 and 68.4 days. These firms also estimate that the productivity loss for workers (when they are at work) ranges between 4–33 percent in the second year before termination and between 22–63 percent in the last year. Similar data can be found for the public sector.

Rosen et al. (2007c) use data from the Zambia Wildlife Authority to show that individuals who likely died from AIDS spent 37 percent less time on patrol three years prior to termination, 51 percent less at two years, and 68 percent less in their final year compared to a set of reference individuals. Adding this up, they estimate that their index subjects lost nearly 1.6 person-years of service delivery compared to the reference population.

Recent studies on the impact of ART (discussed in a later section of this paper) also document the decline in labor productivity in the period preceding the initiation of treatment. Here we discuss evidence from two studies in Kenya and one in Botswana.

In their study from Kenya, following the tea workers setting in Fox et al. (2004), Larson et al. (2008) find significantly lower labor supply among HIV-infected workers. They are absent, on average, four more days per month, which amounts to a 22-percent labor decline in the year before initiating ART. Habyarimana, Mbakile, and Pop-Eleches (2009) examine human resource data from two mines of the Debswana Diamond Company in Botswana, which provides free firm-based ART to its employees. In the five years preceding treatment, HIV-positive workers show no significant difference from other workers. However, 12–15 months prior to treatment, there is a sharp increase in absenteeism, equivalent to an annual rate of about 20 days. This is most marked in the month prior to treatment, when absenteeism peaks at five days, about five times the average of all workers. Thirumurthy, Graff Zivin and Goldstein (2008) find a decline of labor supply in the context of an AIDS treatment program in western Kenya. In this rural population, they find a sharp decline in labor force participation (from about 90 percent to less than 60 percent) and in hours worked (from around 32 to 15 hours per week) in the eight weeks preceding treatment, as CD4 counts decline.

These studies tell us about labor supply and productivity effects of morbidities due to HIV. However, they, as well as the larger literature, have less to say about the more complicated process of occupational choice. It could be that changes in life expectancy associated with the discovery of one's HIV status (phase 1) cause people to change how they earn their living. In addition, the morbidity associated with phase 2 could also be associated with occupational switching as individuals seek less physically demanding work (as was observed in Fox et al. (2004)). Both of these effects are increasingly relevant with the growing availability of treatment, since choices made during these two phases will have longer-term effects, as individuals survive for significantly longer time. We return to this in the final section.

Aside from the impact on own-income and direct costs of medical treatment, there are a number of channels through which HIV/AIDS among employees can affect the bottom line of the firms and government agencies which employ them. These channels vary with HIV/AIDS-related morbidity, mortality, and the provision of ART. We discuss these pathways together, mainly because empirical work on this topic aggregates these costs. First, as noted above, there are the lower levels of productivity of workers with AIDS while they are on the job. From the employer perspective, these are of particular concern when workers' pay is not directly linked to productivity. Second, there is also increased absenteeism (or various forms of leave) which is costly. Third, there are increased supervisory costs as the supervisor has to deal with reallocating labor for lower productivity and absenteeism, provide support for the HIV-infected individual, and possibly interact with the family of the worker and deal with funeral activities (in the case of mortality). Fourth, the funeral often involves leave for other workers in the firm, and in some cases, the organization may bear part of the costs of the funeral ceremony itself. Fifth, in the case of a loss of an employee to HIV/AIDS (due to death or permanent medical leave), the organization will incur costs searching for a suitable replacement and suffer productivity losses until a replacement is identified, particularly in team-based environments. Sixth, the replacement employee, if any, will operate at sub-optimal productivity until training is complete. Finally, the organization will incur increased health and life insurance costs as a result of HIV-related morbidity, and these costs could be particularly large if ART is not provided by the public sector for free. Indeed, even when ART is provided for free by the public sector, costs to the firm may be significant, as accessing medical services entails further absenteeism.

With respect to pre-ART Southern Africa, Rosen et al. (2004) estimate the cost to firms per infection as 0.5 to 3.6 times median salary, with HIV/AIDS adding in total 0.4 to 5.9 percent to firms' annual salary and wage bill. For firms that provided end-of-service benefits, this was a major part of the costs (more than 50 percent). Replacement of an employee was also a significant cost. Looking at a set of small and medium enterprises in a number of African countries, Rosen et al. (2007a) estimate the cost of AIDS-related terminations as $858 per company per year, which for the median company amounts to around a 2.4 percent increase in labor costs. They also provide estimates for the public sector with data from the Zambia Wildlife Authority. In addition to the productivity losses described above, they add in other labor losses—for example, supervisors and managers report spending 11 days taking care of a sick employee, interacting with his family, and other tasks; and then, when the individual dies, an average of 30 people take one day off to attend the funeral. They estimate the total labor losses at 2.0 person-years. Including other costs such as funerals, life insurance, replacing the worker, and care and support, they estimate total costs of $7,869 or 3.3 times typical annual compensation. In 2005, AIDS-related deaths cost the Zambian Wildlife Authority 9.3 percent of its total labor bill.

## III. Impact of AIDS Deaths and Reduced Life Expectancy

In this section, we discuss the economic consequences of the deaths of HIV-infected individuals. This discussion draws mostly on studies that examine prime-age deaths, and in rare cases can attribute the cause of death specifically to AIDS. We center this discussion around three areas which arguably encompass the salient economic consequences of adult deaths: household poverty and livelihoods, investments in children, and gender dimensions. In addition to this look at specific impacts of an individual's death, we include some discussion on how lower life expectancy in general can influence economic behavior.

### *Livelihoods and poverty*

HIV/AIDS-related deaths are expected to have an economic impact on households through the direct loss of an income earner, funeral costs, and disinheritance.[6] Naidu and Harris (2005) review several related studies. The most common empirical approach is to compare households recently affected by the death of a prime-age household member to non-affected households. Several studies find that affected households are not uniformly poorer than non-affected households (for example, see the five country studies in Mather et al. (2004), who then raise the question of the efficacy of targeting on a category of AIDS-affected households thus defined). Using panel data, there is not strong evidence of long-run income declines for households impacted by a prime-age death. Mather et al. (2004) find that rural Kenyan households with an adult death, in general, were not more likely to fall into poverty several years later, although using the same data Yamano and Jayne (2004) find that affected households reduced the amount of land dedicated to cash crops. For households from rural Tanzania, Beegle, De Weerdt, and Dercon (2007) find large negative impacts on income within five years, especially associated with female deaths, but no statistically significant impacts 10–13 years later. Carter et al. (2007) study South African households and find that households below the poverty line are *less* severely affected than somewhat better-off households. Furthermore, these severely affected households are able to recover eventually.

### *Children*

One dramatic consequence of higher rates of prime-age mortality due to AIDS in Africa is the increase in the number of orphaned children. And it is not just the AIDS status of parents that may matter; in settings with high rates of fostering of children, AIDS infections among other co-resident adults can impact children. Children can be affected both before and after a parent's death. Ainsworth,

Beegle, and Koda (2005) and Evans and Miguel (2007) find that school attendance declines in the months *before* the death for children in Tanzania and Kenya, respectively. There are several cross-sectional studies which examine the impact of parental deaths on health and schooling outcomes for children.

Despite widely held assumptions that the impact of mortality of parents will be large and negative, in her review of the literature, Burke (2006) concludes that the findings from these studies are often mixed. Ainsworth and Filmer (2006) emphasize the role of poverty and income over orphan status as a determinant of schooling. Often these studies rely on cross-sectional surveys which confound their interpretation for two reasons. First, the socioeconomic determinants of who gets AIDS may be correlated with schooling outcomes for children. This suggests that comparing children across households is problematic. Case, Paxson, and Ableidinger (2004), for example, compare orphans and non-orphans within the same household to address this. However, a second confounding issue is the placement of children with family networks. To the extent that orphans are found in relatively better-off households in the family network (and ones that also have higher demand for schooling), simple cross-sectional comparisons of enrollment rates between orphans and non-orphans may underestimate the true impact (for example, see Hargreaves and Glynn (2002) and Ksoll (2007)). In their study of orphanhood in Zimbabwe, Nyamukapa and Gregson (2005) describe the system of childcare arrangements as traditionally based in part on both relatives' relationships with the orphan and their ability to assist. They further note that orphan care arrangements are increasingly being influenced by financial considerations.

A handful of researchers are able to use longitudinal survey data, such as Beegle, De Weerdt, and Dercon (2006b) in Tanzania, Case and Ardington (2006) in South Africa, Evans and Miguel (2007) in Kenya, Timaeus and Boler (2007) in South Africa, and Parikh et al. (2007) in South Africa. Several studies conclude that maternal deaths have a greater impact than paternal deaths—and Beegle and De Weerdt (2008) characterize this one clear pattern emerging from empirical studies. Yet, using panel data from South Africa, Parikh et al. (2007) find no disadvantage in school for orphans compared to non-orphans. Likewise, using different data from the same region of South Africa, Timaeus and Boler (2007) find just limited importance of maternal orphanhood and large benefits of residing with fathers for children's schooling. They conclude that it is difficult to generalize results about how AIDS impacts children, given so few and geographically-localized studies.

While there is arguably more empirical work focused on children, with respect to understanding the economic impact of AIDS deaths, most of the panel studies focus on 1–3 years following the death. Long-term effects might be different if children can re-enroll (if the short run shows negative impact), or if they eventually drop out (the short run shows no impact). Secondly, we do not know which causal mechanisms are at work here (e.g., if financial, psychosocial, the movement to another household, stigma, or HIV status among adolescents)—a key element for designing better policy/interventions.

## Gender

There may be important gender dimensions to economic impacts of AIDS on households. Gender inequalities in education, income, and property ownership may play important roles for impacts (as well as the spread of the disease). Women are more likely to be caregivers of both sick adults and foster children in the household. For example, a survey in South Africa showed that two-thirds of care-givers were women with a third of them above age 60 (Steinberg et al. 2002, as cited in UNICEF 2004). Gender inequalities in access to off-farm income oppor-tunities make remittance income and (dis)inheritance of assets more salient issues for women. Women in many African settings have less secure rights to land and assets, raising concerns about women being dispossessed of assets when widowed or when another (male) household member dies.

Evidence of such events often comes from case studies; evidence from sample survey efforts is lacking. One exception from Malawi is somewhat contrary to expectations. Data from the national household survey in 2004–05 showed that less than 15 percent of households suffering a prime-age death in the last two years reported an asset loss, including land, associated with the event (World Bank 2006b). In the same study, it was found that the average value of land and assets lost after a male death in the household was actually lower in the patrilineal North region, where women traditionally have less rights to assets, compared to the South and Central regions (Republic of Malawi and the World Bank 2007). This finding likely reflects rapid changes in national laws and local customs. For exam-ple, Adhvaryu and Beegle (2009) report that of the 51 villages in the Tanzania data they study, in 1991, 39 percent of village informants reported that the norm in the community allowed a woman to inherit land when her husband dies. In 2004, 86 percent report that this is the norm. While male deaths, including husbands and sons, may be more salient for women than men with respect to assets and income, deaths of prime-age women may matter for non-monetary reasons. Adult daugh-ters are more likely to be caregivers to their elderly parents, making older adults potentially vulnerable to a lack of care if they lose daughters.

## Impact of reduced life expectancy, or increased mortality risk

In addition to the impact of HIV/AIDS on incomes, it may be that the large reduction in life expectancy due to HIV/AIDS causes currently infected individ-uals to modify their forward-looking behavior. Moreover, parents may also adjust the levels of investment they make in their children's human capital as a result of reduced expectations about the longevity of their children. These indirect impacts of the disease, it could be argued, could have more long-term implications than some of the direct impacts of the disease on outcomes such as labor productivity and income.

To date, there is limited empirical evidence on the extent to which life expectancy has influenced investment behaviors in the general population. The set of behaviors that could be influenced range from standard measures of investment in human capital, such as schooling and participation in risky health behaviors, to other outcomes such as fertility and investment in physical assets such as land and livestock. Collins and Leibbrandt (2007) find that households respond to the threat of HIV/AIDS deaths by holding a portfolio of funeral insurance, but that this, in turn, crowds out other savings and insurance provisions (such as health insurance). Identifying these impacts can be challenging, as it is difficult to obtain direct measures of (not to mention exogenous variation in) the subjective life expectancy held by individuals. Often this is captured through the sub-national variation in HIV prevalence rates. For example, using Demographic and Health Surveys with regional HIV estimates, some studies explore the differences in sexual behavior across regions and associate that with differences in HIV prevalence. The key assumption here is that individuals' subjective life expectancy is highly correlated with regional HIV prevalence. Using the latter as a proxy for life expectancy when explaining sexual behavior requires assuming that, after controlling for income and other commonly observable characteristics, no variables other than life expectancy are correlated with regional HIV prevalence and also directly influence sexual behavior.

The limited evidence so far, subject to the caveat noted about using regional HIV estimates to approximate perceptions of life expectancy, suggests that life expectancy may play some role in shaping some behaviors. Oster (2009) argues that low life expectancy leads individuals to engage in more risky sexual behavior. She uses the distance to the origin of the disease as an instrumental variable for regional HIV-prevalence rates. While this instrumental variable overcomes some of the endogeneity problems noted above, it, too, is arguably likely to be associated with several characteristics that are correlated with HIV-prevalence rates but also independently influence sexual behavior. Fortson (2008b) also uses data from multiple countries and finds that areas with higher HIV prevalence (and presumably, lower subjective life expectancy) have lower levels of school completion and progress through school. On the other hand, the results from studies of the impact on fertility decisions have been mixed. Fortson (2009) and Kalemli-Ozcan (2008) finds a positive relationship between HIV-prevalence rates and fertility decisions, whereas Juhn, Kalemli-Ozcan, and Turan (2008b) find no impact. Young (2007), on the other hand, finds a fertility decline in response to higher HIV prevalence. The fertility results are especially relevant in studies on the macro-economic consequences of HIV/AIDS; for example, the result that a country's per capita income *benefits* from HIV/AIDS in Young (2005) depends critically on assumptions about population growth rates (or population declines in this case).

## IV. Economic Dimensions of Antiretroviral Treatment

The severe morbidity and high rates of mortality due to HIV/AIDS have led to a rapid growth in the provision of ART in the past five years. Perhaps the most dynamic aspect to HIV/AIDS policy has been the tremendous increase in the coverage of both HIV testing and treatment programs in Africa. Treatment may lessen the direct economic consequences of HIV/AIDS illnesses (Section 2) and also the consequences of AIDS-related mortality (Section 3). A large medical literature has shown that ART has been shown to lower morbidity and prolong the lives of HIV-infected individuals.[7] The evidence gathered to date suggests that these health benefits of ART also result in productivity gains for treated adults. In addition, there are other economic benefits from ART, particularly for families of persons receiving treatment.

Several studies document the impacts of ART on the labor market outcomes of treated adults. Upon initiation of treatment, Thirumurthy, Graff Zivin and Goldstein (2008) show a strong response in both health outcomes and employment outcomes (see Figure 3.1 for the impact of ART on weekly hours worked). The size of the labor supply increases estimated is substantial: over the course of six months, patients who have just initiated ART show a 17-percentage point increase in labor force participation rates and work 7.9 hours more per week. The estimates imply a 26-percent increase in participation rates and a 39-percent increase in number of hours worked. The story that emerges from these data is that in the first six months of ART, there are large increases in labor supply. In the second six months of ART, there are no additional changes in labor supply.[8]

A few of the existing studies also caution that labor productivity may not fully recover to pre-illness levels. Although the productivity gap between comparison and treatment groups narrows significantly once ART is initiated, Larson et al. (2008) find significantly lower labor supply for ART patients for up to 12 months after treatment is initiated. Still, after 12 months on ART, workers worked at least twice as many days in the month as they would have in the absence of ART. Habyarimana, Mbakile, and Pop-Eleches (2009) find that subsequent to ART initiation, there is a rapid decrease in absenteeism rates. In the period from 2–4 years after ART initiation, treated workers have low absenteeism rates that are similar to those of other mining workers at the same company. These workers are quite ill, the average CD4 count at the start of treatment is 163 cells/ml, and 25 percent have CD4 counts below 50. In terms of phase 1 (discovery of status) compared to phase 2 (morbidity associated with moving to later stages of the disease), they

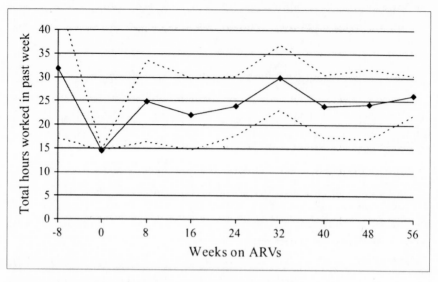

*Figure 3.1*   Weekly Hours Worked Before and After ARV Therapy in Kenya
(Dashed lines are 95 percent confidence intervals)
SOURCE: Thirumurthy, Graff Zivin, and Goldstein (2008), 525, Fig. 4. Originally published in *Journal of Human Resources* 43.3 (Summer 2008): 511–552. © 2008 by the Board of Regents of the University of Wisconsin System. Reproduced courtesy of the University of Wisconsin Press.

find that workers who start treatment as soon as they enroll in the program (an imperfect measure of discovering status) had higher absenteeism rates than those who started treatment after program enrollment. The timing of the start of treatment seems to influence the extent to which treatment offsets productivity declines from HIV-related illnesses.

While these studies of treatment find that the mortality effects are alleviated (patients live longer), not all morbidity effects are alleviated. This may be because these studies occurred in the early stages of treatment availability and at a time when the relevant countries were still pursuing opt-in HIV testing in all avenues of care and, as a result, treated patients were very sick when they began treatment. With a move to some degree of opt-out testing and wider availability of treatment, it is possible that more recent evidence will show much lower levels of pretreatment morbidity with attendant lower effects on labor supply. However, given the low coverage of formal medical care in many areas of Africa, pretreatment morbidity is likely to remain a significant aspect in the economic impact of HIV. Indeed, in discussing the fact that their results show significant effects of morbidity up to three years before termination, Fox et al. (2004) speculate that "the existence of this gap may indicate that HIV/AIDS-related morbidity begins to affect worker performance well before the affected individuals would likely receive an AIDS diagnosis"

(323). If this is the case, then the economic effects of this morbidity suggest using more aggressive testing strategies, especially where treatment is available.

Households in which an adult member falls sick and becomes less able to work may be forced to rely on children to cope with the loss of income and the need for caregiving. Research has begun to address whether ART—when given to adults after they develop AIDS—also improves children's welfare in a manner consistent with the dramatic improvements in adult patient health. In their study conducted in Kenya, Thirumurthy, Goldstein and Graff Zivin (2008) find that ART results in fairly immediate economic benefits to not only the patients being treated but also to the family members of patients. Focusing on several important aspects of children's lives such as schooling and nutrition, evidence suggests that children do benefit when ART is provided to adults in their households. Graff Zivin, Thirumurthy and Goldstein (2009) find large and significant increases in hours of school attended for children between 8–18 years of age. The largest increases in hours of school attended occur for children of ART recipients who are in the early stages of treatment. Attendance levels remain at higher levels after six months of ART. Gains in school attendance are especially large for boys, but they are positive and statistically significant for girls as well. The increases in school attendance are equal to roughly 20–30 percent of pre-ART levels of attendance.

Along with increased productivity and income of treated adults comes the possibility that their households can consume more food. This is especially likely to affect the welfare of very young children, whose nutritional status is highly sensitive to changes in food consumption. Research in Kenya indicates that these children experience large and significant improvements in nutritional status, as measured by weight-for-height, a measure of nutritional status that is sensitive to short-term growth disturbances caused by factors such as inadequate food intake (WHO 1995). Prior to the initiation of ART for adult patients, children in the Kenya study were more malnourished than other children in the clinic's catchment area. Yet this difference was completely erased within six months after ART was initiated, with the weight-for-height measures of children increasing by over 0.5 standard deviations (Graff Zivin, Thirumurthy, and Goldstein 2009). Such nutritional improvements at early ages have significant implications for the cognitive development, future school performance, and employment outcomes of these children (Strauss and Thomas 1995; Glewwe, Jacoby, and King 2001). These may well represent the most long-lasting benefits that society obtains by providing treatment to HIV-infected adults today.

There is continued need for more studies that explore the economic consequences of ART, particularly over the long-term and especially as ART is further scaled up and larger shares of HIV-infected persons are treated. While existing studies may show large, positive impacts over the short-term, it is possible that adherence to medication and retention of patients in treatment programs will decline over time. This would not only lessen the long-term economic impacts of ART, but more importantly might lead to drug resistance and pose larger problems for the future.

As shown, ART has welfare-improving impacts for families, yet changes in sexual behavior in response to treatment availability also have the potential to erode some of these economic benefits. The concern is that for those individuals not in treatment (especially currently uninfected individuals), the availability of ART could result in a lower perceived cost of engaging in risky sexual behavior.[9] If this were the case, scaling up ART could pose a challenge to HIV-prevention efforts. Empirical research on this topic is crucial, as the magnitude of these effects will help assess the need for companion interventions when ART is scaled up. It is reassuring that the evidence to date on the sexual behavior of ART recipients themselves indicates that ART results in *reduced* risky behavior and HIV transmission (Bunnell et al. 2006). Absent more direct evidence on community behavior, the provision of more information and counseling to HIV-negative individuals and those of unknown status seems prudent.

Despite the encouraging evidence on the impacts of ART, there remain a number of other unresolved issues with respect to the policy response to HIV/AIDS. First, while it is clear that mitigating the current and near-term consequences of HIV/AIDS requires the provision of treatment, in the long-term the consequences of HIV/AIDS can best be reduced by achieving large declines in the number of new infections. While this requires a scale-up of effective HIV prevention programs, there are challenges that have to do with a lack of knowledge about effective interventions as well as a lack of resources for scale-up. Second, setting aside issues of resource allocation to treatment as opposed to prevention, on the treatment front alone there remains a large need for more people to access life-saving medications: despite progress over the past five years, only 30 percent of those who need ART are currently receiving the medications. Achieving universal access to treatment (a goal that the international community has committed to) will require even larger funding than what has been recently available which further stresses health delivery systems and other health services. Finally, even for addressing the needs of currently infected individuals, it is vital to look beyond the provision of ART alone, to other interventions such as nutrition and microfinance which may further enable HIV-infected individuals to return to pre-HIV productivity levels. These interventions are starting to be adopted by some treatment programs, but evaluation of them has been limited.

## V. Conclusion

In this chapter, we have sought to summarize some of the large literature on the microeconomic impacts of HIV/AIDS on incomes, livelihoods, and well-being.

The economic impacts of HIV/AIDS on individuals and families stem from various factors: learning one's HIV status, experiencing AIDS-related morbidity, and AIDS-related mortality. Finally, HIV/AIDS can also have an impact on the investment behavior of uninfected individuals by way of the future mortality risk and reduced life expectancy that it causes. In addition to reviewing the various impacts of HIV/AIDS, we have also highlighted the impacts of ART—the leading medical and policy intervention that has been used so far to successfully mitigate many of the health economic impacts of the diseases. Despite the growth in funding for AIDS treatment in recent years, only 30 percent of those who need ART currently receive it. The provision of ART is clearly in a political priority in many HIV-affected countries, and substantial donor support will be needed in order to continue to provide treatment to those already receiving it and to raise coverage rates.

However, there is a need to look beyond ART and consider other interventions that are necessary to reduce the longer-term impacts of HIV/AIDS such as those falling upon families of deceased individuals and orphans, in particular. Unfortunately, there are few evaluations of various candidate interventions such cash or in-kind transfers to HIV-affected families, or programs that target orphans and vulnerable children. It is quite possible that coupled with the provision of ART, these interventions could further lessen the consequences of HIV/AIDS. Evaluating these interventions should be a priority, and lessons from these evaluations could provide better guidance on the allocation of resources.

Assisting those currently suffering from the disease is only one side of the coin—in many countries the number of new infections have continued to grow—thereby ensuring the numbers of people needing ART in the future will also rise. While prevention programs will not address the current labor productivity and welfare consequences, owing to those already infected, they will be of value in reducing the toll taken by HIV/AIDS in future decades. These facts highlight the importance of undertaking more research on effective HIV-prevention programs and increasing donor support for prevention, while ensuring that treatment remains available at high levels. A key limitation in the field of HIV prevention stems from the dearth of rigorous impact evaluations that inform us about the causal effects of various policies on sexual behavior and HIV infection rates. Several main exceptions have been a series of randomized controlled trials that have shown that male circumcision can reduce the risk of HIV infection by over 50 percent. As this intervention is being scaled up in several countries as a major HIV-prevention program, there is a need for similar evaluations of other leading HIV-prevention methods, including some methods that have been promoted and implemented widely (such as ABC programs) but not undergone rigorous evaluation. A number of innovative interventions have also been proposed and piloted in several countries: information campaigns to raise awareness of the risks of unsafe sex and the provision of incentives for remaining HIV negative, for example. Such interventions offer hope for the discovery of effective ways to prevent new HIV infections, but their scalability at the national level can sometimes be debatable. While our understanding of the social and economic consequences of HIV/AIDS has improved considerably in the past few years, and while we now have effective ways to deal with these consequences, much more progress is needed in order to reduce the numbers of people becoming infected each year and thereby lessen the future economic consequences of the disease.

## Notes

1. We are grateful to participants at the UNU-Cornell conference for comments and suggestions. The views expressed here do not necessarily reflect those of the World Bank or its member countries.

2. At the same time, the prevalence and incidence of the disease is influenced by these same factors—poverty, well-being, livelihoods, and investments. The relation between these factors and the *spread* of HIV/AIDS is not the focus of this chapter. Beegle and de Walque (2009) discuss this and reference some of the large literature on this topic with respect to Africa. While there is evidence that HIV infection is not higher among the poor, there is some emerging evidence that economic vulnerability may lead to increased HIV risk, or, in turn, that removing economic vulnerability may reduce HIV risk. Dinkelman, Lam, and Leibbrandt (2007) find that young women respond to negative income shocks by engaging in riskier sex. Robinson and Yeh (2009) look at a broad swath of women engaged in transactional sex in Busia, Kenya. They find that transactional sex responds to household shocks (in particular, the illness of a household member)—they find a 3.1 percent increase in the likelihood that a woman will see a client following a shock. Moreover, with these clients, she is more likely to engage in risky behavior; following a shock, the probability of having unprotected sex increases by 19.1 percent, and the probability of anal sex increases 21.2 percent. While this result may suggest helping mitigate the risks faced by women (many of whom were household heads), recent work in South Africa suggests that economic empowerment of women can have strong effects on HIV risk exposure. Pronyk et al. (2008) examine the effects of providing microfinance and HIV education to 14–35-year-old women. After two years, microfinance beneficiaries were significantly more likely to have accessed testing and were less likely to have had unprotected sex with a non-spousal partner. Part of the reasons underlying this behavior seems to be increased communication by these women about HIV in their homes. While these results are promising, Kim et al. (2008) note that there are other cases in Kenya and Zimbabwe where these results have not been obtained—not least because the microfinance part of the intervention has failed.

3. Beegle and De Weerdt (2008) review the methodological issues that have to be tackled in economic studies of the impact of HIV/AIDS. We discuss these in the last section of this chapter.

4. Progression to AIDS usually takes about nine years from the time of HIV seroconversion and, without any antiretroviral therapy, death usually occurs within nine months after progression to AIDS (Morgan et al. 2002). This progression is often associated with substantial weight loss (wasting) and opportunistic infections such as Kaposi's sarcoma and tuberculosis.

5. The studies discussed here are quite direct estimates of productivity and HIV morbidity. A more indirect approach includes examining the magnitude of worker sickness and death rates in firms, linked with the local rate of HIV prevalence, but not directly assessing the impact of HIV infection of a worker on their actual productivity (such as Biggs and Shah (1996)). A second alternative is to ask households about recent deaths of household members, and ask them to report on the morbidity that preceded the death (as done in some cross-sectional household surveys).

6. In terms of understanding economic impacts cumulatively, being disposed of assets through inheritance systems or land-grabbing is quite different than, for example, less schooling for children or productivity losses due to illness. In the former case, the asset is redistributed in the economy but still exists.

7. Numerous studies have shown that ART dramatically reduces morbidity and mortality among HIV-infected individuals, in both industrialized countries (Hammer et al. 1997; Hogg et al. 1998; Palella et al. 1998) and developing ones (Laurent et al. 2002; Marins et al. 2003; Koenig, Léandre, and Farmer 2004; Coetzee et al. 2004; Wools-Kaloustian et al. 2006).

8. The large impacts of these three ART studies may be upper bounds due to reasons ranging from high supervision and high adherence to medications to high overall quality of care in these facilities.

9. This is considerably less of a concern for those on ART, since these drugs significantly reduce infectivity.

# CHAPTER 4

✕✕✕✕✕✕

## The AIDS Epidemic, Nutrition, Food Security, and Livelihoods:
## Review of Evidence in Africa

*Suneetha Kadiyala and Antony Chapoto*

## 1. Introduction

With a six-fold increase in funding to fight HIV and AIDS this decade, significant advances have been made in combating the intractable AIDS epidemic. Close to three million people received antiretroviral treatment (ART) by the end of 2007—a staggering 10-fold increase in the last six years (UNAIDS 2008a). The annual number of deaths declined from 2.2 million in 2005 to 2.0 million in 2007. At the same time, the multiple drivers, causes, and consequences of the AIDS epidemic have become increasingly evident (Gillespie and Kadiyala 2005a; Chapoto and Jayne 2006; Gillespie et al. 2007). However, significant challenges remain. The empirical record on the effects of HIV and AIDS on nutrition, food security, and livelihoods and the impact of the prevention and mitigation programs remains quite limited, though growing. Despite the massive ART rollout, about two-thirds of Africans living with HIV who qualify for therapy are still not receiving these life saving drugs (UNAIDS 2008a).

Overall, the AIDS epidemic is most severe in sub-Saharan Africa, where pervasive chronic food insecurity and malnutrition are rampant. In Africa, more than 47 million children suffer from stunting (low height-for-age), 11 million children suffer from wasting (low weight-for-height), and about 50 percent of pregnant women are anemic (Hb<11 g/dl). Poor growth is reported in as many as 50 percent of HIV-infected children—they experience slower growth and are at greater risk of severe malnutrition and mortality (Arpadi 2005; Bakaki et al. 2001; European Collaborative Study 2003; Newell et al. 2004).

The United Nations Food and Agriculture Organization (FAO) estimated that 923 million individuals were food insecure globally in 2007, representing an increase of 75 million from 2005. While data are limited on the prevalence of food insecurity among HIV-affected populations in resource-limited settings, a recent summary of 67,038 individuals enrolling in HIV care programs at Academic Model Providing Access to Healthcare (AMPATH) clinics in western Kenya reported that 33.5 percent of enrollees were food insecure, with a range from 20 percent to 50 percent depending on clinic site (Mamlin et al. 2009).

Against this backdrop, although agonizingly slow to take off, there has been an increased recognition of the role of food and nutrition insecurity—often studied through the lens of livelihoods and /or socioeconomic indicators of HIV/ AIDS affected people—as important causes and consequences of AIDS, even as ART is being rolled out. Several frameworks have been advanced to aid the conceptual understanding of and inquiry into these dynamic, complex, and intertwining linkages between the epidemic and food and nutrition security at macro, community, household, and individual levels (Barnett and Whiteside 2006; de Waal and Whiteside 2003; Gillespie and Kadiyala 2005a).[1]

Set against this background, this chapter (a) examines the impact of HIV and AIDS on livelihoods, nutrition, and food security of the affected populations with a focus on sub-Saharan Africa, where the epidemic is most severe; (b) reviews the evidence base on the effectiveness of interventions aimed to mitigate the food and nutrition insecurity impacts of the AIDS epidemic; and (c) concludes with suggestions for a future research agenda to inform action. We focus on the mid and downstream impacts of HIV and AIDS with respect to livelihoods, nutrition, and food security (Figure 4.1). We refer the reader to Gillespie, Kadiyala, and Greener (2007) for a comprehensive review of the impact of poverty, and food and nutrition insecurity on HIV spread.

## 2. Food Security, Nutrition Security, and
## Global Response to the AIDS Epidemic

In the last decade there has been an upsurge in the investigation of the multiple, complex, and dynamic interactions between HIV, nutrition, and food security along

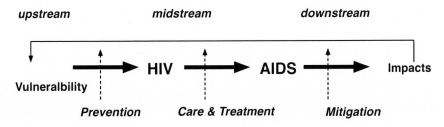

*Figure 4.1*   The HIV Timeline

the HIV timeline (Figure 4.1). The policy environment has shifted significantly, too. The World Health Organization (WHO), in partnership with National Institutes of Health (NIH), held a consultation in Durban, South Africa, in April, 2005.[2] Following this consultation, the Regional Network on AIDS, Livelihoods and Food Security (RENEWAL)/International Food Policy Research Institute (IFPRI) convened a conference in Durban, South Africa, in April, 2005.[3] These consultations resulted in a number of recommendations on integrating food security and nutrition as a critical component of a comprehensive global AIDS response. These consultations culminated in a resolution approved by the World Health Assembly in May, 2006. The e-forum in 2006 leading up to the second partnership forum of the Global Fund to Fight AIDS, Tuberculosis and Malaria urged the Global Fund to consider nutrition as a critical "complementary health product." The UN declaration in June, 2006, represents a significant shift in the global community's approach to combating the epidemic.[4] The policy mandate, with respect to the role of food and nutrition security in the AIDS response, is now clear.

## 3. Concepts and Definitions

At this point, we highlight here three key working definitions of the key concepts (livelihoods, food security, and nutrition security) central to this paper:

*Livelihoods* have become the framework through which food security is usually analyzed and is also often a framework for program interventions. A livelihood "comprises the capabilities, assets (stores, resources, claims, and access), and activities required for a means of living: a livelihood is sustainable which can cope with and recover from stress and shocks, maintain or enhance its capabilities and assets, and provide sustainable livelihood opportunities for the next generation" (Chambers and Conway 1992, 6). While often focusing on food security as an outcome, a livelihoods approach therefore emphasizes understanding people's means of achieving this outcome: their assets, the strategies which they adopt, the constraints they face and the strategies they are forced to depend on to achieve outcomes in terms of food security and accessing other basic requirements (Maxwell et al. 2008). Frankenberger (1996) defines *household livelihood security* as adequate and sustainable access to income and resources to meet basic needs.

*Food security,* here, refers to physical and economic access to food of sufficient quality and quantity. Food security is necessary, but of itself insufficient, for ensuring nutrition security. *Nutrition security* is achieved for a household when secure access to food is coupled with a sanitary environment, adequate health services, and adequate care to ensure a healthy life for all household members. The hungry are a subset of the food-insecure, who in turn are a subset of the nutrition-insecure. Some of the food-insecure are not currently hungry, although they are at risk of becoming so because of their uncertain access to food. Moreover, some of the nutrition-insecure are not food-insecure, as their condition may result from deficits in the health- and care-related determinants of nutrition security.

## 4. Methodological Issues

Evidence from most of earlier microeconomic studies can best be described as anecdotal and speculative, where the impacts of AIDS are hypothesized and conjectured but hardly quantified (see, for example, Haslwimmer (1994); FAO (2003); UNAIDS (1999); Barnett et al. (1995); du Guerny (1999); Drinkwater (1993); Mutangadura and Webb (1999); Topouzis (2000); Stokes (2003); Hall et al. (1998); Kwaramba (1997); Tibaijuka (1997); and Rugalema (1998)).[5] These studies are constrained by the absence of micro-level information on how households respond to HIV/AIDS and the subsequent impacts on household livelihoods, food security, and nutrition security. Fortunately, this has slowly started to change with a number of studies attempting to quantify the impact of prime-age mortality in the era of HIV/AIDS, but the evidence is still modest. (For example, Yamano and Jayne (2004), (2005); Fox et al. (2004); Beegle (2005); Case and Ardington (2006); Evans and Miguel (2007); Beegle, De Weerdt, and Dercon (2007); Chapoto and Jayne (2008); Mather, Donovan, and Jayne (2005); Kadiyala et al. (2009)). However, most of these studies are faced with a number of limitations and methodological challenges that makes it imperative for us to be cautious when assessing the findings. Beegle and De Weerdt (2008) and Murphy, Harvey, and Silvestre (2005) provide an excellent methodological critique and challenges in studying the impact of the epidemic on individuals, households, and economies. In this section, we discuss some of the key shortcomings and methodological issues surrounding the measurement of impact of AIDS epidemic on livelihoods, food security, and nutrition security.

ILLNESS-RELATED MORTALITY AS A PROXY OF AIDS

There are some *a priori* reasons to believe that AIDS-related deaths may have more severe effects than death from other causes, for example, if prolonged illness results in additional burdens associated with extended caregiving and expensive medical treatments. Beegle (2005) and Haddad and Gillespie (2001) provide some insights into why AIDS-related illness and deaths may be different. Being primarily a sexually transmitted disease, HIV infects adults who are economically productive and are of reproductive age. It often clusters within households (and communities)—often more than one person suffers from HIV-related morbidity or mortality within a household, making the traditional safety nets severely strained. Morbidity diminishes labor capacity over the duration of illness. In case of death, however, households will need to adjust to the long-term loss of this individual's labor and related income, in addition to the loss of management skills and acquired human capital investments. In case of AIDS, death is preceded by long and severe illness, thereby increasing medical expenditures and severely limiting daily activities.

Often referred to as the "feminization of AIDS," the situation in many southern and eastern African countries is such that AIDS affects women disproportionately. Another depressing feature of the AIDS epidemic is its silence and invisibility due to stigma, fear, and denial that often prevents those infected and affected from seeking timely assistance. Just as its impacts intensify, with a parallel need for scaled up action, the actual capacity of organizations to respond is eroding. These characteristics of HIV/AIDS-related mortality suggest that we cannot equate it with other short-term health-related or weather shocks facing households.

It is important to take note that almost all the studies measuring the impact of the AIDS epidemic in Africa fail to determine the cause of the illness or death. These studies hence use general illness-related morbidity and mortality as a proxy for HIV/AIDS. This is mainly because of the difficulty and cost of obtaining reliable estimates of AIDS-related mortality as well as the stigma and discrimination that preclude HIV testing and, in general, a more open approach to HIV/AIDS. Also, in the absence of serological data tracking the HIV status of sampled adults over time, a number of studies have used "verbal autopsies" in which medical fieldworkers interview caregivers of the deceased to record information regarding signs and symptoms of the terminal illness, all of which help to reduce the probability of incorrect diagnosis (Garenne et al. 2000; Urassa et al. 2001). However, in population-based samples, verbal autopsies are fraught with problems since there is no generally accepted ideal method of estimating AIDS-specific mortality in most of the population-based samples. It is impossible to get a "gold standard" diagnosis on a true population basis, since the validation of verbal autopsy studies are based on samples that come from clinical samples, and therefore, are not likely to be representative of the population (Gretchen Birbeck, personal communication).[6] Also, an identification of "AIDS' deaths" through diagnoses based on verbal autopsies lacks sensitivity to the extent that certain illnesses will be missed and lacks specificity to the extent that any non-HIV tuberculosis or cancer will also fit the criteria (Doctor and Weinreb 2003). Given these shortcomings, it will be difficult to scale up this approach, hence the need to rely on illness-related mortality.

While not all adult deaths due to illness can be attributed to AIDS in any given country or region, recent epidemiological studies demonstrate that in eastern and southern Africa, HIV is the leading cause of disease-related death among adults between 15 to 49 years of age (Ainsworth and Semali 1998; UNAIDS and WHO 1998; Ngom and Clark 2003). In Kenya and Zambia, Chapoto, Jayne, and Mason (2010) find a strong correlation between prime-age mortality rates and lagged HIV prevalence rates, suggesting that a large proportion of prime-age mortality observed in their household data sets may be due to AIDS-related causes. Therefore, in the absence of widely available diagnostic services in most African countries, the cause of prime-age adult mortality in most studies should be interpreted within the context of a broader complex disease burden.

LIMITED GEOGRAPHIC COVERAGE

The few available micro-level impact studies on the effects of the AIDS epidemic on household livelihoods, and food and nutrition security are almost always drawn from specific geographic sites purposively chosen because they were known to have high HIV infection rates, such as Rakai in Uganda and Kagera in Tanzania. Although these case study panel data sets have generated estimates of the impact of adult mortality and AIDS in particularly hard-hit areas, the studies lack representativeness and could produce overestimates of the impacts of the disease if they are generalized more broadly to the region or continent. Hence, their results cannot provide a comprehensive understanding of the national level impacts.

With few exceptions (for example, Chapoto and Jayne (2008); Kirimi (2008)), the paucity of nationally representative micro-level information remains a critical limitation on the generation of more reliable macro-level projections on the effects of HIV/AIDS. Cross-sectional surveys cannot adequately measure the dynamic effects of mortality or control for unobserved heterogeneity, which are undoubtedly important in this context. Cross-sectional studies do not allow us to measure effects of mortality on outcomes since there is no information prior to the death event; such studies only allow us to compare *ex post* outcomes of afflicted versus non-afflicted households, although this reveals very little about impacts of mortality. Furthermore, for studies with no controls (the comparator group as described by Beegle and De Weerdt (2008)), it is unclear if any observed changes in household welfare for the period before and after death can be attributed to morbidity and mortality apart from other shocks or initial conditions affecting afflicted and non-afflicted households alike.

AIDS MORBIDITY AND MORTALITY MAY BE ENDOGENOUS TO OUTCOMES

Another major difficulty in measuring the impact of adult mortality, especially mortality attributable to AIDS, is that it is influenced by behavioral choices rather than by random events. With some exceptions, the few longitudinal empirical studies measuring the impact of AIDS-related adult mortality on agriculture and rural farm households' welfare acknowledge that the death of prime-age adults, especially mortality attributable to AIDS, may be endogenous to outcomes but nevertheless treat mortality as exogenous (for example, Ainsworth and Dayton (2000); Beegle (2005); Booysen (2003); Yamano and Jayne (2004)). However, with longitudinal data, the endogeneity issue, while still important, is not as critical as with cross-sectional data because fixed effects and/or difference-in-difference models can be estimated to control for time-invariant individual and household characteristics. Nevertheless, time-varying unobserved heterogeneity remains a major problem even with longitudinal data, which may influence both the dependent variables of interest as well as the probability of mortality in the household. Having recognized this problem, instead of relying on parametric approaches (for example, Beegle and De Weerdt (2008); Chapoto and Jayne (2008)), researchers are increasingly employing non-parametric approaches to address endogeneity (for examples, see Mahal et al. (2008); Kadiyala et al. (2009); Mather and Donovan (2008); and Chapoto and Jayne (2008)).

IMPACT BEYOND THE HOUSEHOLD

To date, almost all of the quantitative micro-level studies have investigated the effects of mortality at the household level, even though it is likely that mortality shocks are transmitted across households. This situation, in which a relatively small percentage of households incur a shock, but the shock is spread across households in a community, presents methodological challenges for estimating the full effects of the shock using household survey data. Yet, non-afflicted households are likely to be indirectly affected by the mortality occurring around them; hence, non-afflicted households may not be a valid control group.

In communities hardest-hit by the AIDS epidemic, households not directly incurring a death may nevertheless be affected by taking in orphans, losing access to resources owned by kin-related "afflicted" households, intrahousehold resource transfers to afflicted households, and broader effects of high mortality rates on communities' economic and social structures. With the exception of Jayne et al. (2006) who used the "community" as a unit of observation, the effects beyond the household level seem to be ignored in almost all of the quantitative economic analysis attempting to measure the effects of mortality on livelihoods, and food and nutrition security.

SHORT-RUN VERSUS LONG-RUN IMPACTS

Last, but not the least, most prior micro studies are also unable to estimate the prolonged impact of mortality, starting from the onset of illness, death, and after death short- and longer-term effects. The time periods over which impacts are measured are mostly short-run, which probably understate the full impact on households and communities over time. With the exception of Beegle, De Weerdt, and Dercon (2006a), (2007); and Kirimi (2008), the few existing longitudinal household-level studies have measured the effects of death *in their households* on household-level outcomes, typically over a 2–5 year time frame. Therefore, only short-run effects are measured.

Given the dearth of longitudinal household data over a long time period and methodological limitations, the longer-term effects of AIDS, and particularly the community-level effects, have yet to be rigorously measured. This is especially the case when considering intergenerational effects such as the inability of deceased adults to pass along accumulated knowledge to future generations and the less tangible benefits that children receive from their parents (Bell, Devarajan, and Gersbach 2006; Gertler et al. 2003). The potential persistence of mortality effects beyond the time of death has important implications for policymakers and development practitioners on current and future policies and intervention strategies.

## 5. Evidence of the Impacts

In this section we trace the micro-level impacts of HIV/AIDS on food and nutrition security. The section is organized as follows: We first review the evidence of the interactions between HIV and nutrition at the individual level. Second, with the caveats in methodology of various studies elaborated in the section above, we then elaborate the impact of the AIDS epidemic on food and nutrition security at the household and intrahousehold levels. Here we discuss the evidence of the impact of AIDS on food security-related indicators such as consumption/ expenditures and dietary diversity. Then we present the evidence of the impact of adult mortality of nutrition outcomes of children with in the affected households.

Third, we detail the evidence of the impact of the AIDS epidemic on rural livelihoods. Labor and land are the cornerstones in an agrarian economy. Therefore, we review the evidence on the impact of the epidemic on labor availability, land tenure, and related issues. Although farming is the main source of livelihood in Africa, it rarely is a sufficient means of survival. Practically all rural households juggle a portfolio of activities and income sources. We therefore review the evidence of the impact of AIDS on off-farm income. Finally, we discuss the evidence on "new variant famine" (explained later in the section).

### A. HIV and nutrition: Individual level

Malnutrition and HIV have a few things in common. Both conditions affect the capacity of the immune system to fight infection and keep the body healthy. As shown in Figure 4.2, changes in the immune function due to protein energy malnutrition are very similar to those induced by HIV and AIDS (Beisel 1996).

Figure 4.3 depicts the vicious nutrition-HIV cycle. Lack of nutritious food, loss of appetite, decreased absorption of nutrients due to gastrointestinal complications,

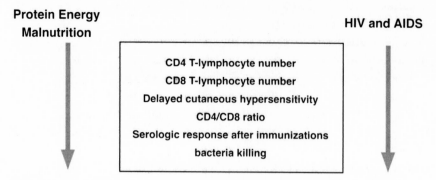

*Figure 4.2*   Some Common Changes in Immune Function due to Protein Energy Malnutrition and HIV
SOURCE: Based on Beisel (1996).

and increased resting energy expenditure play an integral role in HIV-associated weight loss and other micronutrient deficiencies. Poor nutrient status in HIV-infected individuals worsens their immune status, rendering them vulnerable to infections and further deterioration in nutrient status (Scrimshaw and San-Giovanni 1997; Anabwani and Navario 2005). In HIV-infected children, the clinical picture is further complicated by the metabolic demands of growth and development.

The effect of HIV on nutrition begins early in the course of the disease, even before an individual may be aware that he or she is infected with the virus.

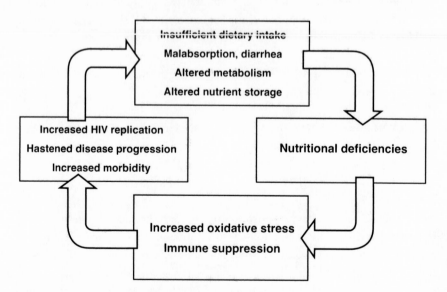

*Figure 4.3*   The Vicious Cycle of Malnutrition and HIV
SOURCE: Adapted from Semba and Tang (1999).

According to the World Health Organization, asymptomatic HIV-positive individuals require 10 percent more energy, and symptomatic HIV-positive individuals require 20–30 percent more energy than HIV-negative individuals of the same age, sex, and physical activity level.

EVIDENCE FROM STUDIES ON ART-NAÏVE PEOPLE LIVING WITH HIV AND AIDS

Studies from the pre-ART era, from both the developed countries and developing countries, show a clear predictive link between macronutrient malnutrition and adverse clinical outcomes. Early studies from the developed countries demonstrated that even modest weight loss (of about 5 percent in four months) and wasting were associated with increased risk of opportunistic infections (Wheeler et al. 1998) and shorter survival time in HIV-positive adults, independent of their immune status (Kotler et al. 1989; Suttmann et al. 1995; Wheeler et al. 1998; Tang 2003).

A similar relationship between macronutrient malnutrition and survival was observed in studies in Africa. In Malawi, among adults with tuberculosis (80 percent of them HIV positive), body mass index (BMI) of less than 17 increased the risk of early death (Zachariah et al. 2002). Among HIV-positive Ugandan children, death before the age of 25 months was nearly five times more likely to occur among those with weight-for-age $z$-scores less than -1.5 than among those with higher $z$-scores (Berhane et al. 1997). In Zambia, low weight-for-age was a strong and independent predictor of poorer survival of ART-naïve children below 14 years of age participating in the Children with HIV Antibiotic Prophylaxis (CHAP) randomized trial (Walker et al. 2006). A multi-country meta-analysis of 10 longitudinal studies (nine African and one Brazilian) confirms these findings (Cross Continents Collaboration for Kids (3Cs4kids) Analysis and Writing Committee 2008).

Deficiencies of vitamins and minerals, which are needed by the immune system to fight infection, are common in people living with HIV in the developed countries and much more so in the developing countries. For example, among HIV-infected and uninfected infants in Uganda, the prevalence of anemia (Hb<11 g/dl) was 90.9 percent and 76.9 percent, respectively (Totin et al. 2002). The evidence from longitudinal observational studies of the effect of declining micronutrient levels on HIV disease progression, in the pre-ART era, has been well documented in developed countries. For example, declining levels of serum vitamin E and B12 were shown to prospectively increase disease progression (Pacht et al. 1997; Tang et al. 1997; Baum 2000); low selenium levels were found to increase the risk of HIV-related mortality by more than 10-fold (Baum and Shor-Posner 1998). Conversely, elevated zinc and iron status have been shown to promote HIV progression (Tang et al. 1993; Tang, Graham, and Saah 1996). Several studies in Africa have prospectively shown anemia to be a strong and independent risk factor for decreased survival during HIV infection among ART-naïve adults (Semba et al. 2002) and children (Walker et al. 2006; Cross Continents Collaboration for Kids (3Cs4kids) Analysis and Writing Committee 2008). However, the causes of these nutrient deficiencies and the effect of reversing them are not yet clearly known.

A large randomized trial on ART-naïve pregnant women in Tanzania examined the effect of micronutrient supplements—vitamin A alone, multivitamins including vitamin B complex and vitamins C and E, and multivitamins plus vitamin A—on the risks of clinical disease progression, HIV-related complications, CD4+ cell counts, viral loads, birth outcomes, and mother-to-child transmission in HIV-positive women in Tanzania. The results are encouraging: daily micronutrient supplementation (without vitamin A) resulted in significantly higher CD4+ and CD8+ cell counts, and significantly lower viral loads, delayed progression to WHO stage 3[7] or higher, delayed death, prevented adverse birth outcomes, and reduced mother-to-child HIV transmission in nutritionally vulnerable women with more advanced HIV disease (Fawzi et al. 2002, 2004). Kumwenda et al. (2002) in Malawi, Coutsoudis et al. (1999) in South Africa, and Friis et al. (2004) in Zimbabwe confirm the role of prenatal micronutrient supplementation in improving pregnancy and birth outcomes which are in turn important determinants of child survival and growth. Studies also indicate that *periodic* vitamin A supplementation reduces morbidity and mortality in HIV-positive children and improves their growth (Coutsoudis et al. 1995; Mehta and Fawzi 2007).

## EVIDENCE FROM STUDIES ON PEOPLE LIVING WITH HIV AND AIDS ON ART

ART dramatically improves survival of people living with HIV/AIDS (Egger et al. 2002). Using data from the Medical Outcomes Study HIV Health Survey (MOS-HIV), Stangl et al. (2007) report that patients in rural Uganda showed large improvements in physical and mental health summary scores within three months of starting treatment, with more gradual improvement in the subsequent nine months. Similarly, results of a cohort of patients receiving ART in Cape Town, South Africa, show that the proportion of these patients reporting no problems in mobility, self care, pain/discomfort, and anxiety/depression increased over the first 12 months of ART, with the most improvement occurring almost immediately after initiation of treatment.

Interactions between these drugs and food and nutrition can significantly influence the success of ART by affecting drug efficacy, adherence to drug regimens, and nutritional status. Management of these interactions is critical to maximizing the benefit of ART to people living with HIV/AIDS in resource-poor settings.

Use of antiretroviral drugs (ARV) can improve nutritional status of children (Verweel et al. 2002) and adults (Silva et al. 1998; Schwenk et al. 1999; Semba et al. 2001; Rousseau et al. 2000). Evidence from cross-sectional and prospective observational studies of micronutrients (almost all of them from developed countries) in HIV-positive persons receiving Highly Active Antiretroviral Therapy (HAART) suggests that some, but not all, micronutrients may increase after HAART initiation.

Yet weight loss and wasting remain significant problems even in the developed countries. For example, weight loss was observed in 48 percent of those on their first HAART regimen after initiation of HAART (Wanke et al. 2000). Early outcomes of patients initiated on ART in African countries show that despite ART, between 10 and 15 percent of individuals die within a median follow-up period of about 15 months (Coetzee et al. 2004; Harries, Schouten, and Libamba 2006; Braitstein et al. 2006). A substantial proportion (about 70 percent) of these deaths occur very early (within the first three months) after starting ART. Zachariah et al. (2006), in a cross-sectional study in Malawi, observed 13 percent of deaths in the first six months among 1,507 people who initiated ART. About 60 percent of these deaths occurred in the first three months.

Compelling evidence from Africa has recently emerged showing that preexisting malnutrition may have adverse implications in outcomes of patients initiating ART. Zachariah et al. (2006), in Malawi, report a linear trend in mortality with increasing grades of malnutrition. Individuals who were severely malnourished at the time of initiating ART [body mass index (BMI) <16.0 kg/m$^2$] had a six times higher risk of dying in the first three months than those with a normal nutritional status. In a prospective cohort study of people starting ART in Tanzania, Johannessen et al. (2008) found severe malnutrition to be an independent predictor of mortality.

More recently, several studies from Africa have shown anemia to be a strong predictor[8] of mortality among patients initiating ART (Moore et al. 2007; Etard et al. 2006; Stringer et al. 2006; Johannessen et al. 2008). In the largest African cohort study published to date, severe anemia (Hb<8 g/dl) was the strongest independent predictor of mortality in 16,198 patients receiving ART in Zambia (Stringer et al. 2006).

We are not aware of any trials assessing the effect of micronutrient supplements on clinical disease progression or mortality in HIV-positive persons receiving HAART. Future research efforts should focus on determining whether certain micronutrients remain depleted after ART initiation and whether micronutrient supplements (and what combination and dosages) would be beneficial in HIV-positive persons receiving HAART. Micronutrients can be an easy and inexpensive adjunctive therapy to decrease the side effects of HIV medications and to improve clinical outcomes in HIV-infected persons in both developed and developing countries.

Reluctance to initiate ART or adhere to the treatment is associated with anxiety regarding being able to maintain consumption of sufficient food and a balanced diet. Indeed, food security or the lack of it is one of the most often cited reasons for poor adherence to ART. Several qualitative studies in sub-Saharan Africa have identified food insecurity as a risk factor for ART non-adherence (Hardon et al. 2007; Au et al. 2006; Olupot-Olupot et al. 2008). For example, among patients surveyed in Rwanda, 76 percent described fear of "having too much appetite and not enough to eat" as a major obstacle to their ART adherence. In contrast, concerns about drug toxicities, disruption of the daily routine, and acceptance of their HIV illness were of concern to only a minority of the study participants (Au et al. 2006).

Once on ART, the side effects of the drugs such as nausea and vomiting may affect adherence to therapy, particularly in the first months of the treatment. Additional metabolic complications such as derangements in glucose, lipid, and bone metabolism, have been associated with the use of certain ARV drugs (McDermott et al. 2001; Carr et al. 1998). Research on the metabolic consequences of ARV therapy and appropriate strategies for their management is a growing field in industrialized countries. Further research is needed in resource-limited settings, where management options and follow-up monitoring are more limited.

## INFANT FEEDING AND MOTHER-TO-CHILD TRANSMISSION OF HIV[9]

The nutrition-HIV nexus first gained prominence with the knowledge that HIV can be passed from mother to child via in utero, intrapartum, or breastfeeding routes. Worldwide, an estimated 2.1 million children live with HIV. In 2008, an estimated 430,000 children became infected with HIV, out of which 390,000 are from Africa (UNAIDS 2009a). The majority of pediatric HIV infections are acquired through mother-to-child transmission (MTCT). In the absence of ART or prophylaxis for the mother or infant, rates of MTCT range from 15 percent to 25 percent when mothers are not breastfeeding to 30 percent to 45 percent in children who are subsequently breastfed up to 24 months of age (WHO, UNAIDS, UNICEF, and UNFPA 2008).

With ART and exclusive formula feeding, the developed countries have successfully reduced the rates of MTCT to less than 2 percent. In Africa, while enormous advances have been made in reducing in utero and intrapartum HIV transmission from mothers to infants through ART, relatively little progress has been made with reducing postnatal HIV transmission through breastfeeding.

There is now substantial evidence that exclusive breastfeeding has substantial child survival benefits, even in the context of HIV (see Coovadia and Kindra (2008) for an excellent review). More recently, exclusive breastfeeding has been found to result in a three-to-four-fold decrease in HIV transmission compared with non-exclusive breastfeeding in several large prospective studies in Africa (Coovadia et al. 2007; Iliff et al. 2005; Kuhn et al. 2007). While some recent studies of HIV-positive mothers and their infants from Africa have shown formula feeding and breastfeeding to have similar risks and benefits (Palombi et al. 2007; Becquet et al. 2007; Thior et al. 2006), exclusive replacement or mixed feeding in most other situations is hazardous (Coovadia and Coutsoudis 2007; Creek et al. 2007).

The current recommendations on infant feeding are now clear (WHO 2006a, 2010): Mothers known to be HIV-infected should exclusively breastfeed their infants for the first six months of life and continue breastfeeding for the first 12 months of HIV-exposed infants' lives.

Following the recent evidence (Obimbo et al. 2004; Johnson et al. 2006; Lunney et al. 2008), early cessation of breastfeeding (before six months), whereas previously recommended by the WHO (2003a), is no longer recommended. WHO also recommends that all HIV-infected infants should be exclusively breastfed for six months and that the HIV-infected infant should continue receiving breast milk for at least two years (WHO 2010).

ART, preferably HAART, for mothers and exclusive breastfeeding for six months in resource-poor settings can efficiently reduce transmission risk.

## PREVENTION OF MOTHER-TO-CHILD
## TRANSMISSION OF HIV PROGRAMS

Despite the introduction of Prevention of Mother-to-Child Transmission (PMTCT) programs in many African countries since 2001, and the availability of efficacious drug regimens, mortality in children, largely due to HIV, is still very high. This is due to the fact that less than 5–10 percent of pregnant women receive any interventions to reduce transmission of the infection to their babies (WHO 2006b).

For a PMTCT program to be successful, pregnant women must follow several sequential steps: (1) attend an antenatal clinic equipped to offer voluntary counseling and testing (VCT); (2) accept pretest counseling and HIV testing; (3) receive their test results; (4) accept ARV prophylaxis; (5) correctly receive and administer therapy; (6) receive infant feeding counseling and enable mothers to make an appropriate infant feeding choice; and (7) participate in postpartum follow-up care (Doherty 2006).

In addition to low-uptake, drop-out from PMTCT services through these key program stages continues to threaten the effectiveness of PMTCT programs (Temmerman et al. 2003; Perez et al. 2004; Manzi et al. 2005). For example, in South Africa, arguably the worst affected country in the world, the PMTCT program has been expanded across the country and is available in over 70 percent of facilities. However, HIV testing of pregnant women remains low at 50 percent, and coverage of nevirapine[10] amongst women identified to be HIV positive continues to be sub-optimal at 45 percent (Doherty 2006).

Infant feeding counseling is clearly one of the most important steps in PMTCT services to prevent postnatal transmission of HIV through breastfeeding. Inadequate training of infant feeding counselors about the relative risks associated with infant feeding and failing to provide them with adequate and sustained support, in the context where mixed feeding is the norm and the prevailing socioeconomic conditions that often make exclusive replacement feeding hazardous and stigmatizing, makes effective infant feeding counseling challenging.

Recent evidence from carefully executed studies shows that in the presence of intense, improved inputs, including intensive training and support to counselors (Bland et al. 2007), improved counseling at health facilities, and frequent home visits by infant feeding counselors (Coovadia et al. 2007), exclusive breastfeeding can be made safe. Reliable information on infant feeding choices and infant outcomes in operational PMTCT settings is sparse. The challenge thus is to translate these successful strategies from research settings to large-scale PMTCT settings and to monitor infant outcomes, including HIV-free survival rates.

## B. HIV and food and nutrition security: Household and intrahousehold level

Few studies have investigated how HIV *per se* impacts food and nutrition security of its household members, as elaborated in the methodology section. Most related studies examine the impacts of disease-related adult illness and mortality (mostly from high HIV-prevalence countries) on a) household consumption and b) nutrition status of children within the household.[11]

### ADULT ILLNESS/DEATH AND HOUSEHOLD CONSUMPTION

Studies estimating the consumption impacts of the AIDS epidemic draw from two strands of literature: one strand flows from the broader literature based on Becker's household economics model introduced in 1965 and the other from Arrow (1964) on consumption smoothing. Becker's model has been used widely to examine the links between household consumption and production decisions and health outcomes (see, for example, Behrman and Deolalikar (1998); Strauss and Thomas (1998); Larson et al. (1995); Jacobson (2000); Strauss (1982)). At the household level, morbidity and mortality is assumed to directly affect household constraints that can be expected to alter time allocation, production decisions, asset management decisions, and final consumption and production outcomes.

The theory of full insurance initiated by Arrow (1964) implies that the growth in household consumption will respond to the growth in aggregate level consumption but not to idiosyncratic shocks such as illness or variation in income. Technically, this means that the functioning of risk-sharing institutions will mitigate the consumption effects of idiosyncratic shocks across households within a village. There is evidence that households are able to smooth consumption over short time horizons such as over the seasons (Townsend 1994). But Gertler and Gruber (2002), in Indonesia, and Cochrane (1991), in the U.S., find that that minor illnesses (that is, illnesses of short duration) are insured, while major illnesses of long duration are not fully insured.

The general narrative in literature is that adult death results in smaller households with higher dependency ratios and increased medical expenditures (especially in case of chronic illness preceding death), thereby leading to increased food insecurity. Although some studies from regions/countries with high prevalence of HIV confirm these outcomes on household size, dependency ratios (Yamano and Jayne 2004; Chapoto and Jayne 2008), and increased medical and funeral expenditures (Tibaijuka 1997; Bechu 1998; Booysen and Bachmann 2002; Mahal et al. 2008), the evidence is much more mixed and nuanced, depending on the gender and position of the deceased in the household.

In Côte d'Ivoire, Bechu (1998) surveyed 107 households with one or more children, and with at least one adult ill with AIDS, and interviewed them six times at two-month intervals. These data were compared with the results of a study conducted in Yopougon in May, 1992, and based on a sample of 2,064 households. The study found per capita consumption of AIDS-afflicted households to be half that of other households. In South Africa, a descriptive study by Booysen and Bachmann (2002) found that the average monthly per capita food expenditures of afflicted households was 70–80 percent that of other households, but no significant difference was found in total monthly expenditures, most likely because of rises in health-related expenditures. In Nigeria, Mahal et al. (2008), using propensity score matching to compare a non-random sample of HIV-positive individuals with a random survey of over 6,400 individuals, find that direct private healthcare costs and indirect income loss per HIV-positive individual were approximately 56 percent of annual income per capita in affected households.

In Ethiopia, Kadiyala (2006), using a three-year panel dataset and controlling for endogeneity of disease-related adult death to outcomes of interest using propensity score matching, find that households with adult death (8.5 percent of households reported death of at least one adult death between 1994 and 1997) were able to maintain monthly total, food and non-food expenditures. However, adult mortality negatively impacted the already alarmingly low dietary diversity, especially among poor households and households with the death of a household head/spouse of the head—a reliable indicator of nutrient adequacy and per capita consumption. Senefeld and Polsky (2006), in a descriptive study of the impact of chronic illness in Zimbabwe, report similar erosive dietary coping strategies.

Beegle, De Weerdt, and Dercon (2007) followed individuals belonging to a baseline set of Kagera Health and Development Survey (KHDS) households reinterviewed more than 10 years—allowing control for household heterogeneity. About 22 percent of the households experienced an adult death between 1991 and

2004. They found significant and robust evidence that the impact of a prime-age death results in a 7 percent drop in consumption in the first five years after the death. This relationship attenuated after five years. The impact death did not differ by the initial poverty status of the household, and neither did it vary by the length of illness.

Based on a computable general equilibrium (CGE) microsimulation model, Jefferis et al. (2008), in a study to measure the impact of HIV/AIDS on economic growth and poverty in Botswana, conclude that HIV/AIDS increases household poverty especially in the short run. The results from their CGE model indicate that the national poverty headcount would be 1.5 percentage points lower in 2021 if there were no epidemic.

The evidence thus far, although not conclusive, is compelling—the AIDS epidemic indeed seems to have a detrimental effect on consumption, having clear implications for food security of AIDS-affected households. However, there is not yet much clarity, given the evidence, on the timing and persistence of these impacts in the short and long run.

## ADULT ILLNESS/DEATH AND CHILD SURVIVAL AND NUTRITION STATUS

Chronic illness and/or death may affect child welfare through a number of pathways. Adult illness and death in the household may result in reallocation of household labor and expenditures. Health expenditures related to the care of the sick household member and expenditures on funerals may both result in reduction in household food security and health expenditures on children. Loss of an adult female may also mean the loss of a caregiver. It may compromise quantity and quality of childcare, since surviving adults divert their attention from health and nutrition-augmenting activities—cleaning, collecting water, hygienic food preparation, adopting optimal child feeding practices—and devote more time to income-earning activities.

Maternal HIV status is also associated with mortality in young children— in Tanzania, for example, the mortality rate among children under two years of age born to HIV-positive mothers was 2.5 times higher than among children of HIV-negative mothers (Urassa et al. 2001). In a 10-year follow-up study in Malawi, Crampin et al. (2003) showed maternal mortality to be associated with child mortality among HIV-positive mothers but not among HIV-negative mothers. Kadiyala et al. (2009) employed propensity score matching with difference-in-difference to control for endogeneity of adult mortality to child survival and growth in Ethiopia. Bereavement (child living in a household with adult mortality) increased the probability of child mortality, with girls faring worse than boys.

Adult mortality also adversely affects children's nutritional status. Ainsworth and Semali (2000) show that the death of the mother was associated with an average decline of one standard deviation in child height-for-age between 1991 and

1994, whereas a paternal death was associated with a decline of one-third of a standard deviation. The impact of maternal death was severe regardless of household assets, while the impact of paternal death was felt only in poor households. In Uganda, orphans' health and nutritional status were worse and their use of public services much lower than those of non-orphans (Deininger, Garcia, and Subbarao 2003).

In the KHDS sample, Beegle, De Weerdt, and Dercon (2006a) found that children who become maternal orphans between the ages of 7 and 15 were 2 cm shorter in adulthood than were similar children whose mother did not die during this age interval. Kadiyala et al. (2009) show that boys living in households experiencing an adult death ("bereaved" households) grew one-third of a standard deviation slower (average change in height-for-age z-score between 1994 and 1997) than matched non-bereaved boys. The authors report similar results for both boys and girls when stratified by economic status—bereaved boys and girls grew approximately one-third of a standard deviation slower than their matched non-bereaved counterparts from poor households.

There is strong evidence of the direct relationship between child mortality rates and fertility rates as well as positive economic growth (Ram and Schultz 1979; Bloom and Canning 2000). Reduced height as a child is correlated with reduced earnings as an adult (Thomas and Strauss 1997; Hoddinott and Kinsey 2001; Hoddinott et al. 2008). Given this, although not yet directly explicated in the literature, the impact of the AIDS epidemic on intergenerational transmission of poverty, earnings capacity, and economic growth of nations through compromised investments in child nutrition may be profound. Indeed, most macroeconomic models endogenizing intergenerational effects on human capital accumulation find large effects on national income per capita (Corrigan, Glomm, and Mendez 2005; Bell, Devarajan, and Gersbach 2006; McDonald and Roberts 2006).

## C. HIV and rural household livelihoods

### IMPACTS ON HOUSEHOLD LABOR AVAILABILITY

Earlier studies have shown that households experiencing premature prime-age mortality due to HIV/AIDS-related causes resulted in households having to adopt a mixture of coping strategies including: an increased in-and-out-migration of household members, an increased rate of fostering, and higher rates of remarriage for surviving spouses (World Bank 1999; Ntozi 1997; Urassa et al. 2001). However, the way in which households adjust to internal labor supply shocks varies according to the resources of the households. For example, better-off households may be able to hire workers or attract additional members to at least partially offset the loss of another (see Yamano and Jayne (2004); Beegle (2005); Ainsworth, Ghosh, and Semali, (1995); Donovan and Bailey (2006), Mather, Donovan, and Jayne (2005)). These demographic changes may have profound short- and long-term consequences for surviving individuals by impacting on a household's labor availability, allocation, consumption (Singh, Squire, and Strauss 1986; Benjamin 1992), and household's ability to insure against risk (Rosenzweig 1988).

Yamano and Jayne (2004) show that households suffering the death of the head of household or spouse were largely unable to replace the labor lost through the death, whereas households suffering the death of another adult were able to attract new household members. Without such adaptation, either through altered structures or roles, and/or through external assistance, families and households may become non-functioning social and productive units and ultimately dissolve (Hosegood et al. 2004). Based on Demographic and Health Surveys from 21 countries across Africa, Beegle et al. (2009) also show that many single orphans do not stay with the remaining parent but are rather sent away to live with other relatives.

Kirimi (2008), using panel data from Kenya, finds that in the year of death, household size, the number of female adults, girls, and young children increase. However, households experienced a decline in household size of more than one person in the third and fourth years after the death of an adult male member, particularly a reduction in the number of girls and young children. The study shows that, in the period one to two years before death, the impact of death does not vary by gender and position of the deceased. While in the year of death, compared to other deaths, a death of a male head of household leads to a decrease in the number of boys and young children. This finding implies that the death of the male head triggers fostering out of boys and young children. However, four years after death, in comparison to other deaths, a male head death is associated with a decrease of more than one adult male in the household. There are indications that changes in household composition take place over time and depend to a limited extent on the gender and position of the deceased member.

Chapoto and Jayne (2008), using national representative survey data from Zambia, find that irrespective of the gender and position of the deceased individual, household size declines by less than one person, implying that households are somewhat successful in replenishing their household sizes. They report that changes in household size and composition depend on initial household conditions. For instance, non-poor households were more likely than poor households to restore their size to pre-death levels, mainly by attracting young boys and girls. However, Mather, Donovan and Jayne (2005) and Peters, Walker, and Kambewa (2008) found low household dissolution rates due to adult mortality.

In addition to changes in household size and composition to maintain household labor supply, households may undertake more erosive strategies. Using panel data from KwaZulu-Natal Income Dynamics Study (KIDS) conducted in the Province of KwaZulu-Natal in 1998 and 2004, Yamauchi, Buthelezi, and Velia

(2008) find that, first, death of prime-age adults significantly increases both the male and female adolescent labor participation at the expense of schooling. In their analysis, the authors find that deaths of prime-age adults in the future decrease female school enrollment, suggesting that girls shift activity, possibly staying at home to take care of the sick or do general chores of the household. Second, since the enrollment of male adolescents is decreased prior to the death of a prime-age adult, their response is different, associated with compensating for an income loss. Third, female adults tend to become a part of the labor force after the death of prime-age adult males. The shift might translate into a decline in their time spent on housework, including child rearing. These findings imply that increased prime-age adult mortality disrupts human capital formation in the society, in turn affecting the future quality of the labor force in hardest-hit countries.

With the rollout of ART, the situation may be changing but it is too early to know, because it is only now that attention has turned from medical benefits to evaluating various socioeconomic impacts of ART on livelihoods and food security. A key medical impact is the ability of ART to restore physical functioning so that an individual can continue with and/or return to normal daily activities after initiating therapy. This then reduces the burden from other family members, who in the absence of treatment, may be required to tend for the sick. However, prolonged illness before ART treatment may mean lower household welfare and food security levels which may take time to rebound even if the health condition of the person improves.

Although the evidence on the impact of ART on individual and household socioeconomic outcomes is limited, the few studies reviewed report generally positive results. Thirumurthy, Graff Zivin, and Goldstein. (2008), in a study of the economic impact of AIDS treatment on labor supply in western Kenya, show that the probability of an HIV-positive adult participating in labor force activities increased by 20 percent in the first six months on ART, and the number of hours worked increased by 35 percent. Larson et al. (2008), investigating the impact of ART on days harvesting tea per month for tea estate workers in Kenya, find that the first year on treatment had a large, positive impact on the ability of workers to undertake their primary work activity. Other studies focusing on individuals and households find positive impacts of ART on schooling of children whose parents receive ART (Graff Zivin, Thirumurthy, and Goldstein 2006) and on the quality of life for ART patients (Wouters et al. 2007). Studies have also reported reduction in worker absenteeism after starting ART (e.g., Eholie et al. (2003), Habyarimana, Mbakile, and Pop-Eleches (2007), and Muirhead et al. (2006)).

IMPACTS ON CROPPING PATTERNS AND CROP OUTPUT

Earlier evidence shows that households affected by AIDS shift their cropping pattern, favoring less capital and labor-intensive crops. These studies, often qualitative or cross-sectional, provide evidence of reduction in area cultivated, shifts to less labor-intensive crops, and reduced weeding (Barnett et al. 1995; Topouzis and du Guerny 1999; Harvey 2004). Other studies have noted that the recent shift in area cultivated with maize to root tubers in much of southern Africa may be reflecting labor shortages and small farmers' attempts to shift to less labor-intensive crops (Barnett 1994; FAO 1993, 1995, 2004; FASAZ 2003). It is possible that the AIDS epidemic has contributed to these shifts, but one has to acknowledge that such shifts may also be due to major changes in agricultural policy, such as market reform programs that eliminated pan-territorial price supports for maize and also reduced fertilizer subsidies (used primarily on maize) in much of eastern and southern Africa, resulting in a shift of household incentives from growing maize to tubers (Jayne et al. 2005). The failure to take account of such policy changes may result in misattributing the shifts in cropping patterns to AIDS-related prime-age morbidity and mortality.

Beegle (2005), using panel data from Kagera, Tanzania, finds that although cash cropping is temporarily scaled back following a male death and wage income falls, afflicted households do not shift towards subsistence crops. Putting these findings in context, Beegle (2005) also notes that the areas of highest AIDS-related mortality in Tanzania (such as Kagera) are in the Lake Victoria basin, an area with high population density and thus, a large labor supply and relatively high labor/land ratios. However, her study lacks measures of aggregate output and does not draw conclusions on changes in total crop production or the composition of crop production. Also, the study evaluated short-term effects during the early years of the epidemic (1991–1993), and the extent to which these findings hold over the longer run is uncertain.

Donovan and Bailey (2006), using panel data from Rwanda, find a significant decrease in coffee and beer banana production among households with a prime-age death. In addition, they report a significant increase in production of sweet potatoes among households with a chronically ill adult. The increase in production of sweet potatoes is likely due to the crop's flexible planting and harvesting schedule, for it allows piecemeal harvesting over a 3–10-month period, an important consideration for labor-constrained households. While the reduction in production of beer banana and coffee is likely due to the labor demands for processing the beer banana and to the loss of male adults and their connections with coffee brokers, these results suggest that when gender is a main determinant of participation in an economic activity, as with many cash crops, the loss of the participating adult (male) may leave the surviving spouse without access to the activity. Addressing the gender bias in agricultural production and marketing knowledge and opportunities could contribute significantly to improved income potential for many households.

In a study using data from the Integrated Household Survey in Malawi, Dorward, Mwale, and Tueso (2006) show that increasingly severe morbidity leads to changing cropping patterns as labor and seasonal capital constraints become tighter—for example, a shift out of hybrid maize and/or tobacco by those (less poor) households initially able to grow these crops. Increasing morbidity was found to increase areas under low-input maize in most households. For the poorest households, the result is an increasing inability to cultivate these crops. Thus, they are forced to decrease their maize area, leaving an increasing amount of land fallow, while maintaining a small area of cassava.

A study in Kenya (Yamano and Jayne 2004) found that rural households suffering a prime-age death between 1997 and 2000 generally experienced a decline in agricultural output relative to non-afflicted households, but the magnitude and statistical significance of this finding was a function of the gender, age, and position in the household of the deceased person, as well as the household's initial level of wealth prior to incurring the shock. The death of a prime-age male household head was reported to be associated with a 68 percent reduction in per capita household crop production value. Adult female mortality caused a greater decline in cereal area cultivated, whereas prime-age male adult death resulted in a greater decline in cash crops (such as coffee, tea, and sugar) and nonfarm income. However, there was little indication that households recovered quickly, though the authors observed that initial asset base does play a role in buffering the shock of adult mortality.

Kirimi (2008), using the extended panel data from the above Kenya dataset collected over a seven-year time period, examined the temporal pattern of the effects of death in the years before and after the occurrence of death. This study shows that small negative impacts of prime-age adult mortality begin to emerge in the period *preceding* death, presumably due to pre-death morbidity, while significant negative impacts are observed in the year of death. Also, the study finds that the impact of prime-age mortality on the households is not just a one-time post-death adjustment but rather persists over time, though in most cases, negative effects are larger in the period closest to the death event. The results on the impact of mortality on land cultivated show, that in the year of death, there is no statistically significant effect on area cultivated, both in total area and by crop type. However, one year after death, area under roots and tubers declined, while two years after death, total cultivated land and area under cultivation with high-value crops, roots, and tubers declined. Also, five to seven years after death, there was a significant decline in the area devoted to high-value crops. This pattern of effects reflects the progression of the severity of disease. Two years before death, illness is relatively mild, and so households are likely to have enough labor and capital to farm their land. As the disease progresses and is followed by

death, households may begin to face labor shortages and cash constraints causing them to cut back the area under cultivation. The decline in area under high-
value crops even five to seven years after death of the male head of household
may signify tighter cash constraints, causing households to shift away from high-
value crops which require larger capital investment and possibly more labor than
other crops.

In Zambia, Chapoto and Jayne (2008) find that the death of a prime-age male
resulted in a 13 percent decline in total land cultivated while the death of a prime-
age female resulted in a 5 percent decline in cultivated land, and the death of male
head of household resulted in a 21 percent reduction in land cultivated. The death
of male heads of households causes the households to cut back more area cultivated, possibly due to their inability to fully replace deceased members. The area
under cultivation with cereals and other food crops was found to significantly
decline as a result of death, with the most severe effects observed in the case of a
male head-of-household death. However, the results show that area cultivated
in total, and the area under cereals in particular, decline more in relatively non-
poor households than poor households after the death of a male household head.
Thus, there is no evidence to suggest that initial poverty exacerbates the impact
of mortality on cultivated land. However, crop output in poorer households was
shown to suffer especially in households experiencing a male head death. Among
this group of afflicted households, the gross value of crop production per hectare
declined by a staggering 49.8 percent relative to non-afflicted households between
the 2001 and 2004 surveys. Evidence suggests that wealthier households incurring
male head-of-household death are able to replenish their household size, while
initially poor households have greater difficulty in doing so. This finding supports
the need for creating and/or strengthening community-based networks to assist
poorer households experiencing mortality of household heads and spouses. Government and donor agencies may also assist with agricultural extension programs
to reach afflicted poor households in order to strengthen their capacity to cope
with the loss of prime-age core members.

There is some evidence that the epidemic may make agrarian communities
more vulnerable and less resilient to drought and other transitory shocks—often
referred to as the "new variant famine" (de Waal and Whiteside 2003). Mason et
al. (2005) regressed change in child underweight prevalence (a measure of malnutrition) on a drought year dummy variable, HIV prevalence, and an interaction term between drought and HIV prevalence. The independent effects of HIV
prevalence and drought were statistically insignificant, but the interaction term
was statistically significant and positive, indicating that the effect of drought is
exacerbated by high HIV prevalence and vice versa. However, the results of this
regression analysis may be biased, because no other factors affecting change in
child underweight were controlled for in the model.

Mason et al. (2010), using nationally representative survey data from Zambia over a 13-year period, estimated the impact of AIDS-related morbidity and mortality on indicators of agrarian livelihoods in Zambia. This study specifically investigated the impact of HIV/AIDS and its interactions with drought and other shocks on district-level crop output, output per hectare, and area cultivated. The results show that the negative impact of drought on crop output and output per hectare is further exacerbated where HIV prevalence rates are relatively high, particularly in the low and medium rainfall zones of the country. In addition, the results show that AIDS reduces the crop production gains associated with fertilizer subsidy increases in the highest rainfall areas.

## EFFECTS ON NON-FARM INCOME AND ASSETS

Farm households are known to rely on remittance and non-farm income as a primary means to afford assets such as oxen, scotch carts, ploughs, and fertilizer, which are used to capitalize farm production (Reardon, Crawford, and Kelly 1995). Unfortunately, such sources of income are often at risk among AIDS-afflicted households, particularly those that were already asset poor and vulnerable (Donovan and Bailey 2006; Mushati et al. 2003). Morbidity and death of a household member tighten cash constraints on agricultural production as medical and funeral expenses rise and caregiving by other members further reduces household income-earning potential.

The evidence on the impacts of AIDS on non-farm income is still limited and inconclusive. For example, Yamano and Jayne (2004) report that death of a male head of household in Kenya results in large reductions in off-farm income. Contrary to the hypothesis that off-farm income sources are at risk among households experiencing prime-age mortality, particularly among those that are asset-poor and vulnerable to begin with, Chapoto and Jayne (2008) find a statistically insignificant relationship for all cases of mortality by gender and position in the household of the deceased. However, there is some evidence, albeit weak, of a decline in off-farm income among households suffering the death of a non-resident male head of household who has come back home to seek terminal care.

Liquidation of assets is cited as one of the erosive coping mechanisms used by households to mitigate the impact of mortality and other shocks (see Barnett and Blaikie (1992)). Asset depletion may allow households to get through crisis periods but may erode their productivity and food security in later years (Mather, Donovan, and Jayne 2005). Qualitative recall data from Mozambique and Rwanda on household responses to adult mortality show that some affected households liquidate assets such as small livestock and cash reserves in response to illness and death (Donovan and Bailey 2006; Mather, Donovan, and Jayne 2005). However, asset depletion can increase households' vulnerability to income shocks and may decrease household use of cash inputs and animal traction in crop cultivation which will tend to result in lower productivity and overall crop production. In addition, prime-age mortality may reduce both the stock and the intergenerational transfer of human capital with respect to location-specific farm management practices.

Impact analysis by Yamano and Jayne (2004) in Kenya shows a decline in mean asset values among all Kenyan households between 1997 and 2000, but larger mean decreases among afflicted households (though insignificant except in the case of small livestock). Within the context of a decline in asset values among non-afflicted households, only part of the (larger) decline in asset values among affected households from 1997 to 2000 was attributed to adult mortality. Generally, the evidence from this study in Kenya shows that households first attempt to dispose of small animals and other assets with the least impact on long-term production potential. Cattle and productive farm equipment are sold in response to severe cash requirements after incurring a death in the family. Such *ex post* coping strategies are costly in the short term and may cause households not to recover from impacts of death even in the long term.

Similar to the Kenyan findings, Chapoto and Jayne (2008) show that, in Zambia, the value of cattle assets appear to suffer greatly from the death of a male head of household. The sale or liquidation of cattle is a relatively extreme coping mechanism, as it may compromise the household's future livelihood (Stokes 2003). Cattle assets are not only a stock of wealth but are also an input into agricultural production (through draft power for land preparation). Fortunately, adult mortality is not associated with significant declines in cattle assets except in the case of male head-of-household mortality which indicates the relative severity of impacts in this case. Another reason why households experiencing male head-of-household death suffer a significant decline in cattle assets is because property of the deceased man (including cattle) is often redistributed to the man's relatives. There is a need to better understand how traditional inheritance rules interact with the HIV/AIDS epidemic to affect the distribution of assets and poverty within rural communities. Government and development agencies may want to understand the effects of targeting households whose capital base is most affected by AIDS-related illness and death as well as encourage change in traditional inheritance institutions to better protect widows and their dependents after their husbands' deaths.

The loss of skilled and unskilled labor due to illness and death has also been shown to lead to a reduction of household income per capita. For example, in a longitudinal study of households affected by HIV/AIDS in the Free State, South Africa, Booysen (2003) found HIV-affected households were poorer, more dependent on non-employment sources of income, and spent less money on food. The total cost of morbidity to households was relatively low where unemployment levels were very high. Ill household members were primarily cared for by family members with no direct loss of income reported. A larger number of children in afflicted households were not attending school, and orphans were found to be sheltered in both afflicted and non-afflicted households.

Similarly, Bachmann and Booysen (2003) found that HIV/AIDS affects the health and wealth of households, aggravating pre-existing poverty. Thirty-five percent of afflicted households needed someone to accompany an ill member to a health service, and the median number of hours that home caregivers spent with ill members was five per day. Also, the study found that over six months, household expenditure decreased significantly more rapidly in HIV-afflicted households than in non-afflicted households, mainly because of increase medical costs and the loss of income of the ill person.

In a more recent student study in Malawi, Dorward, Mwale, and Tueso (2006) report that increasing morbidity led to declining net income per capita, particularly for poor male- and female-headed households. They show that the loss of a skilled household member has a greater impact on income per capita than the loss of an unskilled member. However, as discussed earlier, ART might mitigate this impact if this lifesaving treatment is available and started early, because medical studies have shown that the treatment has the ability to restore physical functioning so that an individual can continue with and/or return to normal daily activities after initiating therapy (Akileswaran et al. 2005; Bekker et al. 2006; Rosen et al. 2008b).

IMPACT ON ACCESS TO LAND

In areas of Africa hardest hit by HIV/AIDS, there are growing concerns that many women lose access to land after the death of their husbands. Many narratives and qualitative studies highlight gender inequalities in property rights and the difficulties that widows face in retaining access to land after the death of their husbands (for example, see Aliber and Walker (2006); Kajoba (2006); Shezongo-Macmillan (2005); Mutangadura (2004); UNECA (2003); Machina (2002); Keller (2000); WLSA (1997)). HIV/AIDS has undoubtedly exacerbated such problems. With the exception of Chapoto and Jayne (2008), there is virtually no other quantitative evidence on the proportion of widows who lose their land after the death of their husbands, whether they lose all or part of that land, and whether certain characteristics of the widow, her deceased husband, and/or her household influence the likelihood of her losing land rights.

Chapoto and Jayne (2008), using national representative survey data from Zambia, find that within one to three years after the death of their husbands, widow-headed households, on average, controlled 35 percent less land than what they had prior to their husbands' deaths. However, there is major variation around this mean, with roughly a third of widow-headed households controlling less than 50 percent of their former land, while over a quarter of widows actually controlled as much or even more land than while their husbands were alive. Factors associated with a relatively large loss in land included the household's wealth prior to the husband's death, the widow's family relationship to the local headman, and the widow's age. Therefore, the view that widows and their dependents face greater livelihood risks in the era of HIV/AIDS is indeed supported by nationally representative survey results from Zambia.

Efforts to safeguard widows' rights to land through land tenure innovations involving community authorities may be an important component of social protection, poverty alleviation, and HIV/AIDS mitigation strategies. These results show the influence of local traditional authorities in affecting the extent to which widows are able to retain land. Government decrees appear to have little impact if local community authorities are not part of the agreement. But certainly national governments, donors, and NGOs have an important role to play in developing programs to work with local authorities to protect widows and orphans against property grabbing by relatives of the deceased, as well as to institute property rights that are more compatible with social protection and anti-poverty objectives in the era of AIDS. Also, enforcing family law which encompasses women's property and inheritance rights, as compared to customary law, may be helpful in reducing vulnerability of households (WLSA 1997; Izumi 2009). These rights generally are secure when legal regimes are committed to enforcing property and inheritance laws and when the general public is conversant with provisions of such laws (ICRW 2004).

In summary, the evidence on household livelihood and food security is mixed as to how AIDS is affecting agricultural systems and cropping patterns and the subsequent impact on household livelihood and food security. There is no doubt that AIDS has taken a huge toll on the agricultural sector in Africa, but the review of findings seem to suggest that there is a need to move away from generalized conclusions about the main factors constraining afflicted households' ability to recover and begin formulating appropriate and programmatic responses based on the specific characteristics of the region, the regional economy, the localized farming systems, the riskiness of alternative crops, and household characteristics and available resources (Jayne et al. 2006). With the medical effectiveness of ART in restoring immune function and extending survival well established, there is no doubt in our minds that the rollout of ART into the rural areas, if scaled up, will help mitigate the impacts of AIDS on their livelihoods, and food and nutrition security. However, there is currently limited evidence on the socioeconomic impacts of ART on households.

## 5. Effectiveness of Interventions

Our growing knowledge of adverse interactions between livelihoods, food and nutrition insecurity, and HIV necessitates a comprehensive and integrated response.

Among HIV care and treatment providers, much of the increased attention to food and nutrition security is being driven by the reality of generalized AIDS epidemics and weak care and treatment programs coexisting with widespread, chronic food insecurity and malnutrition.

Despite this growing recognition and activity in integrating food and nutrition security interventions in the context of HIV, there have been few rigorous studies to evaluate various aspects of these attempts. Below we review what is known about interventions to improve food and nutrition security of HIV-affected populations. Given the wide variety of activities and interventions across Africa in response to the epidemic, it would be impossible to focus on all these efforts. In line with the above section, we focus here on food supplementation programs and programs to improve rural livelihood base.

### A. Food supplementation to improve food and nutrition security

International organizations such as the World Health Organization (WHO), Joint United Nations Programme on HIV/AIDS (UNAIDS), World Food Program (WFP), Food and Agriculture Organization (FAO), and the U.S. President's Emergency Plan for AIDS Relief (PEPFAR) have recommended integration of food assistance into AIDS care and treatment programs (World Bank 2007; UNAIDS 2008a; USAID Bureau for Democracy, Conflict and Humanitarian Assistance, Office of Food for Peace, and the U.S. President's Emergency Plan for AIDS Relief 2007). Health care providers and NGOs involved in HIV care and treatment are increasingly utilizing targeted food assistance. A multitude of objectives are often invoked including delaying initiation of ART; clinical, nutritional, and survival outcomes of people living with HIV on ART or not yet on ART; improving adherence to ART; preventing impoverishment of households; and lowering the incidence of high risk sexual behaviors due to food insecurity. Since integrating food supplementation into AIDS care and treatment is a fairly recent practice, whether it can achieve the multiple objectives set by these organizations in a programming context has not been well tested.

The very basic question is this: Since indicators of malnutrition predict survival rates even among those on ART, does food supplementation improve clinical, treatment, and survival outcomes?

Mahlungulu et al. (2007) reviewed the effect of macronutrient supplementation of various clinical outcomes of people living with HIV. This Cochrane review included eight small clinical trials, all of them in developed countries, where the pre-existing nutrition status of people living with HIV is far superior to those in developing countries. This review offers inconclusive evidence of the effect of macronutrient supplementation (with or without nutritional counseling) on body weight, fat mass, lean mass, or CD4 count. The authors, therefore, support the current WHO recommendations (increased energy intake of 10 percent when asymptomatic and increased energy intake of 20–30 percent when symptomatic), which are *over and above* the Recommended Dietary Allowances (RDA).

The impàct of food supplementation, nestled in a HIV care and treatment program context, on people living with HIV and with pre-existing food and nutrition insecurity is just beginning to emerge. Before we proceed further, it is worth noting the ethical challenges of randomizing food insecure people with HIV to food and control groups. Given this, most studies currently being carried out resort to a) quasi-experimental designs, but with control group, or 2) use retrospective cohorts, or 3) randomize participants to two different types of food supplementation regimens.

In Zambia, Cantrell et al. (2008) report the results of a quasi-experimental food supplementation (in the form of World Food Programme food basket) study, taking advantage of a staggered rollout of Zambia's ART program. The analysis compared adherence, CD4 counts, and weight gain outcomes among food-insecure patients initiating ART and enrolled at the clinics where food was available with those enrolled at the control clinics. They find that while food supplementation improved drug adherence, the authors note that although they ". . . did not observe a statistically significant effect of food supplementation on the clinical outcomes of weight and CD4 cell response, there is a trend toward modest benefit, particularly among men" (193).

While the study makes an important contribution, it does not employ analyses to tease out the causal link between food supplementation and outcomes of interest, given the study design (for example, instrumental variables or propensity score matching). In fact the study shows an *association or the lack of it* between food supplementation and outcomes of interest. For example, it does not account for important bias that may arise if there are unobserved characteristics that affect the probability of participation in the program which are also correlated with the outcome of interest. Two important sources of this selection bias include targeting of the program to recipients or clinics based on characteristics unobservable to the researcher (or on which the researcher did not collect data) and self-selection into the program by eligible recipients.

Using The AIDS Support Organization's (TASO) retrospective cohort data from 2002–2007 in Uganda, Rawat, Kadiyala, and McNamara (2010) estimated the impact of food assistance on weight gain and disease progression. They employed propensity score matching with difference-in-difference to control for endogeneity of food assistance to outcomes of interest. Here, food aid resulted in significant weight gain of people (regardless of receipt of ART) with WHO stage 2 and above at baseline. Food assistance slowed disease progression, but the effect size was small. This study is of course not without its limitations—as is usually the case with program-based retrospective data, loss to follow-up remains an important concern. In addition, the variables used for matching were limited to the variables available in the program database.

In Malawi, a randomized supplementary feeding trial compared the impact on BMI and fat-free body mass of wasted HIV patients starting ART who were supplemented with specialized, energy dense, ready-to-use, fortified spread versus the more commonly used corn-soy blend for 14 weeks (Ndekha et al. 2009). Supplementary feeding with the fortified spread resulted in a greater increase in BMI and lean body mass than feeding with corn-soy blend.

The evidence on the efficacy and effectiveness of micronutrient supplementation is sparse. As reviewed in the above section, while multiple micronutrients and periodic supplementation with vitamin A had beneficial outcomes, we are not aware of any micronutrient supplementation programs, outside of the clinical trial context, specifically investigating their role in delaying disease progression and improving ART outcomes.

Although anemia predicts survival among people living with HIV, iron supplementation is a contentious issue, as high iron levels correlate with faster disease progression (Friis 2005). While supplementation may be appropriate if tests show iron deficiency, we did not identify any studies investigating the efficacy of iron supplementation among iron-deficient people living with HIV. Further studies are needed to explore possible interventions against HIV-associated anemia in resource-limited settings, including the role of iron supplementation. Overall, the optimal formulation of a daily multiple micronutrient supplement for HIV-positive individuals living in chronically food insecure regions requires further study.

Although various food supplementation programs invoke household food security-related objectives, we did not identify studies estimating the impact of food supplementation (supplementary feeding or household food rations) on household food security outcomes.

A study undertaken in Kenya highlights key constraints, opportunities, and challenges relating to interventions aimed at strengthening the nutrition security of people living with HIV on antiretroviral treatment. Through collaboration between AMPATH and RENEWAL, qualitative research was undertaken on a short-term nutrition intervention linked to the provision of free antiretroviral treatment for people living with HIV in late 2005/early 2006 in western Kenya. Recipients of food reported increased dietary diversity and diet quantity and improved health status of other members of their households, especially young children. The majority (61 percent) of clients reported that, as a result of the food supplementation, they regained enough strength to return to their household chores, farming activities, or income-earning activities. The amount of labor available in their household increased as the patient recuperated (Byron, Gillespie, and Nangami 2008).

Brunelli, Kenefick, and Yamauchi (2008) use the World Food Programme's cross-sectional Community and Household Survey (CHS) data on the impact of food aid on child weight in five southern African countries. They find no significant difference in incidence of adult death between households that received food aid and those that did not. Except for Swaziland, all countries show smaller impacts of adult death on child weight among the households receiving food aid than the households not receiving the aid, suggesting that food aid mitigates the shock of adult death on child nutrition.

## B. Agriculture/livelihood interventions to improve food security

Recognizing that food aid is at best a stopgap arrangement, and the limited ability of targeted food assistance to address these complex problems, NGOs, national governments, international agencies, and donor organizations are increasingly being drawn to designing and implementing programs that strengthen the capacity of households to engage in livelihoods that enable them to access adequate food and nutrition resources to meet the basic requirements of all the household members. Since much of this programming to improve long-term food security of households (often referred to as integrated programming) is "cutting edge," organizations are, effectively, learning by doing (USAID Bureau for Democracy, Conflict and Humanitarian Assistance, Office of Food for Peace, and the U.S. President's Emergency Plan for AIDS Relief 2007; Mamlin et al. 2009).

In addition to progressively diminishing an individual's physical capacity and quality of life, HIV alters household dependency ratios, skill structure, time allocation patterns (e.g., as household members reorganize to provide care to the sick and earn income, the person infected with HIV may spend substantial time caring for himself or herself and seeking health care), and resource allocation (including labor) patterns. It affects decision-making in terms of short-term versus long-term investments and norms of reciprocity and trust among community members. Stigma of HIV continues to be a prevalent phenomenon.

While the above list is by no means an exhaustive one, it portrays some key dimensions of the epidemic which have implications for how livelihood interventions are designed and implemented. What are the implications, for example, of mandatory contributions of beneficiaries in an HIV context where households frequently experience surging, often unpredictable, medical expenditures? Formation and use of groups to target services is one of the most universal characteristics of the livelihood programs in the context of HIV (Kadiyala et al. 2009). This approach conforms well to current thinking on the importance of promoting social capital in development interventions. What are the implications for group cohesion and activities when the member is too ill or when the member is overwhelmed with taking care of the sick person so that the member cannot attend business (e.g., lend labor to prepare a garden) or use resources for consumption purposes (e.g., sell the kid goat that had to passed on to another group member)?

While the quest for identifying "best practices" in food security interventions within the context of HIV is growing (AED 2003; RCQHC and FANTA/AED 2008; Project Concern International 2009), insufficient attention has been paid to critical examination of the theory on which such interventions are based and their underlying assumptions. To date, there are no published examples of research that explains how this theory of change (pathways to impact) is conceptualized by program implementers, why these integrated programs do what they do, or that examine the rationale for expecting that doing things this way will improve food security of the target population.

An operations research study employing qualitative in-depth case study approach, conducted by RENEWAL/IFPRI, TASO, and Concern Worldwide in Uganda and Zambia, examined the conceptual foundations and critical program processes of 16 livelihood programs (mainly small scale agriculture and livestock projects) aiming to improve food security in HIV settings with about 70 program participants. This study identified specific weaknesses and lacunae in program conceptualization and program processes that may severely compromise the ability of such programs to achieve their intended outcomes. Kadiyala et al. (2009) report that program personnel across the integrated programs placed heavy emphasis on shortage of funding as the key limiting factor in their project implementation, yet did not on the whole articulate how additional funds would concretely improve the quality of their programs and their likelihood of achieving desired nutrition and food security outcomes. While limited financial resources continue to be a severe constraint in numbers of personnel these programs can hire, areas they can cover, or equipment and materials they can purchase, the authors conclude that that this is only a partial limitation. Chief among these weaknesses identified in this study were insufficient orientation of personnel to project objectives along the impact pathway and the lack of robust monitoring and evaluation systems (together with personnel qualified in their implementation) along the process pathway. A further issue which emerged from this research was a lack of focus: many of these integrated programs studied were mired in excessive multidimensional approaches (and this may also be related to the problems in clearly defining goals and objectives). A better model would simultaneously entail more focused interventions on the part of individual programs, and more formalized, tighter integration between complementary programs. The authors fear that unless these issues are tackled head on, increasing funding alone will not translate into more effective programming. They call upon donors to collaborate by facilitating design of clearly focused, well-defined theory-based programs with realistic coverage goals.

In response to the growing number of orphans as a result of HIV/AIDS, Junior Farmer Field and Life Schools (JFFLS) were developed, supported by FAO to improve children's agricultural and life skills for livelihood support and food security. First piloted in Mozambique in 2003, the program has now expanded to Kenya, Namibia, Swaziland, Zambia, and Zimbabwe. It is reported that over one thousand girls and boys in southern and eastern Africa have acquired new skills for farming, income generation, proper nutrition, the value of medicinal plants, health and hygiene, biodiversity and natural resource conservation, and other topics. These children have also learned about the importance of sound and informed decision-making during the crop cycle as well as in their own lives. Other than self-assessment reports by FAO, the impact of the JFFLS is yet to be assessed.

In addition to the limited funding to these programs, a serious commitment to tackle the AIDS epidemic through the agriculture sector continues to be a serious problem. Of the 33 countries with generalized epidemics (UNAIDS 2008a), 58 percent of them reported including the agriculture sector in their HIV strategies. However, only about 33 percent of these countries' government reports indicate earmarking budgets to address HIV in the agriculture sector (UNGASS 2008). According to UNAIDS (2008a), only six of the 33 countries say that an evaluation of the epidemic's socioeconomic impact has influenced their budget allocations.

To mitigate the impacts of AIDS on household livelihoods and food security, government agricultural policies need to contribute effectively to poverty reduction. To be successful over the long run, Jayne et al. (2006) recommended that greater focus be placed on raising households' and communities' living standards through productivity-enhancing investments in agricultural technology generation and diffusion, improved crop marketing systems, basic education, infrastructure, and governance. However, there remains a gap between desired and available levels of funding and human resources for HIV prevention, treatment, and social and economic programs to mitigate the impacts of AIDS in hard-hit communities. Hence, there is need for governments and donors to continue to search for cost-effective alternative kinds of interventions to simultaneously defeat the AIDS pandemic and the chronic poverty in Africa.

## 6. What Does Evidence of the Impacts Mean for Program and Policy Response?

Even if we were to begin to prevent further spread of the epidemic, as envisioned by the Millennium Development Goals (MDG), by 2015, the long-wave and intergenerational impacts of the epidemic will continue to be overriding challenges for decades to come. In Africa, and other populations where pervasive chronic food insecurity and malnutrition are endemic, the AIDS epidemic, on top of these pre-existing challenges, creates a tremendous burden on people's ability to remain healthy and economically productive.

Rapid advances have been made in science, in characterizing and quantifying the impacts, organizational approaches, and funding to fight the causes and consequences of the epidemic in this decade.

Our review clearly shows that pre-existing macro- and micronutrient status determines clinical outcomes and ultimately survival rates among people living with HIV. Keeping in mind the caveats on methodology and the contextual variations, the AIDS epidemic erodes livelihoods and compromises household welfare. Our review shows that adult mortality (especially from studies in high-prevalence regions) reduces household consumption, at least in the short and medium run and compromises the already alarmingly low dietary diversity. Adult mortality, especially of women (maternal mortality), compromises children's survival and growth. Such loss in human capital has potentially grave consequences in the long run for children as well as the economies. Although not conclusive, the evidence of the negative impacts of the AIDS epidemic on agrarian livelihood is compelling. The evidence shows that the nature and severity of impacts on agriculture often depends on the gender and position of the deceased in the household and the initial wealth status of the household. The review shows that, with the contextual variations, the epidemic impacts cropping patterns as well as crop output, with the poor being the worst affected. It can threaten the very base of livelihoods—access to land, especially in case of women.

ART is a definite and important *part* of the solution. ART results in weight gain and improvement of the status of several micronutrients critical for immunity. ART improves productivity, although earlier unemployment may still be a barrier to re-entry into work force. ART improves household welfare by enabling labor reallocation away from caregiving for the sick to productive activities. ART enables investments in children's schooling and nutrition.

Several barriers continue to exist in the successful rollout of ART. Amuron et al. (2009), in a follow-up of more than 4,300 HIV-positive clients at an AIDS support clinic in Uganda report that about a quarter of subjects eligible for ART did not complete screening, and pretreatment mortality was very high even though patients in this setting were well informed. They conclude that pervasive poverty and lack of funds for transport are significant barriers to successful initiation of ART.

The review of the current evidence base unequivocally shows that food insecurity and malnutrition compromises initiation of ART, and once initiated, adherence to the treatment and survival in the first six months. Even when a person survives past six months, several metabolic complications and side effects to ART exist—implications that African countries are yet to grapple with.

In reflecting on the evidence base for program and policy responses, the following is abundantly clear: addressing food and nutrition security are fundamental to all the four pillars of HIV-response prevention (not revised here), care and treatment, and mitigation along the HIV timeline in Figure 4.1.

What does the evidence of the impacts mean for interventions? Here, the evidence is unacceptably weak. Given the evidence on the interactions between ART and nutrition, delaying the need to initiate ART should be a priority. This means ensuring that people living with HIV consume diets meeting the RDAs. For the already malnourished, reconstituting the nutrition status is critical. Yet, we do not know the extent to which (macro- and micro-) nutrition supplementation meets these objectives in a resource-poor setting.

Rhetoric and experimentation abound; well-thought through, implemented, and evaluated HIV-responsive agricultural interventions are shamefully abysmal. This unacceptable paralysis is pervasive throughout international agencies, donors, governments, and therefore, not surprisingly, NGOs. At the end of the third decade of the epidemic, with a decade's worth of knowledge on the importance and linkages between livelihood security and the AIDS epidemic, we still know very little about the nuts and bolts of the interventions and how to make them effective.

The need for operations research to improve HIV-responsive food and nutrition security programs and enable their scaling up, with rigorous evaluation of these interventions, has never been more urgent.

## Notes

1. Given that the focus of the chapter is to review the evidence of the impacts of the epidemic on food and nutrition security, it is beyond the scope of this chapter to elaborate on all the conceptual frameworks. We refer the reader to Barnett and Whiteside (2006); Gillespie and Kadiyala (2005b); and Gillespie and Drimie (2009).

2. http://www.who.int/nutrition/topics/consultation_nutrition_and_hivaids/en/index .html

3. Highlights of this conference are published in the book, *AIDs, Poverty, and Hunger*. Available at : http://www.ifpri.org/publication/aids-poverty-and-hunger-0

4. Two more recent examples of the commitment were the i) World Health Assembly resolution WHA57.14 passed in 2005 that *"urged Member States, as a matter of priority, to pursue policies and practices that promote, inter alia, the integration of nutrition into a comprehensive response to HIV/AIDS"*; and ii) the Africa Forum 2006 *Declaration on the Dual Epidemics of HIV and AIDS and Food Security* calls for the scaling up of effective integrated programming to improve food and nutrition security for those affected by HIV and AIDS.

5. For a comprehensive review, see Gillespie and Kadiyala (2005b).

6. Gretchen Birbeck is a professor in the department of Neurology and Epidemiology at Michigan State University.

7. For details about WHO clinical staging of HIV disease in adults and adolescents, see http://www.avert.org/stages-hiv-aids.htm

8. Like the complicated relationship between micronutrients in general and HIV, it is uncertain whether the association between anemia and mortality is causal or whether

anemia is rather a marker of progressive HIV disease. It is known that the incidence of anemia increases with progression of HIV infection. Furthermore, anemia can be a feature of certain opportunistic diseases, like disseminated mycobacterial infection. Several other etiologic factors may be involved in the development of HIV-associated anemia, including other micronutrient deficiencies, immunological myelosuppression, impaired erythropoietin production, and blood loss from intestinal opportunistic disease.

9. Given the wide scope of this chapter, and the rich and extensive literature on this topic, we discuss HIV and infant feeding issues and challenges in improving prevention of mother-to-child transmission programs only briefly. For further reading we recommend: Coovadia and Coutsoudis (2007); Coovadia and Kindra (2008); Jackson et al. (2009); WHO (2010).

10. The first guidelines for PMTCT intervention were issued by WHO in 2000 recommending the use of single dose nevirapine (200 mg) for the mother at least 4 hours before delivery, as well as applying a single dose of 0.6 ml nevirapine to the baby within the first 72 hours after birth. Since then, considerable evidence has accumulated showing advantages, safety, and effectiveness of using more potent ARVs for prophylaxis. Based on the evidence, the most recent 2009/2010 WHO PMTCT guidelines recommend moving away from the use of single dose nevirapine to using more efficacious ARV regimens. (For the most recent WHO guidelines on PMTCT, see http://www.who.int/hiv/pub/mtct/advice/en/index.html).

11. Of course there is substantial literature on the nutrition-related complications and growth faltering of HIV-exposed and infected children. (See Arpadi (2005) for an excellent review.)

# CHAPTER 5

XXXXXX

The Relationship between HIV Infection and Education:
An Analysis of Six Sub-Saharan African Countries[1]

*Damien de Walque*[2] *and Rachel Kline*[3]

## 1. Introduction

Sub-Saharan Africa has been disproportionately impacted by the HIV/AIDS epidemic, with two-thirds of all HIV positive people living in the region and 32 percent of both new infections and AIDS-related deaths in the world (UNAIDS 2007a). In the face of this crisis, trying to understand the specific dimensions of the epidemic can help in deciding where to focus resources. In the absence of a vaccine for HIV, there is enormous motivation to find reliable methods of preventing infection. One logical place to look to prevent HIV has been in the realm of education. Recently, there is some evidence that national HIV prevalence has stabilized or started to decline (UNAIDS 2007a); though it is difficult to know if this is because fewer people are contracting HIV or more people have died. Could education be helping to change the infection rate?

General education, which may include, but is by all means not limited to, HIV-specific education, is believed to impact many different behaviors related to HIV infection. Jukes, Simmons, and Bundy (2008) describe various ways education may influence sexual behavior and therefore the level of risk of HIV infection. Some factors could be preventative. More educated individuals may be more likely to be exposed to prevention information, understand the connection between their actions and their exposure to HIV, and also feel that they have more control over their own behavior than less educated individuals. This may result in situations such as educated women being more able and likely to negotiate safer sex. More education has also been linked to a greater likelihood of using condoms (de Walque 2007, 2009).

However, other behaviors may be considered risk factors for HIV infection. More education often translates into a wider social/sexual network, which can imply a higher risk of HIV infection. Increased education also often means having a higher socioeconomic status. For men with higher levels of disposable income, this may provide greater freedom in sexual behavior. For women, it may mean delaying marriage but having more sexual partners during the longer period that they are single. More education also has been shown to have a positive association with extramarital sex for women (de Walque 2009). It is also important to note that these relationships between education and different sexual behaviors are not necessarily causal.

In line with these varied potential influences of education, the evidence on the association between education and HIV infection has also been mixed. Several studies using data from different contexts in sub-Saharan Africa have found that more educated people are also more likely to be infected with HIV. However, most evidence shows no association between education and HIV infection. Still other research concluded that indeed more educated people have a lower risk of HIV infection.

This study will review the research on the topic and build on previous analyses to help to determine the type of relationship between HIV and education with data from six of the most recent Demographic Health Surveys (DHS) completed in sub-Saharan Africa, which included HIV testing. The data sets, which use nationally representative samples of the adult population, are from Ethiopia (2005), Guinea (2005), Ivory Coast (1998/99), Malawi (2004), Rwanda (2005), and Zimbabwe (2005/06). It will also examine some examples of impact evaluations that identify successful school-based HIV prevention interventions.

The paper will proceed as follows. Section 2 reviews relevant literature, starting with studies examining changes over time and following with cross-sectional studies. Section 3 explains the results of the analysis of the association between HIV and education in the six countries. Section 4 reviews and examines the causal relationships between certain school-based interventions and behaviors related to HIV. Section 5 concludes.

## 2. Background and Literature Review

There have been different conclusions reached about the association between HIV infection and education in studies done using data from Africa. There are various reasons the association may be different, including the specific context and ways of analyzing the data, but the factor that seems to have the biggest influence is the time the data was recorded relative to the stage of the HIV/AIDS epidemic in the country.

There is also some debate in the literature about whether, given the positive correlation between education and wealth, one should control for wealth separately when analyzing the association between education and HIV infection, yielding the effect of education net of wealth, or only control for education and not wealth, giving the gross effect of education. One example of these contrasting approaches is in the different methodologies used by de Walque (2006, 2009) and Fortson (2008a) when analyzing the same data. Both used data from the Demographic Health Surveys from the same five African countries; however, Fortson found a positive association between education and HIV infection looking at the gross effect of education, i.e., not controlling for wealth, while de Walque did not find any association when looking at the net effect of education, controlling for wealth. De Walque argues that using the net effect of education is more interesting, because wealth and education, even if positively correlated, are sufficiently different. In light of this debate, the description of each study in the literature review section will indicate whether the author(s) controlled for wealth when looking at the association between education and HIV status in their methodology.

To make comparisons between studies easier, the literature review will be divided into two sub-sections. The studies that focus on the change in the association between HIV and education over time will be reviewed first. Following that, studies that look at the cross-sectional relationship between education and HIV infection will be explained. It should be noted that the cross-sectional studies described below do not allow for establishing whether the relationship between education and HIV is causal. Indeed, the relationship between education and HIV could be driven by self-selection or unobservable variables such as heterogeneous preferences, ability, or the discount rate. To complement the literature review, Appendix Table 5.A.1 gives a brief summary of the basic characteristics of each study explained in the following sections.

## The evolution of the association between HIV infection and education over time

Hargreaves and colleagues completed two systematic reviews of the literature and studies with individual data in general population groups relating to the association between educational attainment and risk of HIV infection in sub-Saharan Africa. The first review (Hargreaves and Glynn 2002) concluded that there was either no association between educational attainment and HIV infection (16 studies), or that there was a positive association between education and HIV infection (15 studies) with the exception of one case in Uganda where the response to the epidemic was the most developed. Only one of the 27 studies reviewed controlled for wealth separately, so most showed the gross effects of education.

Hargreaves et al. (2008a) published an updated version of the review, combining additional data published between 2001 and 2006 with the previous data. Overall, 44 populations did not show any statistically significant association between

HIV infection and education, 20 populations showed a positive association, and in only eight populations was there a negative association. In this updated version, there is evidence that the HIV epidemic is changing, as shown by the fact that a larger proportion of studies conducted from 1996 onwards identified a lower risk of infection associated with the most education than studies from before 1996; seven studies showed a negative association with post-1996 data compared to only one study showing a negative association with pre-1996 data. In addition, studies from after 1996 (5/40 populations) were less likely to show a positive association between HIV infection and the highest level of education than studies from before 1996 (15/32 populations). In studies from 1996 onwards that showed changes over time, there seemed to be a shift from strong positive associations towards weaker or negative associations between the highest levels of educational attainment and HIV infection. Additionally, HIV prevalence seemed to fall more consistently among the higher educated groups. Hargreaves et al. (2008a) also refer to evidence that levels of self-reported condom use were consistently higher among individuals with more education in a variety of settings. However, results were more mixed for other safer-sexual behaviors. Only two of the studies included control for wealth separately, so these are the only two with the effect of education net of wealth.

Michelo, Sandøy, and Fylkesnes (2006) also note a shift towards a more negative association between HIV and education between 1995 and 2003 based on analysis, controlling for wealth, of data from serial population-based surveys in both urban and rural Zambia. Urban young people with higher education illustrated this shift towards reduced risk of HIV infection, and the pattern was similar among rural young men, though not among rural young women. Conversely, the prevalence rates among the less educated remained stable during the same time period.

Jukes, Simmons, and Bundy (2008) analyze literature reviews and recent randomized evaluations relating to the role schools play in protecting girls from HIV in southern Africa. They discuss theories about why education may influence sexual behavior and HIV infection specifically relating to social-cognitive determinants, the size and nature of social networks, the changes in socioeconomic and demographic characteristics that can result from education, and how school attendance can change sexual behavior. They also review research on the relationship between education and HIV and evaluations of HIV prevention education, ending with policy recommendations for girls' education in Africa. They conclude that there is a need to increase the evidence regarding the nature of the impacts of education on HIV but, in the meantime, work towards education for all and include anti-discrimination messages paired with HIV prevention programs in school curriculum.

In terms of the association between education and HIV infection, Jukes, Simmons, and Bundy (2008) explain that most of the studies show that as educational level rises, so does HIV infection, but there are also many that find no significant relationship between HIV and education, and a few population-based studies that show a negative association. Referring to the Hargreaves et al. (2008a) literature review, Jukes, Simmons, and Bundy highlight the theory that the nature of the relationship between education and HIV infection is changing over time, whereby the early positive association between education and HIV is weakening as the epidemic matures in a particular country, though they also say that there is no hard evidence that these shifting associations can be attributed to a causal effect of education on HIV infection rates.

De Walque (2007) found that there is a negative association between HIV and education among young women in his analysis of an individual level longitudinal data set in rural Uganda. By using the type of housing as a proxy for wealth, de Walque measures the effect of education net of wealth. He explores the evolution of this association over a period of 12 years and finds it changes over time. He found no robust association between HIV/AIDS and education in 1990, but then found a negative association for young females in 2000. De Walque (2007) confirms this finding that educated females also have been more responsive to HIV/AIDS information campaigns by also showing that condom use is positively associated with education.

### Cross-sectional relationships between HIV infection and education

Glynn et al. (2004) found either a negative association or no association between HIV infection and schooling in data gathered in two-stage cluster sampling from four African cities in Benin, Cameroon, Kenya, and Zambia. They did not control for wealth to obtain their results. In addition, they report finding that the more educated in all the cities tended to report less risky sexual behavior.

Hargreaves et al. (2008b) published a study focused on school attendance in rural South Africa giving evidence that, controlling for wealth, school attendance is negatively associated with HIV infection among young males. They also found that some behaviors believed to lower the risk of HIV infection were also associated with school attendance. Both men and women attending school reported significantly fewer sexual partners than those not attending school. In addition, young women attending school were less likely to have an older male partner, had sex less often, and were more likely to use condoms than those not attending school.

It is interesting to note that this study highlights the benefits, in terms of risk of HIV infection, of going to school, even if those attending school did not have greater exposure to information about HIV prevention, life skills, or sexual health education as this curriculum was poorly developed in South Africa at the time.

The study produced little evidence that students who attended school had better knowledge of HIV, used testing services, or communicated more about HIV than those who did not attend school.

Smith et al. (1999) found a statistically significant positive association between education and risk of HIV infection for residents of rural villages (though not in main road trading centers and intermediate trading villages) based on a cross-sectional analysis of a population-based cohort in rural Uganda, even after controlling for socio-demographic and behavioral variables, including a proxy for socioeconomic status, yielding a effect of education net of wealth. Later, Fortson (2008a) also found a positive association between HIV and education. Using data from the nationally representative DHS surveys from five African countries (Burkina Faso, Cameroon, Ghana, Kenya, and Tanzania), she concluded that the relationship is nonlinear with the level of schooling corresponding to different rates of HIV. She found that individuals in the study with more than 12 years of schooling had lower HIV infection rates than those with between six and 12 years of schooling, but, in turn, that those with six years of schooling were as much as 50 percent more likely to be HIV positive than those with no education.

De Walque (2006, 2009) analyzes the same data set as Fortson to examine the socioeconomic determinants of HIV infection and associated sexual behaviors. In contrast to Fortson's results, de Walque found no significant association between HIV and education. Earlier in this section, we discussed how and why controlling or not for wealth might explain those different results. Although he found no association between education and HIV, de Walque (2006, 2009) did show that education is a very consistent predictor of both behavior and knowledge that relate to HIV infection. Schooling is strongly associated with risk factors such as higher levels of extramarital sex and lower levels of abstinence. However, it is also strongly positively associated with protective behaviors such as condom use, use of counseling and testing, and discussion about HIV among spouses.

In contrast, based on another analysis of socioeconomic determinants of HIV in Africa, Corno and de Walque (2007) find that, in Lesotho, education is negatively associated with HIV infection for men who have attended primary school. They also find that education strongly predicts preventative behaviors such as condom use and fidelity for females. Using the Lesotho DHS, their methodology includes controlling for wealth separately, giving the education effect net of wealth.

Based on the above information, we conclude that we have no clear-cut evidence showing that the association between HIV and education goes in one or another direction. The direction of the association appears to be context- and time-specific. The next section will extend the work in de Walque (2006) and Corno and de Walque (2007) to a larger set of countries.

## 3. Empirical Analysis

The six data sets used are very similar: they are all standard DHS surveys which also include HIV testing for a subsample of the population. In the analysis, we have used variables that were defined similarly across the six surveys. With such cross-sectional data, while we can establish an association between education and the risk of HIV infection, we cannot establish causality. Indeed, the association between education and HIV could be driven by self-selection or by omitted variables such as ability, heterogeneity in preference, or time-discounting rather than by a causal relationship. The independent variables used in the regressions are almost always the same: education, wealth quintiles, urban location, and marital status, including polygamy and the existence of successive marriages. Not shown in the tables but included in the regression are dummies for each year of age, regional dummies, and ethnicity dummies.

The variables describing marital status are defined as follows. The omitted category is composed of individuals who have never been married. Marriage is defined as being legally married or living with a partner with the intention of staying together, and therefore, covers both formal and informal marriage. The formerly married category includes widowed, divorced, and separated individuals. The proportion of widows and widowers is calculated as the fraction of all formerly married individuals and should be understood in the regressions as an interaction term with that variable. Being in a polygamous union is also calculated as a fraction of all currently married individuals and is used as an interaction term in the analysis. But the mean for the variable for having been in successive marriages, which should not be confused with polygamy, is taken on the entire sample and can apply to both currently married and formerly married persons.

Table 5.3 includes individuals younger than 30 years old to see if there are different results for young people.

Widowhood is defined as having lost one spouse and not being remarried. Widows and widowers constitute a substantial portion of the formerly married individuals, and there are usually more widows than widowers, either because women have longer life expectancies and often marry older men, or because it is easier for males to remarry after the death of their spouse.

As a measure of wealth, we include in the regressions a set of dummies for the quintiles of a wealth index calculated by the data provider and based on assets. Our coefficients on the education variable should therefore be understood as net of wealth.

Table 5.1 reports unadjusted means for HIV prevalence by education and wealth for each country. These unadjusted means are usually reported in the DHS (Ethiopia Government and ORC Macro 2005; Guinea Government and ORC Macro 2005; Ivory Coast Government and ORC Macro 1998/99; Malawi

Government and ORC Macro 2004; Rwanda Government and ORC Macro 2005; Zimbabwe Government and ORC Macro 2005/06). We use them as a starting point for the analysis and in order to compare and contrast them with regression coefficients in multivariate analyses. From the bivariate analysis in Table 5.1, it appears that in most countries, there is a tendency for HIV prevalence to increase (in particular among women in Ethiopia, Guinea, and Rwanda) or to be stable with education. Only in Zimbabwe does it seem that males with no education are more at risk. However, these results should be viewed with caution as they do not take into account the impact of other variables that could change the association. The remaining tables analyze the relationship of HIV with education further by controlling for other explanatory variables.

*Table 5.1a*  HIV prevalence by education and wealth: unadjusted means

|  | Ethiopia 2005 | | Guinea 2005 | | Ivory Coast 1998/99 | |
|  | (1) males | (2) females | (3) males | (4) females | (5) males | (6) females |
| --- | --- | --- | --- | --- | --- | --- |
| Overall | 0.9 | 1.9 | 0.9 | 1.9 | 2.9 | 6.4 |
| No education | 0.8 | 1.0 | 1.2 | 1.3 | 2.9 | 5.2 |
| Primary education | 0.5 | 2.5 | 0.6 | 2.5 | 1.6 | 8.2 |
| Secondary education | 2.0 | 5.5 | 0.7 | 5.1 | 3.6 | 7.0 |
| Poorest quintile | 0.7 | 0.3 | 2.1 | 1.4 | 1.7 | 3.6 |
| Second quintile | 0.3 | 1.0 | 0.6 | 0.7 | 3.4 | 3.8 |
| Middle quintile | 0.9 | 0.4 | 0.4 | 0.6 | 4. 3 | 6.5 |
| Fourth quintile | 0.4 | 0.2 | 1.0 | 2.8 | 2.1 | 8.0 |
| Richest quintile | 2.2 | 6.1 | 0.7 | 3.6 | 2.7 | 8.8 |
| Observations | 4804 | 5736 | 2616 | 3772 | 4413 | 4023 |

*Table 5.1b*  HIV prevalence by education and wealth: unadjusted means

|  | Malawi 2004 | | Rwanda 2005 | | Zimbabwe 2005/06 | |
|  | (7) males | (8) females | (9) males | (10) females | (11) males | (12) females |
| --- | --- | --- | --- | --- | --- | --- |
| Overall | 10.2 | 13.3 | 2.3 | 3.6 | 14.5 | 21.1 |
| No education | 10.7 | 14.0 | 3.0 | 3.3 | 24.2 | 20.0 |
| Primary education | 9.1 | 12.7 | 1.8 | 2.8 | 15.7 | 22.4 |
| Secondary education | 12.9 | 15.1 | 3.2 | 6.4 | 14.2 | 20.5 |
| Poorest quintile | 4.4 | 10.9 | 1.3 | 2.6 | 13.4 | 17.7 |
| Second quintile | 4.6 | 10.3 | 1.7 | 2.2 | 15.1 | 21.1 |
| Middle quintile | 12.1 | 12.7 | 2.0 | 3.6 | 12.2 | 22.7 |
| Fourth quintile | 11.7 | 14.6 | 2.1 | 3.4 | 17.1 | 26.8 |
| Richest quintile | 14.9 | 18.0 | 4.1 | 6.5 | 13.5 | 17.1 |
| Observations | 2465 | 2686 | 4361 | 5656 | 5848 | 6947 |

SOURCE: Data from Demographic and Health Surveys (Ethiopia 2005, Guinea 2005, Ivory Coast 1998/99, Malawi 2004, Rwanda 2005, and Zimbabwe 2005/06).

Table 5.2 shows the results from regressions for each country in which HIV status is the dependent variable for male and female individuals of all ages. Out of the six countries analyzed, there are only a few cases where education is significantly associated with HIV. For males from Ivory Coast, primary education is negatively associated with HIV at the 5 percent significance level. However, for females from Ethiopia, primary school is positively associated with HIV, also at the 5 percent significance level. Secondary school is positively associated with HIV in only two countries. For females from Guinea, having a secondary education is associated with a 1.8 percentage point increase in risk of HIV infection with a 5 percent

*Table 5.2a* Determinants of HIV prevalence in six Demographic and Health Surveys. All ages. Analysis by country.

|  | Ethiopia 2005 | | Guinea 2005 | | Ivory Coast 1998/99 | |
|---|---|---|---|---|---|---|
|  | (1) | (2) | (3) | (4) | (5) | (6) |
|  | males | females | males | females | males | females |
| Primary | 0 | 0.0078** | −0.0049 | 0.0091 | −0.0085** | 0.0018 |
|  | [0.0014] | [0.0039] | [0.0039] | [0.0073] | [0.0037] | [0.0099] |
| Secondary | 0.003 | 0.006 | −0.0016 | 0.0180** | −0.0005 | −0.0002 |
|  | [0.0038] | [0.0047] | [0.0048] | [0.0086] | [0.0056] | [0.0089] |
| 2nd quintile wealth | −0.0019 | 0.0115 | −0.0059* | −0.005 | 0.0114 | 0.0028 |
|  | [0.0012] | [0.0103] | [0.0034] | [0.0034] | [0.0093] | [0.0095] |
| 3rd quintile wealth | 0.0007 | 0.0051 | −0.0045 | −0.0064** | 0.0113 | 0.0285** |
|  | [0.0020] | [0.0065] | [0.0035] | [0.0030] | [0.0101] | [0.0140] |
| 4th quintile wealth | −0.0017 | −0.0005 | −0.0008 | −0.0024 | 0.0027 | 0.0367** |
|  | [0.0014] | [0.0032] | [0.0043] | [0.0038] | [0.0092] | [0.0178] |
| 5th quintile wealth | 0.0017 | 0.0272 | −0.0015 | −0.0080** | 0.0088 | 0.0508*** |
|  | [0.0025] | [0.0179] | [0.0073] | [0.0038] | [0.0103] | [0.0188] |
| Urban | 0.0007 | 0.0088* | 0.0014 | 0.0206*** | 0.0024 | −0.0063 |
|  | [0.0024] | [0.0053] | [0.0056] | [0.0069] | [0.0043] | [0.0072] |
| Currently married | 0.0025* | 0.0055*** | 0.0052 | 0.0045 | −0.0031 | −0.0385*** |
|  | [0.0014] | [0.0021] | [0.0047] | [0.0042] | [0.0054] | [0.0110] |
| Formerly married | 0.0056 | 0.0219* | (*) | 0.0097 | 0.0071 | −0.0165* |
|  | [0.0082] | [0.0113] |  | [0.0147] | [0.0122] | [0.0090] |
| Widow | 0.0409 | 0.0108 | (*) | 0.0634 | 0.0774 | 0.0856** |
|  | [0.0587] | [0.0096] |  | [0.0538] | [0.0811] | [0.0414] |
| > 1 marriage | (*) | 0.0127** | 0.0083 | 0.0097* | 0.0049 | 0.0424** |
|  |  | [0.0053] | [0.0068] | [0.0052] | [0.0056] | [0.0174] |
| Polygamous | 0.0052 | 0.0039 | −0.0022 | −0.0002 | −0.0090*** | 0.0002 |
|  | [0.0090] | [0.0054] | [0.0037] | [0.0031] | [0.0034] | [0.0101] |
| Observations | 3715 | 4854 | 2565 | 3691 | 3852 | 4419 |

*Table 5.2b* Determinants of HIV prevalence in six Demographic and Health Surveys. All ages. Analysis by country.

| | Malawi 2004 | | Rwanda 2005 | | Zimbabwe 2005/06 | |
|---|---|---|---|---|---|---|
| | (7) | (8) | (9) | (10) | (11) | (12) |
| | males | females | males | females | males | females |
| Primary | −0.0056 | 0.0178 | −0.0015 | 0.0056 | 0.008 | 0.0541 |
| | [0.0163] | [0.0148] | [0.0034] | [0.0044] | [0.0319] | [0.0354] |
| Secondary | 0.009 | 0.04 | −0.0008 | 0.0085 | 0.0047 | 0.0601* |
| | [0.0216] | [0.0313] | [0.0038] | [0.0090] | [0.0317] | [0.0344] |
| 2nd quintile wealth | −0.0141 | 0.0324 | 0.0033 | −0.0035 | 0.03 | 0.0475** |
| | [0.0178] | [0.0272] | [0.0054] | [0.0062] | [0.0240] | [0.0209] |
| 3rd quintile wealth | 0.0494* | 0.0590** | 0.0031 | 0.0085 | 0.0167 | 0.0591** |
| | [0.0276] | [0.0267] | [0.0043] | [0.0077] | [0.0199] | [0.0258] |
| 4th quintile wealth | 0.0487* | 0.0853*** | 0.006 | 0.0081 | 0.0325 | 0.0646** |
| | [0.0284] | [0.0277] | [0.0048] | [0.0078] | [0.0232] | [0.0271] |
| 5th quintile wealth | 0.0702* | 0.1193*** | 0.0078 | 0.0149 | 0.01 | −0.0288 |
| | [0.0379] | [0.0371] | [0.0055] | [0.0096] | [0.0265] | [0.0268] |
| Urban | 0.0295* | 0.0294 | 0.0279*** | 0.0305*** | 0.0157 | 0.0382 |
| | [0.0173] | [0.0212] | [0.0080] | [0.0081] | [0.0224] | [0.0254] |
| Currently married | 0.0476*** | 0.014 | −0.0035 | −0.0035 | 0.0580** | 0.0203 |
| | [0.0145] | [0.0297] | [0.0040] | [0.0062] | [0.0274] | [0.0186] |
| Formerly married | 0.1288* | 0.1535*** | 0.0039 | 0.0534*** | 0.1993*** | 0.1749*** |
| | [0.0681] | [0.0553] | [0.0096] | [0.0162] | [0.0551] | [0.0324] |
| Widow | 0.0155 | 0.0718* | 0.0338 | 0.0156 | 0.1694** | 0.2038*** |
| | [0.0729] | [0.0429] | [0.0356] | [0.0106] | [0.0665] | [0.0304] |
| > 1 marriage | 0.0680*** | 0.0798*** | 0.0091* | 0.0247*** | 0.0981*** | 0.1594*** |
| | [0.0178] | [0.0183] | [0.0051] | [0.0085] | [0.0216] | [0.0206] |
| Polygamous | −0.0252** | 0.0418* | −0.0045 | 0.0124 | 0.0633* | 0.0424* |
| | [0.0112] | [0.0220] | [0.0035] | [0.0096] | [0.0337] | [0.0257] |
| Observations | 2362 | 2853 | 4724 | 5613 | 5549 | 7278 |

NOTES: HIV prevalence is the dependent variable. Marginal effects of probit estimates. Robust and clustered standard errors in brackets.
* Significant at 10%; ** significant at 5%; *** significant at 1%.
(*): not applicable or the variable predicts the outcome perfectly. Controls for age, region, religion and ethnicity are also included. For education, the omitted category is no education, "primary" means "at least some primary," and "secondary" means "at least some secondary."
SOURCE: Data from Demographic and Health Surveys (Ethiopia 2005, Guinea 2005, Ivory Coast 1998/99, Malawi 2004, Rwanda 2005, and Zimbabwe 2005/06).

significance level. There is a 6 percentage point increase for females in Zimbabwe associated with attending secondary school but only at a 10 percent significance level. Based on this analysis, there appears to be no strong or consistent association between education and HIV in these countries for males and females of all ages.

The conclusions from Table 5.3 are similar. Table 5.3 includes regressions with HIV status as the dependent variable for male and female individuals younger than 30 years old. Examining the association between HIV and education for younger people is important because this age group is more likely to have started

*Table 5.3a* Determinants of HIV prevalence in six Demographic and Health Surveys. 30 years and under. Analysis by country.

| | Ethiopia 2005 | | Guinea 2005 | | Ivory Coast 1998/99 | |
| | (1) | (2) | (3) | (4) | (5) | (6) |
| | males | females | males | females | males | females |
| --- | --- | --- | --- | --- | --- | --- |
| Primary | −0.0005 | 0.0013 | −0.0007 | 0.0326 | −0.0031 | 0.0045 |
| | [0.0009] | [0.0014] | [0.0047] | [0.0221] | [0.0022] | [0.0080] |
| Secondary | 0 | 0.0023 | 0.0019 | 0.0307** | 0.0027 | 0.005 |
| | [0.0012] | [0.0025] | [0.0054] | [0.0153] | [0.0021] | [0.0078] |
| 2nd quintile wealth | −0.0004 | 0.0097 | −0.0037 | (*) | 0.0002 | 0.0061 |
| | [0.0008] | [0.0102] | [0.0035] | | [0.0016] | [0.0090] |
| 3rd quintile wealth | 0.0005 | 0.0079 | −0.0062* | −0.0019 | −0.0001 | 0.0142 |
| | [0.0012] | [0.0069] | [0.0037] | [0.0076] | [0.0015] | [0.0124] |
| 4th quintile wealth | 0.0001 | 0.0089 | 0.0023 | −0.0009 | 0.0004 | 0.0371* |
| | [0.0016] | [0.0076] | [0.0068] | [0.0087] | [0.0023] | [0.0201] |
| 5th quintile wealth | −0.004 | 0.0495* | 0.0168 | −0.0206** | 0.0005 | 0.0365* |
| | [0.0027] | [0.0281] | [0.0280] | [0.0095] | [0.0019] | [0.0190] |
| Urban | 0.0062 | 0.0014 | −0.0138** | 0.01 | −0.0021 | −0.0082 |
| | [0.0063] | [0.0018] | [0.0067] | [0.0075] | [0.0020] | [0.0062] |
| Currently married | −0.0008 | 0.0050*** | 0.0147 | 0.0104 | 0.0022 | −0.0153*** |
| | [0.0009] | [0.0019] | [0.0136] | [0.0068] | [0.0024] | [0.0057] |
| Formerly married | 0.0104 | 0.0114 | (*) | 0.0115 | 0.0217 | −0.0107*** |
| | [0.0115] | [0.0086] | | [0.0227] | [0.0215] | [0.0041] |
| Widow | (*) | 0.0234 | (*) | 0.0457 | (*) | 0.0597 |
| | | [0.0225] | | [0.0801] | | [0.0861] |
| > 1 marriage | (*) | 0.004 | (*) | −0.0021 | −0.0007 | 0.0776** |
| | | [0.0050] | | [0.0074] | [0.0018] | [0.0324] |
| Polygamous | 0.0096 | −0.0014** | (*) | −0.0029 | (*) | −0.0080* |
| | [0.0255] | [0.0006] | | [0.0054] | | [0.0044] |
| Observations | 1437 | 2872 | 753 | 1269 | 1863 | 2740 |

*Table 5.3b* Determinants of HIV prevalence in six Demographic and Health Surveys. 30 years and under. Analysis by country.

| | Malawi 2004 | | Rwanda 2005 | | Zimbabwe 2005/06 | |
|---|---|---|---|---|---|---|
| | (7) males | (8) females | (9) males | (10) females | (11) males | (12) females |
| Primary | 0.013 [0.0081] | 0.0123 [0.0182] | −0.0061 [0.0040] | 0.0014 [0.0043] | 0.0151 [0.0602] | 0.1386 [0.0952] |
| Secondary | 0.0127 [0.0143] | 0.0038 [0.0274] | −0.0024** [0.0012] | 0.0034 [0.0090] | 0.001 [0.0541] | 0.1172** [0.0544] |
| 2nd quintile wealth | −0.0119*** [0.0045] | 0.0082 [0.0258] | 0.0109 [0.0126] | −0.0069 [0.0048] | 0.002 [0.0157] | 0.0328* [0.0191] |
| 3rd quintile wealth | 0.0025 [0.0078] | 0.0413 [0.0279] | 0.0086 [0.0099] | 0.0017 [0.0065] | 0.0004 [0.0153] | 0.0314 [0.0215] |
| 4th quintile wealth | 0.0073 [0.0096] | 0.0472 [0.0289] | 0.0136 [0.0123] | −0.004 [0.0052] | 0.0179 [0.0183] | 0.0268 [0.0228] |
| 5th quintile wealth | 0.012 [0.0133] | 0.0589* [0.0357] | 0.0136 [0.0113] | 0.0008 [0.0066] | 0.0338 [0.0262] | −0.0516** [0.0233] |
| Urban | 0.0057 [0.0076] | 0.0565** [0.0263] | 0.0159** [0.0069] | 0.0183** [0.0084] | −0.0091 [0.0175] | 0.0388 [0.0253] |
| Currently married | 0.0156* [0.0086] | 0.0155 [0.0258] | 0.002 [0.0029] | 0.0008 [0.0048] | 0.0442** [0.0217] | 0.0298* [0.0160] |
| Formerly married | 0.0469 [0.0403] | 0.1135** [0.0502] | 0.0007 [0.0046] | 0.0321** [0.0164] | 0.1604*** [0.0571] | 0.1556*** [0.0380] |
| Widow | (*) | 0.1288 [0.0965] | (*) | (*) | 0.0655 [0.0883] | 0.2030*** [0.0565] |
| > 1 marriage | 0.0369** [0.0188] | 0.0363 [0.0230] | −0.0001 [0.0032] | 0.0238 [0.0168] | 0.0436 [0.0276] | 0.1417*** [0.0372] |
| Polygamous | 0.0061 [0.0139] | 0.0348 [0.0292] | (*) | 0.0193 [0.0160] | 0.1909* [0.1018] | 0.0611* [0.0345] |
| Observations | 1322 | 1758 | 1935 | 3012 | 3486 | 4534 |

NOTES: HIV prevalence is the dependent variable. Marginal effects of probit estimates. Robust and clustered standard errors in brackets.
* Significant at 10%; ** significant at 5%; *** significant at 1%.
(*): not applicable or the variable predicts the outcome perfectly. Controls for age, region, religion and ethnicity are also included. For education, the omitted category is no education, "primary" means "at least some primary," and "secondary" means "at least some secondary."
SOURCE: Demographic and Health Surveys (Ethiopia 2005, Guinea 2005, Ivory Coast 1998/99, Malawi 2004, Rwanda 2005, and Zimbabwe 2005/06).

their sexual life after the start of the epidemic. They also would be more likely to have received HIV/AIDS prevention messages. In addition, de Walque (2007) found a negative association between HIV and education only among young women in Uganda. In this analysis, the only negative association is for males in Rwanda who have attended secondary school at the 5 percent significance level. Alternately, there is a positive association for females who attended secondary school from Guinea and Zimbabwe at the 5 percent significance level. Because these are the only statistically significant associations out of the 12 regressions, it seems that, overall, there is not a strong or consistent association between education and HIV even for the younger age group.

Tables 5.4 and 5.5 may explain a possible reason for the lack of association between education and HIV. Table 5.4 looks at condom use, a preventative measure, and Table 5.5 looks at extramarital sex, a more risky behavior. When viewing these results, it is important to take into account the fact that condom use and extramarital sex are self-reported behaviors, and therefore, prone to reporting bias that may vary with education. For example, Glick and Sahn (2008), using data from repeated rounds of DHS surveys in Africa, found evidence of changes in the way people answer questions relating to HIV-related behavior. Based on the regression analysis in which the dependent variable is whether the individual used a condom during his/her last sexual intercourse, there is a strong positive association with attending secondary school in almost every country. The only exceptions to this positive association at the 5 percent significance level are males from Rwanda and males and females from Ethiopia. In general, it seems that having secondary education means that one is more likely to have used a condom during the last sexual intercourse. The analysis suggests education reinforces this preventive measure.

However, Table 5.5 shows the association between education and having had extramarital sex in the last 12 months among a sample of married people. In five of the six countries, there is a positive association of varying levels of significance for males and/or females. It seems that in some countries, while education reinforces important preventive measures such as condom use, education can also push individuals towards more risky behaviors such as extramarital sex. Possible reasons for these risky behaviors include having more opportunity for this type of behavior with the larger social network that comes with having attended school, increased travel, and more disposable income than those not having attended school. Each of these behaviors, one risky and the other preventive, could act as a balance for the other, resulting in no association between HIV and education.

Overall, based on these analyses, it is difficult to generalize across countries that there is any pattern in the association between education and HIV in Africa. Most frequently, there is no significant association between education and HIV. One possible reason for this is that more educated individuals engage in preventative

*Table 5.4a* Determinants of condom use during last sexual intercourse in six Demographic and Health Surveys. Analysis by country.

|  | Ethiopia 2005 | | Guinea 2005 | | Ivory Coast 1998/99 | |
|  | (1) males | (2) females | (3) males | (4) females | (5) males | (6) females |
|---|---|---|---|---|---|---|
| Primary | 0.0005 [0.0020] | 0 [0.0019] | 0.0295 [0.0207] | 0.007 [0.0050] | 0.0768** [0.0365] | 0.0770*** [0.0193] |
| Secondary | 0.0075 [0.0058] | −0.0004 [0.0021] | 0.0922*** [0.0241] | 0.0385*** [0.0118] | 0.1111*** [0.0331] | 0.1597*** [0.0271] |
| 2nd quintile wealth | −0.0009 [0.0036] | −0.0048* [0.0026] | −0.0166 [0.0235] | 0.0057 [0.0074] | 0.0285 [0.0386] | −0.0108 [0.0121] |
| 3rd quintile wealth | 0.0014 [0.0044] | (*) | −0.0058 [0.0235] | 0.015 [0.0114] | 0.0441 [0.0439] | 0.0022 [0.0156] |
| 4th quintile wealth | −0.0021 [0.0031] | (*) | 0.0411 [0.0336] | 0.0163 [0.0118] | 0.0707 [0.0471] | 0.0319 [0.0229] |
| 5th quintile wealth | 0.0134 [0.0109] | −0.0008 [0.0024] | 0.0793* [0.0454] | 0.0201 [0.0181] | 0.0939* [0.0508] | 0.0366* [0.0209] |
| Urban | 0.0053 [0.0061] | 0.0096 [0.0078] | 0.0169 [0.0251] | 0.0086 [0.0056] | 0.0597* [0.0334] | 0.0270** [0.0121] |
| Currently married | −0.2485*** [0.0633] | −0.2092*** [0.0811] | −0.0983*** [0.0297] | −0.0814*** [0.0184] | −0.2742*** [0.0357] | −0.0909*** [0.0259] |
| Formerly married | −0.0031** [0.0015] | −0.0033** [0.0016] | −0.0247 [0.0197] | −0.0032 [0.0037] | −0.0291 [0.0619] | −0.0186 [0.0151] |
| Widow | 0.0992 [0.0746] | 0.0055 [0.0126] | (*) | 0.001 [0.0084] | 0.1277 [0.2061] | −0.0263 [0.0365] |
| > 1 marriage | (*) | −0.0003 [0.0028] | 0.0157 [0.0265] | 0.0077 [0.0051] | −0.0088 [0.0518] | 0.0236 [0.0233] |
| Polygamous | −0.0039** [0.0018] | 0.0008 [0.0044] | −0.0163 [0.0213] | −0.0025 [0.0031] | −0.0676 [0.0925] | −0.0176 [0.0184] |
| Observations | 3133 | 2184 | 2376 | 5139 | 3030 | 3567 |

behaviors but also risky behaviors that can negate these preventative measures. However, causality between this behavior and the lack of association between education and HIV cannot be established with this cross-sectional data.

# 4. Discussion

It is important to note that while the results from the analysis above help us understand how general schooling and HIV infection relate, they can only be interpreted

*Table 5.4b* Determinants of condom use during last sexual intercourse in six Demographic and Health Surveys. Analysis by country.

| | Malawi 2004 | | Rwanda 2005 | | Zimbabwe 2005/06 | |
|---|---|---|---|---|---|---|
| | (7) males | (8) females | (9) males | (10) females | (11) males | (12) females |
| Primary | 0.0328 [0.0242] | 0.0079 [0.0051] | −0.0054 [0.0060] | 0.0028 [0.0027] | 0.1254** [0.0592] | 0.0231 [0.0186] |
| Secondary | 0.0935** [0.0393] | 0.0211** [0.0108] | 0.0141 [0.0095] | 0.0215** [0.0093] | 0.1490*** [0.0410] | 0.0384** [0.0150] |
| 2nd quintile wealth | −0.009 [0.0231] | 0.0042 [0.0076] | −0.0016 [0.0071] | 0.0005 [0.0050] | 0.0625 [0.0382] | 0.008 [0.0125] |
| 3rd quintile wealth | −0.0277 [0.0209] | 0.0123 [0.0076] | 0.0012 [0.0076] | 0.0087 [0.0063] | 0.0726* [0.0426] | 0.0085 [0.0132] |
| 4th quintile wealth | −0.0188 [0.0202] | 0.0106 [0.0080] | 0.0026 [0.0073] | 0.0036 [0.0051] | 0.0831** [0.0382] | 0.0559*** [0.0195] |
| 5th quintile wealth | 0.0113 [0.0262] | 0.0264** [0.0115] | 0.0198 [0.0124] | 0.0120* [0.0071] | 0.1144** [0.0475] | 0.0569** [0.0233] |
| Urban | 0.0028 [0.0212] | 0.0003 [0.0073] | 0.0217* [0.0111] | 0.0127** [0.0052] | 0.0253 [0.0278] | −0.0118 [0.0095] |
| Currently married | −0.3639*** [0.0424] | −0.2109*** [0.0242] | −0.2799*** [0.0525] | −0.1133*** [0.0243] | −0.6560*** [0.0276] | −0.4163*** [0.0318] |
| Formerly married | −0.0466* [0.0267] | −0.0279*** [0.0037] | −0.0100*** [0.0030] | −0.0059*** [0.0022] | −0.0702*** [0.0254] | −0.0238*** [0.0062] |
| Widow | (*) | 0.0187 [0.0207] | −0.0013 [0.0165] | 0.0205 [0.0144] | −0.0909** [0.0387] | −0.002 [0.0125] |
| > 1 marriage | 0.0174 [0.0234] | −0.0001 [0.0057] | 0.0011 [0.0065] | 0.0026 [0.0041] | 0.0022 [0.0237] | −0.002 [0.0092] |
| Polygamous | 0.0114 [0.0330] | −0.0148*** [0.0052] | 0.0022 [0.0117] | −0.0007 [0.0039] | −0.0454 [0.0404] | 0.0325** [0.0164] |
| Observations | 2585 | 9150 | 2629 | 5800 | 4613 | 5605 |

NOTES: HIV prevalence is the dependent variable. Marginal effects of probit estimates. Robust and clustered standard errors in brackets.
* Significant at 10%; ** significant at 5%; *** significant at 1%.
(*): not applicable or the variable predicts the outcome perfectly. Controls for age, region, religion and ethnicity are also included. For education, the omitted category is no education, "primary" means "at least some primary," and "secondary" means "at least some secondary."
SOURCE: Data from Demographic and Health Surveys (Ethiopia 2005, Guinea 2005, Ivory Coast 1998/99, Malawi 2004, Rwanda 2005, and Zimbabwe 2005/06).

*Table 5.5a* Determinants of extramarital sex in six Demographic and Health Surveys. Analysis by country with sample of only those currently married.

| | Ethiopia 2005 | | Guinea 2005 | | Ivory Coast 1998/99 | |
| | (1) males | (2) females | (3) males | (4) females | (5) males | (6) females |
|---|---|---|---|---|---|---|
| Primary | 0.0001 | −0.0005 | 0.0679** | 0.0138 | −0.0019 | 0.0901** |
| | [0.0018] | [0.0008] | [0.0280] | [0.0096] | [0.0371] | [0.0364] |
| Secondary | 0.0002 | 0.01 | 0.0950*** | 0.0517*** | 0.0528 | 0.0324 |
| | [0.0023] | [0.0106] | [0.0290] | [0.0135] | [0.0468] | [0.0678] |
| 2nd quintile wealth | 0.0032 | −0.0008 | 0.0107 | −0.0072 | 0.0175 | −0.0472 |
| | [0.0039] | [0.0007] | [0.0246] | [0.0055] | [0.0386] | [0.0362] |
| 3rd quintile wealth | 0.0052 | −0.0001 | −0.0215 | 0.0052 | 0.0422 | −0.0099 |
| | [0.0042] | [0.0009] | [0.0226] | [0.0068] | [0.0452] | [0.0476] |
| 4th quintile wealth | 0.0008 | −0.0016* | 0.0136 | 0.0035 | 0.1069 | 0.0359 |
| | [0.0029] | [0.0009] | [0.0306] | [0.0071] | [0.0720] | [0.0608] |
| 5th quintile wealth | −0.0023 | −0.0016* | 0.0218 | −0.0048 | 0.0212 | 0.0132 |
| | [0.0016] | [0.0009] | [0.0472] | [0.0097] | [0.0760] | [0.0604] |
| Urban | 0.0035 | 0.0061 | 0.0379 | 0.0001 | 0.0238 | −0.0449 |
| | [0.0051] | [0.0055] | [0.0331] | [0.0074] | [0.0382] | [0.0532] |
| > 1 marriage | (*) | 0.0095** | 0.0582** | 0.0306*** | 0.0671 | 0.0021 |
| | | [0.0041] | [0.0240] | [0.0079] | [0.0499] | [0.0418] |
| Polygamous | 0.0832** | 0.0056 | −0.0048 | −0.0063* | −0.0819** | 0.0960** |
| | [0.0337] | [0.0046] | [0.0183] | [0.0038] | [0.0395] | [0.0382] |
| Observations | 2465 | 3338 | 1758 | 6157 | 1607 | 2654 |

as statistical associations, not as causal relationships. Rigorous impact evaluations of interventions, whether those are interventions to increase school enrollment and attendance generally or school-based specific HIV/AIDS interventions, give us a better chance at looking at the causal effect of those interventions that may help inform and improve the effects of schooling. Though educational interventions aimed at HIV/AIDS prevention through increased knowledge and sexual behavior change have been implemented in many African schools, there is generally little evidence of their effectiveness based on rigorous randomized trials. However, we have identified some of these rigorous evaluations and summarized their results below. Though we find no consistent association between education and HIV in our study, these other interventions can provide additional depth to our results by giving specific insights into ways education may be able to impact knowledge of HIV/AIDS and sexual behavior.

One recent randomized study (Baird et al. 2009) provides empirical evidence of the causal link between general schooling and self-reported sexual behavior.

*Table 5.5b* Determinants of extramarital sex in six Demographic and Health Surveys. Analysis by country with sample of only those currently married.

| | Malawi 2004 | | Rwanda 2005 | | Zimbabwe 2005/06 | |
|---|---|---|---|---|---|---|
| | (7) males | (8) females | (9) males | (10) females | (11) males | (12) females |
| Primary | 0.0167 [0.0161] | 0.0019 [0.0019] | 0.0125 [0.0099] | 0.0019** [0.0009] | −0.0076 [0.0301] | −0.0011 [0.0039] |
| Secondary | 0.0521* [0.0315] | 0.0024 [0.0041] | 0.0045 [0.0161] | 0.0018 [0.0027] | −0.0143 [0.0362] | −0.0009 [0.0041] |
| 2nd quintile wealth | 0.0281 [0.0238] | −0.0029 [0.0019] | −0.0063 [0.0109] | −0.0004 [0.0009] | 0.0193 [0.0200] | −0.001 [0.0024] |
| 3rd quintile wealth | 0.0416 [0.0253] | −0.0031* [0.0019] | −0.0047 [0.0118] | −0.0015* [0.0009] | 0.03 [0.0235] | 0.0045 [0.0054] |
| 4th quintile wealth | 0.0447* [0.0260] | −0.0023 [0.0021] | −0.0180* [0.0099] | −0.0002 [0.0012] | 0.0214 [0.0236] | −0.0012 [0.0029] |
| 5th quintile wealth | 0.0078 [0.0225] | −0.0035 [0.0023] | −0.0122 [0.0114] | 0.0006 [0.0013] | 0.0059 [0.0273] | −0.0056** [0.0025] |
| Urban | 0.0145 [0.0169] | −0.0018 [0.0032] | 0.0322 [0.0265] | 0.0022 [0.0018] | 0.0484** [0.0219] | 0.001 [0.0046] |
| > 1 marriage | 0.0199 [0.0125] | 0.0075** [0.0035] | −0.0017 [0.0119] | 0.0088** [0.0038] | 0.0431*** [0.0151] | 0.0232*** [0.0070] |
| Polygamous | 0.0115 [0.0233] | 0.003 [0.0028] | 0.0051 [0.0200] | 0.0015 [0.0016] | 0.0364 [0.0267] | 0.0139*** [0.0050] |
| Observations | 2095 | 8021 | 2471 | 5209 | 3325 | 4848 |

NOTE: HIV prevalence is the dependent variable. Marginal effects of probit estimates. Robust and clustered standard errors in brackets.

* Significant at 10%; ** significant at 5%; *** significant at 1%.

(*): not applicable or the variable predicts the outcome perfectly. Controls for age, region, religion and ethnicity are also included. For education, the omitted category is no education, "primary" means "at least some primary," and "secondary" means "at least some secondary." The sample is individuals currently married.

SOURCE: Data from Demographic and Health Surveys (Ethiopia 2005, Guinea 2005, Ivory Coast 1998/99, Malawi 2004, Rwanda 2005, and Zimbabwe 2005/06).

The study measures the impact of a conditional cash transfer program in rural Malawi whereby unmarried girls in school or unmarried girls who had dropped out of school between the ages of 13 and 22 were given both a monthly cash incentive and school fees if they maintained an 80 percent attendance record as an incentive to either stay in or return to school. The impacts of staying in school and the cash incentives were measured by comparing treatment and control groups (randomly selected) after one year of the program.

In addition to a large increase in school enrollment (61.4 percent of treatment group dropouts at baseline returned to school vs. 17.2 percent of control group dropouts and more treatment schoolgirls at baseline stayed enrolled), the marriage rate of initial dropouts in the treatment group was reduced by 40 percent, and the pregnancy rate was reduced by 30 percent. The treatment group also reported reducing their sexual activity by delaying the initial sexual act (one-third of beneficiaries) and reducing the number of sexual partners (significant for the initial dropouts in the treatment group). There was no apparent difference in self-reported condom use between the treatment and control groups; however, the likelihood of having an older partner was significantly lower for baseline schoolgirls.

The authors attribute these impacts to attending school and the incentives to stay in school rather than what was specifically learned at school, based on the finding that there was no significant improvement in knowledge of HIV or the likelihood of getting tested for HIV. Using the same conditional cash transfer experiment in Malawi, Baird, McIntosh, and Özler (2009) also find that the program led to significant declines in risk of HIV and HSV-2 infection after one year. However, they cannot yet conclude that keeping girls in school, as opposed to an exogenous income shock, is the reason for the decline in HIV risk, since the program effect was similar regardless of schooling status in follow-up.

In addition to years of schooling, education and the school environment might offer a useful platform to deliver HIV information and prevention messages. To help understand specific ways to impact students' behavior so they will have less risk of contracting HIV, we will review the results from some impact evaluations.

Duflo et al. (2006) analyze results from a randomized evaluation comparing two different HIV prevention interventions and one economic intervention and their impact on the students in certain behaviors considered to be risk factors for HIV infection. They tested three different types of school-based interventions in rural Kenya. One intervention involved training teachers in the national HIV/AIDS curriculum for them to present to their students. The second intervention consisted of students being encouraged to debate the benefits of using condoms and write essays on ways to protect themselves against HIV. The third intervention involved lowering the cost of schooling by providing school uniforms to students attending school as a way to get students to stay in school longer. To measure effectiveness, the authors primarily evaluated teenage childbearing as a proxy for unprotected sex, the main risk factor for HIV/AIDS in Africa. They also collected information on knowledge, attitudes, and behavior regarding HIV/AIDS.

The results from the different interventions provide interesting insights into the types of interventions that seem to be effective in this rural Kenyan context. The teacher training was found to have little impact on teen childbearing, students' knowledge, and self-reported sexual activity and condom use. It did seem that girls exposed to the program who became pregnant were more likely to marry the fathers of their children and students had increased tolerance toward HIV-positive people. The debate and essay intervention increased self-reported condom use, but not self-reported sexual activity. Paying for uniforms reduced dropout rates by 15 percent and resulted in an almost 10 percent decrease in teen childbearing; girls were 12 percent less likely to be married, and boys were 40 percent less likely to be married. Similar to the conditional cash transfer intervention in Malawi discussed earlier, these results show that being able to afford to stay in school created incentives for teenagers to avoid teen pregnancy more than direct information given about the dangers of unprotected sex. Though there were no biomarkers in this study, a lower rate of teen pregnancy is likely to mean less HIV infection among these teenagers.

Another randomized controlled trial in rural Tanzania of a specific HIV/AIDS intervention aimed at changing the knowledge and sexual behavior of adolescents produced mixed results. The DFID (United Kingdom Department for International Development) trial (2004) evaluated the impact of the intervention on HIV rates, other STIs, unintended pregnancy and adolescents' knowledge, reported attitudes, reported behaviors, and cost effectiveness. The intervention included an in-school, teacher-led, peer-assisted sexual and reproductive health education component, training for health workers to make reproductive health services at the clinics more youth-friendly, community-based condom promotion, and periodic community activities promoting sexual health.

Comparing the communities that received the interventions with the control communities showed that the intervention communities had statistically significant improvement in knowledge and reported sexual attitudes for both males and females. Males also reported delayed sexual debut, fewer sexual partners, and more condom use at last sex. However, there was no evidence of a consistent impact of the intervention on biological outcomes including HIV incidence, other STIs, and unintended pregnancies.

A review (Gallant and Maticka-Tyndale 2004) of 11 quasi-experimental designs that measured the impacts of a variety of school-based HIV-prevention interventions in sub-Saharan Africa reinforce the finding from the DFID (2004) trial that behavior is more difficult to change than knowledge. While the authors note that the evaluations should be viewed with caution as only one is a rigorous study, they show that all studies resulted in a positive change in knowledge and attitudes related to HIV, though attitudes towards abstaining from sex and condom use were less consistent. While fewer studies targeted behavior changes as a desired outcome, still only one out of four studies included a reported increase in condom use. Common to most studies involving discussion of condom use was opposition by teachers or community members.

In addition to results, the review provides insight into program elements that seemed to be more successful, including targeting younger children (before they were sexually active), integrating the program throughout the regular curriculum, using peer educators, implementing multiple participatory activities, using cascade training (where one teacher is trained and that teacher trains others), and having at least a one- to two-year program period. This review also emphasizes the need for monitoring, as most of the programs were not uniformly implemented, and that access to resources needs to be considered in resource poor schools.

While general HIV knowledge may not often result in behavior change, another study (Dupas 2009) shows that specific information that distinguishes levels of HIV risk may be more useful in changing behavior. Dupas rigorously tests an information campaign aimed at changing teenagers' sexual behavior. She studies the impacts of telling teenagers about the relative risks of different types of partners, based on their HIV infection rates. The context for this campaign includes a common practice of teenage girls having older sexual partners who negotiate having sex with the younger girls in exchange for some sort of material support. The intervention consisted of a 40-minute presentation, a survey, and a 10-minute video. Information in the campaign included comparing a 4 percent HIV-prevalence rate for 15–19-year-old males to 13 percent for 20–24 year olds, 28 percent for 25–29 year olds, and 32 percent for 30–39 year olds. The idea of the campaign was to make teenagers aware of relative risks of different aged partners, in the hopes that they will take these different levels of risk into account when choosing a partner. This campaign is in marked contrast to most campaigns that generally give the average risk of having sex with any individual and also often only promote abstinence.

As a result of the campaign, the incidence of cross-generational pregnancies among the treatment group decreased by 61 percent, while intragenerational pregnancies remained stable. This type of information on the relative risks of different partners resulted in a sizable decrease in unprotected sex between older men and teenage girls but without an increase in unprotected sex between teenage boys and girls. In contrast, another program that only gave general information about HIV risk had no impact on the incidence of unprotected sex (measured by pregnancy rates).

While this chapter looks at the effects of general schooling on HIV prevalence, the studies included in this section provide instructive nuance to these results. We see how schooling may help change behavior, especially if paired with a financial incentive, and how HIV-specific programs can impact the level of knowledge and also provide some insights into how to impact behavior. This type of information can help policymakers to shift the relationship between HIV and education towards a negative association by clarifying how education and school-based interventions can be effective in lowering the risk of HIV.

## 5. Conclusion

This analysis builds on previous studies by using data from the most recent DHS surveys in sub-Saharan Africa in order to continue to examine the relationship between education and risk of HIV infection. The countries included were Ethiopia, Guinea, Ivory Coast, Malawi, Rwanda, and Zimbabwe. Based on the evidence from the data from these six African countries, there is no significant or consistent association between education and HIV infection, though education is a strong predictor of certain behaviors relating to HIV infection. These behaviors, some protective and some more risky in terms of HIV, could potentially balance each other, resulting in the neutral relationship between HIV risk and education.

However, as explained in detail earlier in the chapter, evidence exists for all different types of associations between education and HIV infection in sub-Saharan Africa, depending on the specific context and time period. Therefore, it is very difficult to generalize about the nature of the relationship between education and HIV throughout sub-Saharan Africa. An additional limitation to understanding this issue is the small number of studies that show a causal effect of education or a school-based intervention on HIV-related behaviors.

This is not to say that the relationship between education and HIV infection seems static in the region or in any one context. The apparent change over time in the data is one reason to hypothesize that the nature of the association is shifting from a positive gradient towards a more negative gradient whereby more educated individuals are less likely to contract HIV. Initially, more educated people were more at risk for HIV because of their way of life. They often travel in a wider radius from home, live in a more urban area, and have more disposable income. These are all factors that could increase the opportunity for behaviors associated with higher risk of HIV infection, such as extramarital sex and having more sexual partners. However, as the epidemic matures and information about the risks associated with unsafe sex is disseminated more widely, educated people may respond earlier and faster. This response to prevention information may result in this evolution in the HIV/education gradient over time. This hypothesis would explain the disparity of results across countries because different countries might be at different stages of their epidemic or at different stages of their response to it.

Research establishing causal relationships between education, or school-based interventions, and a decrease in teenage pregnancies or other risky sexual behaviors (and, hopefully, HIV infection) can help reinforce this shift towards more educated people being at less risk for HIV. These impact evaluations can help to clarify the types of educational programs that can reduce HIV infection rates.

# Notes

1. We thank Sowmya Srinivasan for excellent research assistance. The findings, interpretations, and conclusions expressed in this paper are entirely those of the authors. They do not necessarily represent the view of the World Bank, its Executive Directors, or the countries they represent.

2. Development Research Group. The World Bank. Email: ddewalque@worldbank.org

3. The World Bank. Email: rachelkline@post.harvard.edu

*Appendix Table 5.A.1* Characteristics of studies described

| Study | Sample Characteristics | Location | Urban/ Rural |
|---|---|---|---|
| Baird et al. (2009) | Baseline surveys were conducted with 3,805 girls in 176 Enumeration Areas (EAs) randomly selected from the EAs used in 1998 Census. The 3,805 girls were all the never-married, 13-22 year-old females in the 176 EAs. Out of these 3,805 young women, 1,230 girls (all drop-outs and 75-100% of current school girls) in 88 randomly selected EAs were sampled to be part of the CCT program. A household questionnaire was administered to treatment and control groups at baseline and follow-up, which were conducted 12 months apart. | Zomba District, Southern Malawi | Urban and rural |
| Corno and de Walque (2007) | Lesotho Demographic and Health Survey, nationally representative repeated cross-sections of demographic, economic, and fertility micro-data linked with HIV test results. | Lesotho | Urban and rural |
| De Walque (2006) | Demographic and Health Surveys, nationally representative repeated cross-sections of demographic, economic, and fertility micro-data linked with HIV test results. | Burkina Faso, Cameroon, Ghana, Kenya, and Tanzania | Urban and rural |
| De Walque (2007) | Individual level data set from a longitudinal survey, the General Population Cohort (GPC) of the Medical Research Council (MRC) Programme on AIDS in Uganda, which follows the general population of a cluster of villages over 12 years. | Masaka District, Southern Uganda | Rural |

| Study | Sample Characteristics | Location | Urban/ Rural |
|---|---|---|---|
| | Compares those who started their sexual life before the arrival of the information and those who initiated their sexual activity afterward. Compares HIV outcomes for the better and the less well educated. | | |
| Duflo et al. (2006) | A sample of 328 schools was divided into 6 treatment groups, each selected randomly after stratifying for particular characteristics depending on the treatment for that group. The baseline sample consisted of 74,000 students enrolled in grades 5 through 8 in any of the 328 schools. 3000 upper primary school teachers were also involved in the study. | Bungoma, Butere-Mumias Districts, Western Kenya | Rural |
| Dupas (2009) | The study involved 328 primary schools. After stratifying for particular characteristics depending on the treatment, 163 schools were randomly selected for the HIV/AIDS teacher training treatment and 71 were sampled to receive the relative risk information campaign treatment given to $8^{th}$ graders. | Western Kenya | Rural |
| Fortson (2008a) | Demographic and Health Surveys, nationally representative repeated cross-sections of demographic, economic, and fertility micro-data linked with HIV test results. | Burkina Faso, Cameroon, Ghana, Kenya, and Tanzania | Urban and rural |
| Gallant and Maticka-Tyndale (2004) | A critical review and synthesis of the results of 11 evaluated programs designed to reduce HIV transmission to youth and delivered in schools. | Sub-Saharan Africa | Urban and rural |
| Glick and Sahn (2008) | Demographic and Health Surveys, nationally representative repeated cross-sections of demographic, economic, and fertility micro-data linked with HIV test results. | Benin, Burkina Faso, Ghana, Kenya, Mozambique, Nigeria, Uganda, and Zambia | Urban and rural |
| Glynn et al. (2004) | Two-stage cluster sampling was used to identify approximately 1000 men and 1000 women as part of the Multicentre Study on Factors Determining the Differential Spread of HIV in four African Cities. | Cotonou (Benin), Yaounde (Cameroon), Kisumu (Kenya) and Ndola (Zambia), two have relatively low HIV prevalence and two have relatively high prevalence. | Urban |

| Study | Sample Characteristics | Location | Urban/ Rural |
|---|---|---|---|
| Hargreaves et al. (2008a) | A systematic review of published peer-reviewed articles that reported original data comparing individually measured educational attainment and HIV status among at least 300 individuals representative of the general population of countries or regions of sub-Saharan Africa. 36 articles were included in the study, containing data on 72 discrete populations from 11 countries between 1987 and 2003. | 13 populations from five countries: Malawi (1 population), Tanzania (2 popula-tions), Uganda (3 populations), Zambia (6 popula-tions) and Zimbabwe (1 population) | Urban and rural |
| Hargreaves and Glynn (2002) | A survey of studies with individual level data in general population groups. | Africa, Thailand | Urban and rural |
| Hargreaves (2008b) | A random population sample of unmarried young people (916 males, 1003 females) aged 14–25 years. | Limpopo, South Africa | Rural |
| Jukes, Simmons, and Bundy (2008) | A review of studies related to education and HIV. | Africa | Urban and rural |
| Medical Research Council (MRC)/ DFID | 20 trial communities were randomly allocated to receive the intervention either immediately or at the end of the trial. 9645 adolescents aged at least 14 years and about to enter Years 5, 6 and 7 of primary school were divided equally between intervention and comparison communities. | Mwanza, Tanzania | Rural |
| Michelo, Sandøy, and Fylkesnes (2006) | Data from serial population-based HIV surveys conducted in selected communities in 1995 (n 1/4 2989), 1999 (n 1/4 3506), and 2003 (n 1/4 4442). | Kapiri Mposhi, Chelstone, Zambia | Urban and rural |
| Smith et al. (1999) | A cross-sectional analysis of a population-based cohort. | Rakai district, Uganda | Rural |

# CHAPTER 6

×××××××

## Back to Basics: Gender, Social Norms, and the AIDS Epidemic in Sub-Saharan Africa

*Susan Cotts Watkins*[1]

## 1. Introduction

For more than a decade, multilateral and bilateral organizations have provided policy guidance, funds, and technical expertise to support national governments in their response to the AIDS epidemic. The outpouring of humanitarian assistance to sub-Saharan Africa has been particularly intense, and for good reason: it is there that the epidemic has also been most intense. This chapter provides an example of how good will and money may be misdirected when insufficient attention is paid to evidence.

In what follows, I examine the evidentiary foundation for the international HIV prevention community's presentation of women as particularly vulnerable to HIV infection, said to be due to social and cultural norms that disadvantage women. I define "particularly vulnerable" in terms of the magnitude of gender differences in HIV prevalence and incidence, rather than in less measurable terms such as assumed lack of ability to protect themselves from potential infection. While many of the points made below have been made by others, they have largely been ignored. I thus begin by going back to the basics of research, the first question that should be asked: what is it that needs to be explained? I begin with a simple graph of gender differences in prevalence at the younger ages, 15–24, for multiple countries in sub-Saharan Africa, since it is these differences that are often used to advocate for programs that address the particular vulnerability of women to HIV. Such programs include teaching women to negotiate condom use, microfinance programs that are meant to empower women economically, and changing social norms. I then use simple graphs of HIV prevalence by age, gender, and marital status in rural Malawi to show that disaggregating the data by marital status provides a different perspective on the vulnerability of young women to HIV. Since this perspective may be surprising to some, I show that it is consistent with rich survey and qualitative data from rural Malawi, as well as published data on the epidemiology of HIV. I then use data on prevalence and incidence from other countries in the region to show that the picture of the greater vulnerability of women than men is distorted by 1) basing conclusions about the vulnerability of women on data on young men and women but ignoring older men and women; and 2) using data on prevalence but ignoring incidence.

I do not, however, disagree with the view that women, both young and old, are often disadvantaged, sometimes severely so, on other dimensions of their lives than HIV infection: importantly, they typically have less access to economic resources than men and lower educational attainment. Here I choose to focus on the claim that women are particularly vulnerable to infection, because as a feminist, I am particularly concerned about women (Watkins 1993); and because over the course of many years conducting research in sub-Saharan Africa, I have come to believe that the misconceptions about women and AIDS there have been barriers to effective HIV-prevention programs (Watkins, Rutenberg, and Wilkinson 1997; Watkins 2004; Tawfik and Watkins 2007; Swidler and Watkins 2007; Watkins and Swidler 2009).

## 2. Policy Documents

International policy documents are important because they guide the spending—or misspending—of substantial resources on AIDS prevention programs, not only in Malawi but elsewhere in the region. In this section, the description of the conventional wisdom on the particular vulnerability of women to HIV infection is drawn primarily from two sets of policy and program documents collected by Anne Esacove and Joanna Watkins. One set consists of 386 international documents; the other set consists of 124 documents produced in Malawi, although usually with financial and/or technical support from an international agency. The international policy documents represent predominantly large organizations such as UNAIDS, the United States Agency for International Development (USAID), and the World Bank that have provided influential policy guidance and massive funding for AIDS: many of these documents were located on the Web, but some were obtained directly from the organization.[2] Overall, this section suggests that misconceptions gain their force by constant repetition, from the documents produced by the United Nations to newspaper articles in Malawi.

For the purposes of this chapter, it is not necessary to analyze all these documents systematically: this would lead to pages and pages of quotes and counts. Rather, I select examples from a variety of types of sources to show that the depiction of women as particularly vulnerable to HIV infection is widely shared, despite evidence to the contrary, as are the common claims that there is a causal bridge between gender norms and HIV infection.[3]

In 2001, the United Nations addressed the special vulnerability of women and girls (UN Declaration of Commitment 2001). The Declaration is important because it draws on the authority and the global reach of the United Nations; it provides guidance for national policymakers; and it establishes benchmarks. While the benchmarks are unlikely to be met, the bureaucratic machinery of the UN requires regular reports of progress in meeting its goals, thus ensuring that the UN's priorities are not forgotten (Kardam 1991). The Declaration begins:

> We, Heads of State and Government and Representatives of States and Governments, assembled at the United Nations, from 25 to 27 June 2001, for the twenty-sixth special session of the General Assembly convened in accordance with resolution 55/13, as a matter of urgency, to review and address the problem of HIV/AIDS in all its aspects as well as to secure a global commitment to enhancing coordination and intensification of national, regional and international efforts to combat it in a comprehensive manner (UN 2001, 1).

The Declaration then proceeds to list 103 articles, the fourth of which addresses women's particular vulnerability: "Noting with grave concern that . . . people in developing countries are the most affected and that women, young adults and children, in particular girls, are the most vulnerable" (UN 2001, 1–2). No numbers are presented, suggesting that the authors of Article 4 assumed that their audience was familiar with the empirical basis for this statement.

Subsequent articles of the Declaration construct the causal bridge connecting the AIDS epidemic with gender and social norms: "Stressing that gender equality and the empowerment of women are fundamental elements in the reduction of the vulnerability of women and girls to HIV/AIDS" (UN 2001, Article 14, 3) and "The vulnerable must be given priority in the response. . . Empowering women is essential for reducing vulnerability" (Articles 62–64, 9–10). Articles 62–64 fall under the heading "Reducing vulnerability;" the vulnerable here being women, girls, and boys—men are not mentioned at all (and little is said about boys). The Declaration then moves to recommend action and sets benchmarks. By 2003, all nations are expected to ". . . address those factors that make individuals particularly vulnerable to HIV infection, including . . . lack of empowerment of women." Thus, the Declaration directs that all strategies, policies, and programs "should address the gender dimension of the epidemic, specify the action that will be taken to address vulnerability, and set targets for achievement" (Article 62, 9–10).

Although the Declaration of Commitment does not present empirical data on the special vulnerability of women to HIV, many other policy documents do. Often, two numbers are the only data: the percent of the HIV positive worldwide who are women and the percent of infected people, aged 15–24, who are women and girls.[4]

> Nowhere is the epidemic's 'feminization' more apparent than in sub-Saharan Africa, where 57% of adults infected are women, and 75% of young people infected are women and girls. Several social factors are driving this trend. Young African women tend to have male partners much older than themselves—partners who are more likely than young men to be HIV-infected. Gender inequalities in the region make it much more difficult for African women to negotiate condom use. Furthermore, sexual violence, which damages tissues and increases the risk of HIV transmission, is widespread, particularly in the context of violent conflict.

> In countries where the general population's prevalence is high and women's social status is low, the risk of HIV infection through sexual violence is high. A survey of 1366 women attending antenatal clinics in Soweto, South Africa, found significantly higher rates of HIV infection in women who were physically abused, sexually assaulted or dominated by their male partners. The study also produced evidence that abusive men are more likely than non-abusers to be HIV-positive (Dunkle et al. 2004).

Figure 6.1 shows HIV prevalence by gender for young people, based on data from Demographic and Health Surveys (DHS). Across the countries in which female prevalence is higher than male, prevalence for both men and women vary, as does the magnitude of the gender ratio.

Figure 6.1 is certainly striking, but it says nothing about causal factors. Nor does the U.N. Declaration, other than its calls for changing social norms to reduce their vulnerability. Other policy and program documents, however, are more specific. Below is an explanation provided by three UN agencies that presumably played a role in drafting the Declaration:

> At its heart, this is a crisis of gender inequality, with women less able than men to exercise control over their bodies and lives. Nearly universally, cultural expectations have encouraged men to have multiple partners, while women are expected to abstain or be faithful. There is also a culture of silence around sexual and reproductive health. Simply by fulfilling their expected gender roles, men and women are likely to increase their risk of HIV infection (UNAIDS, UNFPA, and UNIFEM 2004, 7).

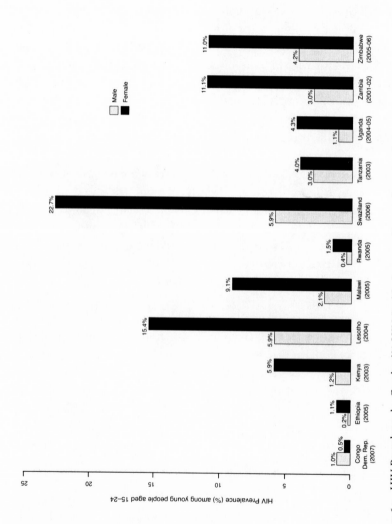

*Figure 6.1* HIV Prevalence by Gender (% HIV-Positive) among Respondents Aged 15–24

SOURCE: Based on DHS data. Information about each survey is available at http://www.measured hs.com/aboutsurveys/search/search_survey_main.cfm?srvyTp=type&listtypes=1, and the data for each survey can be accessed at http://www.measuredhs.com/accesssurveys/

Similar explanations are provided by the European Union, in its remarks on AIDS Day in 2005, and by USAID, one of the major funders of HIV intervention programs:

> Every year the number and proportion of women living with HIV increases. Globally more than half of all adults who are infected are women. In Africa the proportion is reaching 60%. In sub-Saharan Africa 75% of young people infected are women and girls. Gender power imbalances and inter-generational sex are important factors, along with biological factors, that place girls at higher risk than boys. In sub-Saharan Africa, girls are having sex at an earlier age than boys and their sexual partners tend to be older. Knowledge and information and access to services are the first lines of defence for young people. The percentage of girls who have access to information is very low in most regions. Women living with HIV or AIDS often experience greater stigma and discrimination because of gender inequality (European Union 2005).

> It is important to recognize special circumstances related to youth sexuality, including sexual violence/rape as part of sexual debut; age differences between partners; and sexual exchange behaviors (exchanges of gifts or favors as opposed to monetary exchange in commercial sex) (USAID 2002, 8).

Nor are the explanations provided by African leaders different: In 2006, a meeting of the Southern African Development Community (SADC) listed the main "drivers" of the epidemic, including gender inequality which makes "young women particularly vulnerable" (SADC PF 2006, 3). At a Parliamentary Forum in 2008, SADC recommended to members of parliament from Africa the promotion of "known strategies such as use of condoms, reduction in the number sexual of partners, reduction in gender based violence, poverty and empowerment of women beyond education in order to succeed in the fight against HIV and AIDS" (SADC PF 2008).

And from Malawi, there were echoes of the international rhetoric: "The low socio-economic status of girls and women render them unable to negotiate safe sex in a society which still promotes male dominance" (United Nations System in Malawi 2001, 73).

A newspaper article in one of the two leading newspapers in Malawi, *The Nation*, published on AIDS Day 2004, begins with the statement that infection rates are higher for women, and provides numbers: the National AIDS Commission reports that in 2003 there were 36,000 new female AIDS cases (i.e., new HIV infections (incidence)), compared to 25,000 male cases in 2003. The journalist then asks: Why are women and girls being infected more than men and boys? In this case, the answers include both women's particular biology and social norms. Women's sexual organs allow HIV entry more easily them men's, such that while men can have unprotected sex without becoming infected, this is "not so for a woman or girl," especially girls whose sexual organs are immature. In addition, sexually transmitted infections in women "grow slowly." Socioeconomic status makes things worse: "men control the economy," thus women and girls "succumb to unreasonable sexual demands of men and boys. . . Men and boys expect to have their sexual demands met" (Mkolokosa 2004). This article does not mention intergenerational sex or sexual violence, although others do: the Executive Director of the National AIDS Commission told a reporter that there was survey data showing the young girls were particularly at risk because of "intergenerational sex with adults" (Ntonya 2005, 19).

The list of causal explanations for young women's higher HIV prevalence is varied and long, but the rhetorical depiction of males as dominant and females as subordinate is ubiquitous. It is said that males see it as their prerogative to have multiple partners, they refuse to use condoms, they may prevent their women from accessing VCT, or they may perpetrate violence (from rape to beatings). Intergenerational sex—better known in popular speech as sex with "Sugar Daddies"—is said to be a major contributor to the epidemic. Correspondingly, women are presented as powerless in the face of their male partner: they have been taught to suffer in silence when they learn that their husband has another partner; they are unable to negotiate condom use. If women do act by accepting, or seeking, premarital or extramarital partners, it is because they have no other option to support themselves and their children.[5]

In general, however, there is widespread consensus among international and Malawian actors in HIV prevention that women are particularly vulnerable, and on the causes of this vulnerability: it appears that the space connecting the United Nations and Malawi's National AIDS Commission is a giant echo chamber. There is much less consensus about the particular vulnerability of women in the academic literature, with some researchers finding that women are less vulnerable than usually portrayed (for example, Susser and Stein (2000); Campbell (2000); Luke and Kurz (2002); Schatz (2005); Tawfik and Watkins (2007)). It appears, however, that academic research has had little influence on policies.

### 3. Other Possible Explanations for Women's Particular Vulnerability to HIV

Before addressing the social and cultural factors that are said to make women more vulnerable to HIV infection than men, it is useful to briefly note other possible influences on the estimated sex ratio of infection among young people living through a mature epidemic. Some of the studies cited below precede many of the documents referred to in the previous section, and thus would have been available to the authors of the studies.

Most important is the accuracy of the estimates. Initial evidence for UNAIDS's authoritative figures on HIV prevalence by gender were based on testing pregnant women at antenatal clinics; the data were then adjusted to take men into account by assuming a sex ratio of infection based on a relatively small number of studies in which men were also tested (Stover 2004). Nationally representative HIV testing was rare until 2004: it is now frequent and has been the basis of revised estimates. These typically show that HIV prevalence had been overestimated in the earlier studies based on pregnant women (Montana, Mishra, and Hong 2008; Boerma, Ghys, and Walker 2003; Hertog 2009). More relevant for this paper, an analysis of refusal bias in the population-based figures produced by the DHS showed that these surveys tend to overestimate the female-to-male ratio of infections (Reniers and Eaton 2009).

Two other explanations for the striking differences in the gender ration of infection among young people that are unrelated to social norms are the stage of the epidemic and the demography of the population. First, as the epidemic matures, the gap in male-female prevalence usually increases, making women appear to be even more vulnerable than early in the epidemic (Carpenter et al. 1999; Gregson and Garnett 2000). Second, demography matters, because in a growing population (fertility is higher than mortality), each birth cohort is larger than the one that preceded it. As we will see later, women are infected with HIV at younger ages than men: thus, it would be expected that at ages 15–24, more women would be infected than men even in the absence of norms or any physiological differences that made women particularly vulnerable.

A final explanation for the particular vulnerability of women that is proffered is that the male-to-female transmission of HIV is more efficient than vice versa. Many studies of heterosexual transmission have shown that the former was more efficient than the latter (Abimiku and Gallo 1995; Mastro and Vicenzi 1996; Bolan, Ehrhardt, and Wasserheit 1999). This has been attributed to the greater area of exposure in the genital tracts of women than men, to higher concentrations of the virus in semen than in vaginal fluids, to the larger amount of fluid exchanged from men to women than vice versa, to the greater fragility of the woman's vagina than the man's penis and, in some groups, to male circumcision (Moss et al. 1991; Pettifor et al. 2005; Donoval et al. 2006; Hertog 2009). The evidence on this is contradictory, however. Some studies using data from developing countries have found greater transmission from women to men (Mastro et al. 1994; O'Farrell 2001; Gray et al. 2001), although not in Malawi (Galvin and Cohen 2004). Lastly, sexually transmitted infections are known co-factors of HIV infectiousness and infectivity and may multiply transmission by two to five times, occasionally more

(Fleming and Wasserheit 1999; Rottingen, Cameron, and Garnett 2001; Aral et al. 2006). Clearly more research is needed before the argument that women are particularly biologically more vulnerable to HIV infection can be used as an explanation for gender differences in HIV prevalence.

### 4. Misunderstood Women in Rural Malawi

Gross national income per capita was $750 in 2007, compared to an average of $1,870 for sub-Saharan Africa (World Bank 2008a). Total adult HIV prevalence is estimated at 11.8 percent nationally by the Malawi Demographic and Health Survey (MDHS), which tested a representative sample of the adult population in 2004; rural prevalence was 10.8 percent (Malawi and ORC Macro 2005, Table 12.3, 230 and Table 12.4, 232).

Figure 6.2 presents a bar graph for prevalence by gender for young males and females aged 15–24 in rural Malawi; it demonstrates that in terms of the gender ratios at ages 15–24, Malawi is similar to the other countries in the region that were shown in Figure 6.1.

Below, I begin by examining differences in HIV prevalence for unmarried males and females in rural Malawi. After presenting and interpreting these differences, I assess the role of marriage by comparing HIV prevalence by gender and marital status. I draw primarily on previous analyses of data collected in villages in rural Malawi by the Malawi Diffusion and Ideational Change Project (MDICP), which has conducted five rounds of a panel survey (1998, 2001, 2004, 2006, 2008) and

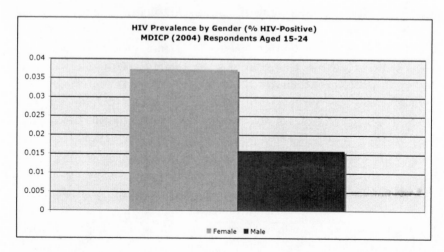

*Figure 6.2*    HIV Prevalence by Gender (% HIV-Positive) MDICP among Respondents Aged 15–24

SOURCE: Based on data from the Malawi Diffusion and Ideational Change Project (MDICP, 2004).

collected an unusually rich set of other types of data to augment the surveys, including qualitative data (semi-structured interviews, ethnographies), Global Positioning System data (roads, health facilities, village structures), and biomarker data
(HIV, other sexually transmitted infections). The MDICP is described in detail at
http://www.malawi.pop.upenn.edu.[6]

In 2004, when the MDICP first offered tests for HIV and other sexually transmitted diseases, the sample size was approximately 4,000, including approximately
1,500 adolescents age 15–24, male and female, married and single. Of the sample
respondents who could be located (some had moved or died since the first round in
1998, or were temporarily away), 91 percent agreed to be tested, with no significant
differences by age or gender (Obare et al. 2009). Prevalence in the MDICP sample
was approximately 7 percent.[7]

### HIV prevalence among 15–19 year old men and women

Figure 6.3 shows HIV status by gender for MDICP respondents, aged 15–19. Although again the prevalence for young women is higher than young men, what
may be surprising to those who emphasize the particular vulnerability of young
women is that, while they are more likely to be infected than young men, only a
small proportion are HIV positive. "Only," of course, is relative to the usual rhetoric: in terms of the lives the young women who are infected, knowledge that they
are going to die from AIDS is knowledge of an absolute, not a relative, fate.

The most plausible explanation for the low prevalence at ages 15–19 is an interaction of biology and behavior. The likelihood that an HIV-negative individual

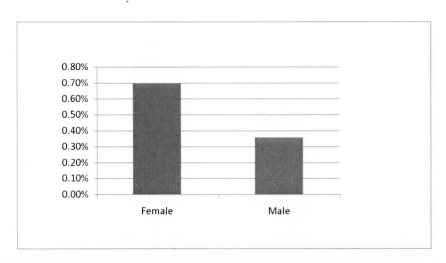

*Figure 6.3*    HIV Prevalence by Gender (% HIV-Positive) among Respondents Aged 15–19
SOURCE: Based on data from the Malawi Diffusion and Ideational Change Project (MDICP, 2004).

will become HIV-positive from a single act of unprotected intercourse is substantially lower than is generally perceived. A recent meta-analysis of epidemiological studies that estimated transmission probabilities per act of unprotected intercourse with an HIV-positive partner found that for low-income countries, the likelihood was well below a 1 percent chance per act. Female-to-male transmission was 0.38 percent per act; male-to-female transmission was 0.30 percent per act (Boily et al. 2009, Table 1, p.120).[8] Transmission probabilities are higher in some circumstances, such as the presence of sexually transmitted infections (especially, genital ulcer disease), lack of male circumcision, and exposure to commercial sex work. When these were taken into account, there was no statistically significant difference in the risk of infection of males and females. Even when such factors act in combination, the probabilities of transmission are still far lower than most other sexually transmitted infections (Holmes et al. 1999; Santow, Bracher, and Watkins 2008).

Because transmission probabilities for a single act of unprotected intercourse are so low, it is not only the number of partners, but also the frequency of sex, that matters for the likelihood that an individual will become infected over time.[9] Many youth between 15 and 19 may not yet have entered a sexual relationship. Even when they have begun a relation, for young unmarried couples in rural Malawi, both circumstances and expectations of proper behavior *inhibit* coital frequency. Qualitative data collected in rural Malawi by Michelle Poulin show that the young people may live too far from each other to walk to regular assignations and may be too poor to pay for a minibus; they want to hide their relationships from their families; and they are concerned about out-of-wedlock pregnancy as well as AIDS. Moreover, relationships among young unmarried sexual partners are often of short duration—a few months with sporadic sex, then the relationship ends, often because either the young woman or the young man has found a more attractive partner—young single women exercise considerable agency in ending a relationship, as well as instituting it (Poulin 2007; see also Clark (2004) for Kenya and Zambia). The discarded partner then seeks a replacement, which can take months, or even longer: Shelley Clark, using data for Kenya and Zambia, found that one-quarter of non-virginal young women reported no penetrative sex in the previous year (Clark 2004, 154). Also inhibiting coital frequency for young people in Malawi is a widespread belief that doing well in one's studies and having a sexual relationship are incompatible (Poulin 2009; Grant 2008). Analysis of the MDICP survey data show that school girls, compared to their peers who left school but have not yet married, are less likely to report having ever had sex; those who have had sex report fewer partners and less frequent sex within a partnership (Poulin 2009).[10]

Another possible explanation for the low HIV prevalence among 15–19-year-old women in rural Malawi is that most of their partners are their peers, among whom HIV prevalence is 0.364 percent (Figure 6.2, above). Income is positively associated with HIV prevalence among men in Malawi and elsewhere in the region

(Malawi and ORC Macro 2005; Montana, Mishra, and Hong 2008), suggesting that the poverty of young men is protective, simply because they cannot afford the gifts to their partners that men are normatively expected, and expect themselves, to provide. Nor can young men afford sex workers, who are more costly and more likely to be HIV positive than girlfriends. Once they are able to afford sex workers, however, they are also able to marry, thus putting their brides at risk of HIV infection.

Survey data collected in rural southern Malawi, near the MDICP southern site, provide unusual information about the characteristics of the partners of sexually active young single women (Mensch et al. 2008). The aim of the study was to evaluate the quality of self-reports of sexual behavior. Some of the respondents were randomly selected to be interviewed face-to-face, the others to audio computer-assisted self-interview (ACASI), which presumably reduces any social desirability bias as well as the effects of interviewer characteristics.[11]

Table 6.1 below is taken from Mensch et al. (2008) who compared study results from Kenya and Malawi, but here I show only those for Malawi. The largest categories of reported partners are boyfriends and expected spouses.

Note that although a higher percentage of the young single women reported sexual experience in the face-to-face interviews than in the ACASI interviews, further questions added more partners in specific categories in the latter than in the former; thus, lifetime sexual partners were higher in ACASI than in the face-to-face interviews.

*Table 6.1* Predicted percentages of respondents by sexual behavior and mode of interview, Malawi 2004

|  | Interview Mode | |
|---|---|---|
|  | FTF | ACASI |
| Sexual behavior | (236) | (211) |
| Ever had sex | 47.9** | 34.8 |
| Ever had sex with: |  |  |
| Boyfriend | 30.9** | 21.0 |
| Expected spouse | 27.5 | 29.4 |
| Friend or acquaintance | 6.8 | 17.1** |
| Family member | 1.3 | 7.1 |
| Stranger | 2.5 | 3.3 |
| Teacher | 1.0 | 1.4 |
| Employer | 1.0 | 1.9 |
| More than one sexual partner in lifetime | 16.5 | 27.2** |
| Composite: sex with any partner | 47.4 | 50.7 |
| Composite: ever had sex or sex with any partner | 48.3 | 57.8* |

SOURCE: Adapted from Mensch et al. (2008, Table 2, 326).
NOTE: *Significant at $p < 0.05$; **$p < 0.01$; represents significance of interview mode variable in logistic regression, controlling for background characteristics.

What about categories of partners who are likely to be substantially older and thus more likely to have money, and thus, more likely to be HIV positive? While Mensch et al. (2008) do not report the age differences between partners, the qualitative data collected by Poulin shows that the age difference between young girls and their boyfriends and expected spouses is small (Poulin 2006). The Mensch et al. data do, however, provide an opportunity to see how common intergenerational sex might be. In Table 6.1, sex with strangers, teachers, and employers account for a very small proportion of the behaviors reported, even through ACASI. These reports are probably underestimates, since some older men may have been reported as friends/acquaintances, relatives, or strangers. Nonetheless, their contribution to the HIV prevalence of young women in Malawi (and elsewhere) has probably been exaggerated. For example, a study of men's non-marital sexual partners conducted in Kenya found that in only 4 percent of the relationships were the men Sugar Daddies, defined as 10 or more years older than their sexual partner and relatively wealthy compared to the other men in the sample: this percentage is only slightly higher than the percentage of young women reporting sex with teachers and partners in Table 6.1 (Luke 2005; Luke and Kurz 2002; for a review of the literature on intergenerational sex, a broader category of partnerships, see Hope (2007)).[12]

Even if there were more Sugar Daddy relationships, how risky are they for young women? A study in rural Uganda found that there was no effect of the age difference between partners on HIV incidence among women (Kelly et al. 2003). This result is consistent with findings from mathematical modeling that show that while limiting intergenerational sexual partnerships would decrease the risk of infection, at the population level, this may do little to limit the spread of HIV unless it were accompanied with wider-ranging behavioral changes that reduced the number of risky sexual contacts (Hallett et al. 2007).

And what about the significance of rape or other versions of forced sex for young women's vulnerability, another item of conventional wisdom (Center for Women's Global Leadership 2007; Greig et al. 2008; Gupta et al. 2008; Jewkes et al. 2006a)? One mechanism that has been postulated is that forced sex, and perhaps, particularly rape, is believed to tear women's genital tissues in a way that increases their likelihood of becoming infected (Glynn et al. 2001). Data on sexually active unmarried adolescents (15–24) from the 2004 round of the MDICP speak to this issue. Respondents were asked "Did your partner ever want to have sex when you did not?" The 58 percent who said "Yes" were then asked "What happened?" The responses were precoded: "I refused and then I accepted," "[He] persuaded me," and "[He] physically forced me." Seven percent of the girls reported having been physically forced. This is likely an underestimate: not all sexually active girls report this to the interviewer, and of those, some may not wish to report that the sex was forced. The MDICP figures are similar in magnitude to reports on the prevalence of forced sex based on surveys with large samples in South Africa, which may also reflect underreporting (Hallman 2004; Pettifor et al. 2005; Jewkes et al. 2006a; Jejeebhoy, Shah, and Thapa 2006), but both sets may be subject to underreporting.

The literature cited above does not mean that young women are not infected through intergenerational or forced sex: it may well be that some of the 1 percent of women aged 15–19 who tested HIV positive in the MDICP, or the 6 percent that were infected in the Mensch et al. (2008) data, were infected as a consequence of such relationships. Concern for these young women is justified. While women can, and do, actively choose to make partnerships with older and wealthier men (both as Sugar Daddies and as husbands), by definition they do not choose forced sex, which may be quite devastating emotionally as well as physically. However, HIV prevalence is an aggregate figure, and the low HIV prevalence for men and women, 15–19, in the MDICP data and the few reports of sexual relationships with categories of sexual partners in which the men are likely to be substantially older (and thus substantially more likely to be HIV positive) suggests that they make a minor contribution to Malawi's epidemic.

Lastly, what about the claim that women are particularly vulnerable because they are too powerless to negotiate condom use? Women in rural Malawi have a considerable amount of agency, which is deployed to accept or refuse men's proposals for a sexual partnership, and to terminate or continue a relationship. Perhaps they could even negotiate condom use. But in Malawi, women have the same objections to condom use as men (Tavory and Swidler 2009): as long as women do not want to use condoms, the issue of negotiating condom use is moot.

In summary, behavior and biology appear to protect young women (and young men) in rural Malawi. The social patterns of premarital sexual relationships, including intergenerational and forced sex, in rural Malawi may be unusual, but that has yet to be demonstrated. The burden of proof is on those who claim Malawi is *so* different that the evidence presented here is not useful for concluding that the misconceptions about young women's particular vulnerability to HIV are not also prevalent elsewhere in the region. Convincing evidence about the consequences of intergenerational and forced sex will be difficult to generate. It is obviously even more difficult to provide evidence to support the presumed causal bridge between norms (e.g., "Men are expected to dominate women") and women's HIV status, either at the individual or aggregate level. [13]

*HIV prevalence among married and single women, 15–24, in rural Malawi*

Just as the epidemiology of HIV interacts with behavioral patterns to reduce the likelihood of infection among young unmarried women and men in Malawi, epidemiology and behavior appear to raise the likelihood of infection for young married women. To examine this, I expand the age range to 15–24, the one most often used to demonstrate the particular vulnerability of young women. We would expect HIV prevalence to be higher in this age group than among younger women, simply because they are older and have had more time to have sexual relationships, and even their partners, who are peers, have had more time and money to become infected. Overall HIV prevalence in this age group is 2.7 percent, (3.7 percent for women, 1.6 percent for men), compared to a prevalence of 7 percent in the total MDICP sample, which includes adolescents and adults of all marital statuses.

Figure 6.4 shows that when we take marital status into account, there is a striking difference in infection status between single and married women aged 15–24: 1.4 percent of single women are HIV positive compared to 5.0 percent of married women; the highest prevalence, 14.3 percent, is found among those women who, before age 24, have divorced, separated, or become widowed. Widowhood is obviously related to AIDS, but divorce may also be: in Malawi, either women or men may initiate and justify divorce on the grounds that a spouse's behavior suggests that he or she will become infected (Watkins 2004; Reniers 2003, 2008; Boileau et al. 2009).

That marriage is a risk factor for HIV has previously been documented elsewhere in the region (Auvert et al. 200l; Glynn et al. 2001; Kelly et al. 2003; Clark 2004; Clark, Bruce, and Dude 2006; Gavin et al. 2006). The low transmission rate of HIV, coupled with the considerably higher frequency of intercourse within marriage, takes us a long way to understanding why married women 15–24 are

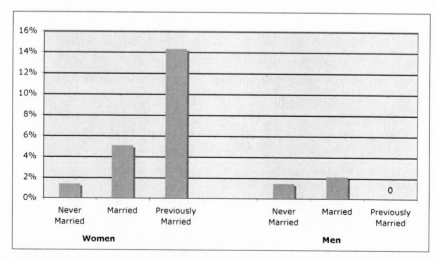

*Figure 6.4*   HIV Prevalence by Gender and Marital Status (% HIV-Positive) among Respondents Aged 15–24
SOURCE: Based on data from the Malawi Diffusion and Ideational Change Project (MDICP, 2004).

much more likely to be infected than their still-single peers. In rural Malawi, one of the major reasons for marriage is to have a regular sexual partner. An analysis of the MDICP data shows a striking difference between the frequency of sex with their fiancée(s) and with their spouse: both men and women report more frequent contact with their spouses, as well as a much lower likelihood of using condoms with them (Clark, Poulin, and Kohler 2009). Qualitative data collected by another study in rural Malawi suggests that intercourse occurred about four or five times a week, although this could be interrupted by menstruation, childbirth, funerals, or the husband's absence (Hickey 1999).[14] Older respondents recalled that, shortly after marriage, intercourse was likely to be daily, sometimes several times a day; their frequency is much less now, they said.

Because coital frequency is relevant for HIV infection, and it is greater in marriage, the age at marriage of men matters for the likelihood that HIV will be transmitted to their wife.[15] Microsimulations using parameters from the MDICP survey data showed little variation by age at marriage in the likelihood that brides were infected at marriage, but substantial variation by age at marriage in the likelihood that grooms were infected (Bracher, Santow, and Watkins 2003). Although divorce is common, it is typically rapidly followed by remarriage (Reniers 2003). Moreover, women themselves may introduce infection into the marriage through extramarital partnerships. These are motivated not only by economic need but by a woman's desire for a more satisfactory sexual relationship, or for revenge when a woman finds her husband has a sexual partner (Tawfik and Watkins 2007). As with single women, married women have considerable agency in accepting, refusing, continuing, or terminating extramarital relationships.

## 5. HIV Prevalence by Gender and Age and Marital Status in High HIV-Prevalence Countries in Sub-Saharan Africa

The previous presentation has shown that in rural Malawi young single women are more likely to be HIV positive than men, a typical finding that led to the attribution of a causal relation between gender norms and HIV prevalence in policy and program documents as well as in newspapers and some academic articles. I also showed a graph that is rarely presented in these documents: the sex ratio of infection between ages 15–24 by marital status as well as gender. We see there that the disproportionate vulnerability of young women is among married, not single, young women, and especially among those who are divorced, separated, or widowed. Below I expand the range of age groups to examine whether what might appear to be the greater vulnerability of women to HIV infection persists at the older ages. For this analysis I focus on the age and gender pattern of prevalence and incidence; the latter is particularly relevant here since it represents new infections, whereas prevalence is the accumulation of as long as a decade of infections.[16] I begin with Malawi but then examine prevalence and incidence by gender for other countries in the region in order to assess whether the gender patterns of prevalence and incidence in Malawi appear to be unusual.

The figures shown below are produced by modeling data from Demographic and Health Surveys in the region. The DHS surveys typically cover the age range 15–50, and thus do not provide information on the oldest ages; however, in this analysis the models incorporate patterns based on data from two DHS surveys (Niger and Swaziland) that interviewed and tested people of all ages. The modeling was done for the United Nations Population Division by Patrick Gerland and others; the figures were produced for this chapter by Gerland.

Figure 6.5 shows prevalence at all ages above age 15 for Malawi, rural and urban combined. As expected, due to the association of marriage and infection and the later age of marriage of men in Malawi, the age at which prevalence begins to rise is later for men. The peak prevalence, however, is about the same magnitude, and prevalence declines at approximately the same rate for both men and women.

The next figure shows incidence: it illustrates, better than the previous figure on prevalence, the importance of looking beyond ages 15–24. Incidence among

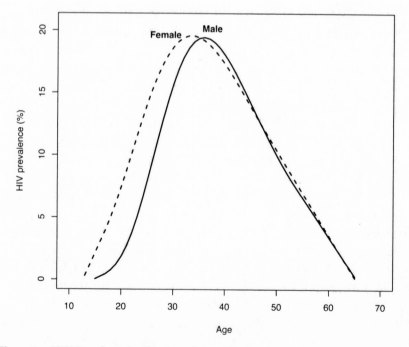

*Figure 6.5*   HIV Prevalence by Gender and Age, All Ages above Age 15, Rural and Urban, Malawi, Demographic and Health Survey data, 2004
SOURCE: Prepared by Patrick Gerland, United Nations Population Division, from DHS survey data.

women rises earlier and perhaps somewhat more steeply, but after about age 30, incidence is higher for men than for women, and peak incidence is higher for men than for women.

Thus, in Malawi, women appear to be particularly vulnerable to HIV infection at the younger ages, men at the older ages. This is likely due to widespread expectations that men will provide money and/or the things that must be bought with money, such as soap and clothing, to wives, girlfriends—and bar girls and freelance prostitutes, who are more likely to be HIV positive. Indeed, in rural Malawi, it is sometimes said that, ". . . the money was forcing him to have many partners" (Swidler and Watkins 2007, 152).

How similar are the sex ratios of prevalence and incidence in other countries in sub-Saharan Africa where prevalence is high? Although there are few studies of transmission probabilities, it is reasonable to assume that the basic transmission probability of HIV in a single act of intercourse varies little across countries in the region. There are, however, likely to be differences in behavioral factors that may hinder transmission, such the extent of male circumcision (Weiss et al. 2008) or facilitate transmission, such as the extent to which sexually transmitted infections are untreated (Fleming and Wasserheit 1999). There are also likely to be differences in exposure to HIV related to the proportion married by age, which is

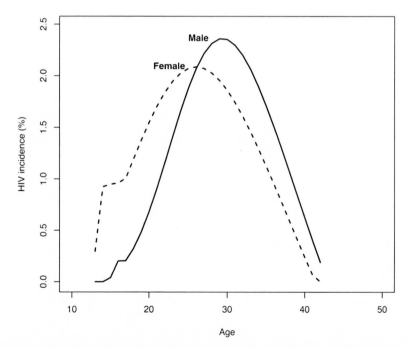

*Figure 6.6*   Incidence by Gender and Age, All Ages above Age 15, Rural and Urban, Malawi, Demographic and Health Survey data, 2004

SOURCE: Prepared by Patrick Gerland, United Nations Population Division, from DHS survey data.

influenced by, among other things, social norms of age at marriage, the acceptability of divorce, and the desirability of remarriage, as well as patterns of sexual
mixing and prevalence among potential partners of the opposite sex (for an extended discussion, see Hertog (2009)).

I begin with Zambia (Figures 6.7 and 6.8) and Tanzania (Figures 6.9 and 6.10),
both of which share a border with Malawi across which there is considerable
movement for marriage and work; thus, social norms are likely to be more similar
to those in Malawi than more geographically distant countries. Figures 6.7–6.10
show that both countries are similar to Malawi in that there is a crossover in incidence, an age after which men are more likely to become infected than women.
There are differences across the three countries in behavior that affect prevalence,
such as the timing and pace of rises and declines in incidence by gender; these
produce different gender prevalence ratios by age.

To examine whether Malawi is also similar to countries with which it is not
contiguous, and thus where any social norms that could affect incidence might be
different, I show two more graphs of incidence, one of Zimbabwe (Figure 6.11)
and one of Kenya (Figure 6.12). Although they differ from Malawi, Zambia, and
Tanzania in some aspects, such as the timing of the rises and declines in incidence

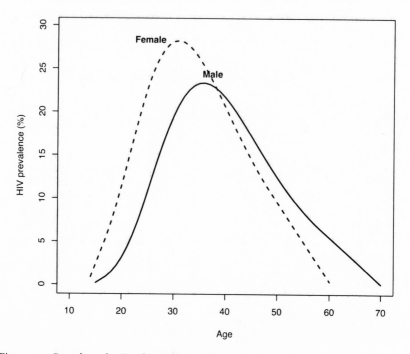

*Figure 6.7*  Prevalence by Gender and Age, All Ages above Age 15, Rural and Urban,
Zambia, Demographic and Health Survey data, 2001-02
SOURCE: Prepared by Patrick Gerland, United Nations Population Division, from DHS survey data.

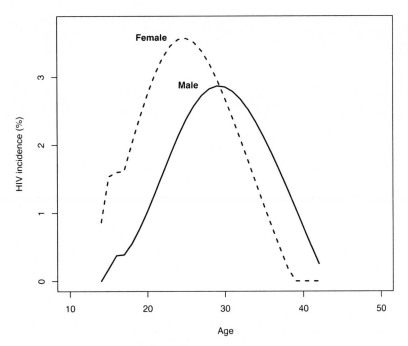

*Figure 6.8*  Incidence by Gender and Age, All Ages above Age 15, Rural and Urban, Zambia, Demographic and Health Survey data, 2001–02

SOURCE: Prepared by Patrick Gerland, United Nations Population Division, from DHS survey data.

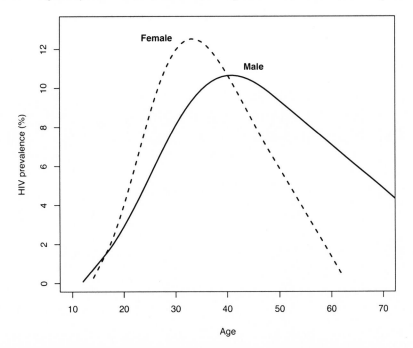

*Figure 6.9*  Prevalence by Gender and Age, All Ages above Age 15, Rural and Urban, Tanzania, Demographic and Health Survey data, 2004–05

SOURCE: Prepared by Patrick Gerland, United Nations Population Division, from DHS survey data.

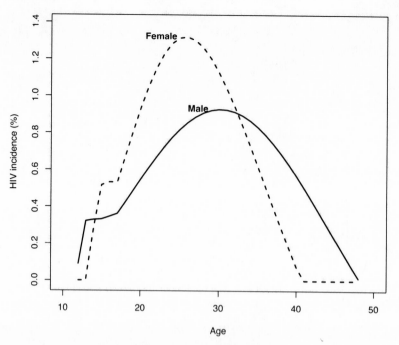

*Figure 6.10*    Incidence by Gender and Age, All Ages above Age 15, Rural and Urban, Tanzania, Demographic and Health Survey data, 2004–05

SOURCE: Prepared by Patrick Gerland, United Nations Population Division, from DHS survey data.

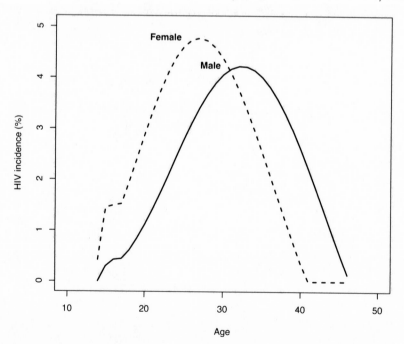

*Figure 6.11*    Incidence by Gender and Age, All Ages above Age 15, Rural and Urban, Zimbabwe, Demographic and Health Survey data, 2005–06

SOURCE: Prepared by Patrick Gerland, United Nations Population Division, from DHS survey data.

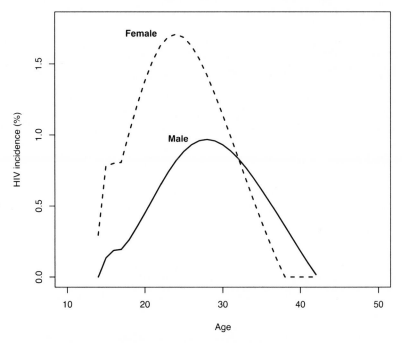

*Figure 6.12*    Incidence by Gender and Age, All Ages above Age 15, Rural and Urban,
Kenya, Demographic and Health Survey data, 2003
SOURCE: Prepared by Patrick Gerland, United Nations Population Division, from DHS survey data

and the ages of peak prevalence, in both we see again that at the older ages men
are more likely to become infected than women.

In summary, in the five high-prevalence countries of Africa shown above,
young women are more vulnerable to HIV infection than young men (earlier
onset of infection for women, more new infections for older men than for older
women). In all, however, when we expand our view to consider all ages at which
women and men become infected, rather than truncating our gaze at age 24, the
greater vulnerability of young women is considerably less striking.

A final, more precise, and more meaningful measure of the relative vulnerability of males and females to HIV infection is the lifetime probability of infection.
Although transmission probabilities in any single act of unprotected intercourse
are low, the accumulation of these acts over years represents a substantial loss
of life. Data that permit estimating the lifetime probability of infection are rare,
but they show that although crude prevalence is typically higher for women, the
*lifetime* risk for men is similar or higher (Gregson and Garnett 2000; Bärnighausen et al. 2008).

## 6. Discussion

The rhetoric in policy documents about the particular vulnerability of women and girls to HIV infection is ubiquitous: claims made in policy documents produced by international donors are echoed in the prevention community and media in Malawi. This rhetoric and the accompanying simple, but striking, gender ratios of infection at the younger ages are used to justify urgent interventions to reduce young women's particular vulnerability. Some of the rhetoric is quite heated, as in this excerpt from a speech given by the special Envoy of the former Secretary General of the UN for AIDS in Africa:

> There is one factor more than any other that drives me crazy in doing the Envoy job: it's the ferocious assault of the virus on women. We're paying a dreadful and inconsolable price for the refusal of the international community, every member of the community without exception, to embrace gender equality. And in so many parts of the world, gender inequality and AIDS is a preordained equation of death. . . . There's nothing new in that. It's irrefutably documented in encyclopedic profusion. The culture, the violence, the power, the patriarchy, the male sexual behaviour . . . it's as though Darwin himself had stirred this Hecate's brew into a potion of death for women (Lewis 2004, 4).

The evidence to support these claims and many others like it is almost invariably limited to female and male prevalence at age group 15–24. In this chapter, I criticized this evidence on two grounds. First, it ignores the role of marital status in determining whether a young woman will or will not be infected; second, it does not consider the evolution of incidence and prevalence over all ages. These points have been made previously by other researchers using data from other countries in the region (e.g., Clark (2004) and Auvert et al. (2001) for marriage, and Gregson and Garnett (2000) and Bärnighausen et al. (2008) for gender patterns of infection at the older ages), but without the advantage of the unusual variety of data available for Malawi that permit assessing some of the behavioral patterns that are not evident in the numbers alone.

Data from rural Malawi show that interactions of behavior and biology (coital frequency) appear to protect young single Malawian women (and young men) in rural Malawi, but expose married women and older men to greater risk. Thus, unless sex is unusually frequent, even when a young unmarried woman's partner is infected, the young woman is highly likely to be lucky since intercourse is infrequent; while married women may escape infection, there are fewer who are so fortunate.

It has been said that, "In Africa, AIDS has a woman's face" (Annan 2002). If we look only at the youth, either married or single, both HIV prevalence and incidence are consistently higher for women than for men. Estimates of incidence after age 30 or so, however, show new infections for women declining but new infections for men increasing (Gerland 2008): the face of AIDS morphs from that of a young woman to that of an older man. If infection at all ages is considered, men are as, or more, likely to become HIV positive than women (Gregson and Garnett 2000; Bärnighausen et al. 2008).

It is puzzling that policymakers and donors mobilizing effort and funds on behalf of vulnerable women did not ask a simple question: what happens after age 24? Some of the evidence used in this paper was previously available. Certainly academics have previously noticed the gender crossover in HIV prevalence: an article published in *AIDS*, a prestigious journal, in 2001, reported results from an important multi-country study in sub-Saharan Africa that showed that HIV prevalence was higher among women than men in the age group 15–24, but not afterward (Glynn et al. 2001). Similarly, analyses of prevalence by marital status for ages 15–24 have shown for at least a decade that prevalence is higher for young married women than young single women (Auvert et al. 200l; Glynn et al. 2001; Kelly et al. 2003; Clark 2004; Clark, Bruce, and Dude 2006; Gavin et al. 2006). These findings, however, did not echo around the prevention community.

In this chapter, I also examined some of the claims made in policy documents about the role of social norms in accounting for women's vulnerability to HIV, again using the unusually rich data for rural Malawi. I did not attempt to examine the effects of difficult-to-measure constructs such as patriarchy, subordination, and discrimination on HIV prevalence among women. However, on two measures that are often seen to be related to these constructs, intergenerational sex and sexual violence, there is little evidence that these are frequent enough to contribute significantly to Malawi's epidemic, however damaging they may be to individual women.

In an era when the term "evidence-based policy" is routinely invoked, did any policymakers and funders ask how complete the evidence for women's particular vulnerability was, or how solid the bridge between women's subordination and HIV prevalence was? Apparently, not. While some of the evidence presented above comes from Malawi, much does not. Certainly the age and gender patterns of HIV infection are quite similar in some other countries in the region; in interpreting the data, I drew on research conducted in other settings. The evidence needed for evidence-based policy is not hidden—many of the articles cited were published in major journals with an international circulation, such as *The Lancet, AIDS,* and *Sexually Transmitted Infections*. It would seem that the burden of proof should be on those who make the claims for women's particular vulnerability to

HIV, and then, if the claims are supported, for concluding that it is social norms that make them so.

There would be less justification for the argument of this chapter that women's vulnerability to HIV has been misunderstood, if interventions based on the assumption of social norms that subordinated women actually did reduce the likelihood that women would become HIV positive. For example, perhaps programs that attempted to empower women to negotiate condom use or programs to change men's attitudes towards women did lead to measurably lower incidence of HIV (or even other sexually transmitted infections, which are evident more quickly). The ratio of successful interventions to money, however, is extremely modest. A compilation of 300 evaluations of AIDS-related programs targeting adolescents in sub-Saharan Africa found that 92 percent of these had no objective outcome measures (HIV, other sexually transmitted infections, pregnancy)–impact was measured only by self-reports: of the 8 percent that did have objective outcomes, only one-quarter were successful (World Bank 2008a). It is clear that self-reports are deceptive measures of program success (Minnis et al. 2009).

An instructive example comes from an article published in a special issue of *The Lancet* published to coincide with the 2008 International AIDS Conference in Mexico City. The article describes the Intervention with Microfinance for AIDS and Gender Equity (IMAGE) project in South Africa. Compared to many interventions, this was unusually well designed—the intervention was of a much longer duration than is typical and included testing for HIV, thus providing an objective outcome measure (Pronyk et al. 2006; Jewkes et al. 2008). The intervention, funded by USAID, aimed to change gender norms by training males in gender equitable norms. The authors call IMAGE a success and visually emphasized the results by presenting them in a box apart from the general text (Gupta et al. 2008). The evaluation was said to increase the proportion of men who reported that they held gender equitable norms (e.g., they disagreed with statements such as "There are times when a woman deserves to be beaten" and "A man should have the final word about decisions in his home.") In addition, ". . . the study team estimated that levels of intimate partner violence were reduced by 55% in the intervention group relative to the comparison. Additionally there was evidence that the intervention improved household wellbeing, social capital and empowerment." They then speak to the issue of the objective outcome measure: "Disappointingly, however, there appeared to be no direct effects on HIV incidence" (Gupta et al. 2008, 767). (For similar contradictions between self-reports and biological outcomes in well-designed interventions, see Auvert et al. (2001); Ross et al. (2007).) It is clear that unless we take self-reports of changes in behavior at face value, there is little evidence that our attempts to help women avoid HIV infection have been successful.

I end with the perspectives of those women whom our policies and programs are intended to help. This suggests that women might be better served if we ask them what policies and programs they would like, rather than deciding ourselves what they need.

On a survey in rural Malawi in 2008, approximately 4,000 respondents were asked to rank their preferences for programs that would address the following issues: agricultural development, health services in general, AIDS programs, clean water, and education. An analysis of the data shows that the demand for clean water is highest, the demand for AIDS programs least (Dionne, Gerland, and Watkins 2009). It might be expected that those who are HIV positive would rank services for AIDS higher than those who are HIV negative. This is not the case: AIDS services rank low even for those who are positive (a T-test of difference in mean rank between HIV positive and HIV negative is statistically significant at: ˙˙p<0.01; ˙p<0.05).

The low demand for AIDS programs is not a sign that women are not profoundly worried about dying with AIDS: survey and qualitative data show that they are, as are the members of their social networks, their friends, relatives and neighbors (Watkins 2004; Smith and Watkins 2005; Kohler, Behrman, and Watkins 2007). Rather, other policy priorities appear to them to be more urgent. The response of rural Malawian women is not unusual. Analyses of data from two multi-country surveys in sub-Saharan Africa, the Gallup World Poll and the Afrobarometer, show a similar disconnect between the policy priorities of policymakers and those of Africans (Dionne, Gerland, and Watkins 2009; Tortora 2008; Kharas 2008).

It may be that the prevention community does know what is best for rural Malawian women living in the midst of an AIDS epidemic, who attend three to four funerals a month of people they know who did not survive. Still, we have not done well in mounting evidence-based interventions or in providing evidence that interventions aimed at changing norms are effective. Perhaps it takes longer, perhaps it's just too difficult to change norms, or perhaps it's a mistake to think that norms are drivers of the epidemic. So how else should the money be allocated? Perhaps it would be better to focus on addressing problems that women themselves see as more important than their vulnerability to AIDS. Resources spent on the policy priorities of rural Malawian women might have an indirect effect on their vulnerability to HIV, but even if they do not, clean water is a public good—and at least those mounting programs to provide clean water can measure the number of wells dug, the quality of the water, and, if the Ministry of Health keeps proper records, changes in illness and death due to waterborne illnesses.

## Notes

1. *Acknowledgements:* I am grateful to Anne Esacove, Patrick Gerland, Paul Hewett, Michelle Poulin, and Joanna Watkins for providing me with unpublished data and with

documents; to Philip Anglewicz, Kim Dionne, Patrick Gerland, and Tara McKay for transforming data into figures and tables; and to the excellent research by members of the Malawi Research Group that provides much of the information—some published, some not—in this paper. I am also grateful to Shelley Clark, Kim Dionne, Deborah Minsky, Michelle Poulin, and Ann Swidler for insightful comments on earlier drafts. Lastly, I acknowledge funding from NIH for the collection of survey and qualitative data by the Malawi Longitudinal Survey of Families and Households.

2. The collection of Malawi documents was put together by Esacove and J. Watkins going in person to various government departments, the National AIDS Commission, and offices of NGOs, and is less comprehensive, since the documents were produced for a specific purpose and many appear to have been subsequently discarded or lost. (For more detail, see Esacove (2010)). These documents are in the process of being made publicly available on The Malawi Social Science and HIV/AIDS Research (MaSoSHA) Database, at http://malawiresearch.org. MaSoSHA is maintained by a consortium of researchers at Chancellor College (University of Malawi), the University of Pennsylvania, and the University of California-Los Angeles. MaSoSHA was built in 2008 with the support of a grant from the University of Pennsylvania's Population Studies Center and in partnership with an NGO, Global Medical Knowledge.

3. Policy documents on gender and HIV often refer to social norms in a way that suggest they are long-standing, rigid, and uniform in a given community. The literature in anthropology and sociology, the two disciplines most concerned with norms, has long abandoned this understanding of norms, and indeed, rarely uses the term. Rather, this literature provides evidence that the social and cultural environment is complex; it varies not only across cultural and social contexts but within these contexts: since there may be contradictory norms relevant to a particular situation, sometimes one may be called on, sometimes another, or sometimes different participants in the same social interaction may enunciate contradictory norms at different points in the interaction, or even at the same time (e.g., Swidler (1986) who uses the metaphor of a tool kit; Greenhalgh (1988) who uses the metaphor of a spice rack; Moore, S.F. (1994); and Moore, H. L. and Sanders (2006)).

4. These numbers vary slightly from document to document.

5. One of the few documents I have found that does *not* assume a causal relationship between women's subordination and HIV is a "Guide to Indicators for Monitoring and Evaluating National AIDS Prevention Programmes for Young People," published by the World Health Organization (WHO 2004c), one of the agencies that constitute UNAIDS. The Guide also includes indicators "that are not causally related to HIV infection, but which contribute to young people's vulnerability to it, e.g., forced sexual relations, and cross-generational sexual partnerships (especially among young women)" (WHO 2004c, 7). This is also one of the few documents to call for evaluating the effects of HIV prevention programs using new HIV infections as evidence.

6. The Malawi Longitudinal Study of Families and Households (MLSFH) continues the research of The Malawi Diffusion and Ideational Change Project (MDICP) described in this chapter.

7. This is lower than the national rural prevalence of 10.8 percent in the Malawi Demographic and Health Survey conducted at the same time (Malawi and ORC Macro 2005). Analyses of the non-response showed that this did not appear to be an important factor; the difference is probably largely due to the inclusion of rural trading centers, which are known to have higher prevalence than village samples, in the MDHS category "rural" but not in the MDICP (Obare et al. 2009). Urban prevalence in Malawi is 17.1 percent.

8. These estimates are higher than the often-cited estimates based on data from Rakai, Uganda, which estimated transmission probabilities as .001 (Gray et al. 2001).

9. Few studies have distinguished between the different effects of number of partners and frequency of sex; among those few studies, the evidence for gender differences in the effect of coital frequency on infection is contradictory (Hertog 2009, 152).

10. An analysis of school participation of the children of the MDICP respondents shows that at age 15, 70 percent of girls are still in school, and about 80 percent of boys (Grant 2008, Figure 1, 1611). By age 15, over two-thirds of the girls had experienced sexual debut, and slightly more boys (Tawfik 2003, Fig 5.2A and 5.2B, 66).

11. The questionnaire used was the 2004 MDICP questionnaire; the respondents assigned to ACASI were interviewed face-to-face for most of the questions, but by ACASI for sexual behavior and sensitive questions related to AIDS. The computer itself was hidden; the respondent heard both the question and the response categories through headphones and answered by pressing a number on a keypad of computer keyboard. The questions and the response categories were recorded; thus, all respondents heard the same phrasing and intonations. The precise question to determine initial sexual experience was "How old were you the first time that you had sex?" This is the figure reported in the first row of the table. Even if a respondent replied that she had not had sex, the next question asks about partners, and some who had said they had not had sex answered this question. When all responses are combined, 57.8 percent of the ACASI respondents had had sex compared to 48.3 percent of those interviewed face-to-face. Even this, however, underestimates the proportion of the sample who had ever had sex, since a notable proportion of those who had not had sex were found to have a sexually transmitted infection (either HIV or Chlamydia, gonorrhea or trichomonas): 8.3 percent of those who said they never had sex in the face-to-face interviews had a sexually transmitted infection as well as 9.6 percent of the ACASI respondents (Mensch et al. 2008, Table 6, 330). The prevalence of HIV in the Mensch et al. study sample of women 15–21 was higher than the prevalence among women 15–19 in the MDICP sample (6 percent and 1 percent, respectively). Unpublished tabulations from the Mensch et al. data show that this difference diminishes only somewhat when the comparison between the two samples is made for women in the same age group (15–19);[2] most of the difference was associated with differences in the location of the respondents—rural villages in the MDICP, trading centers in the Mensch et al. study.

12. In the Kenya study, the mean age difference between non-marital sexual partners was 5.5 years, and 47 percent of men's female partners were adolescents (Luke 2005, 6). For age differences between sexual partners and HIV risk, see Kelly et al. (2003) and Gregson et al. (2002).

13. Maman et al. (2002) found that HIV-infected women reported significantly more sexual violence in their relationships than did HIV negative women. They do not claim that the sexual violence caused the HIV infection, nor should they. This is a cross-sectional survey, so the authors cannot know if the women were HIV positive before the sexual violence occurred. A study reported in Jewkes et al. (2008) had a much better study design. It was a cluster randomized controlled trial of an intervention, Stepping Stones, with an unusually long follow-up period. They found that the intervention had no impact on HIV, although it did reduce the number of new HSV-2 infections. Men reported less perpetration of sexual violence, less transactional sex, and less problem drinking at 12 months. Women did not report changes in the behaviors addressed by the intervention; indeed, those in the intervention arm reported more transactional sex at 12 months.

14. These estimates come from my analysis of interview transcripts from a study conducted by Claire Hickey of the Centre for Social Research, University of Malawi (Hickey 1999).

15. In rural Malawi, age at marriage varies substantially across three regions that also differ in lineage and residence patterns, ethnicity, and religious affiliation. Since brides and

grooms are typically not tested before marriage, Bracher, Santow, and Watkins (2003) used microsimulation techniques with input parameters drawn from the MDICP to estimate the impact of age at marriage on variation in the proportion of brides and/or grooms who were infected at marriage. The average age at first marriage is lowest in the southern region and highest in the northern region: while the proportion of women who were estimated to be HIV positive at first marriage did not vary significantly across the three regions (all were under 2 percent), the proportion of their grooms who were HIV positive did. In the North, an estimated 18.1 percent of grooms were infected, in the South, 11.9 percent, and in the Center, 16.0 percent (Bracher, Santow, and Watkins 2003, Table 7, 229). The much higher proportion of grooms than brides who are infected does not mean that the fates of their brides are determined. Although their risk is greater than when they were single because intercourse is more frequent, brides may escape infection, because some infected men die or their marriages end by divorce before their wives become infected.

16. Measures of prevalence are measures of current infection, whereas incidence is the rate of new infections. Prevalence estimates thus do not include those who were infected but died before the time of the survey. This is not a significant problem when prevalence figures are confined to ages 15–24, since the typical time from infection to death is approximately 10 years; and, as we saw earlier, relatively few are infected before age 15, and thus relatively few would have died before reaching age 25. When the age range is extended, however, deaths that reduce prevalence are more likely to occur.

# CHAPTER 7

ⵝⵝⵝⵝⵝⵝ

## The Fight against AIDS in the Larger Context: The End of "AIDS Exceptionalism"

*Roger England*

HIV has been promoted as an exceptional disease, a concept encompassing HIV as a disease of poverty, a developmental catastrophe, and an emergency demanding special measures, including interventions beyond the health sector and beyond leadership by the World Health Organization. This led to the creation of UNAIDS, making HIV the only disease to have its own United Nations organization. Under UNAIDS, the "exceptionality" argument was used to raise international political commitment and large sums of money for HIV from, among others, the World Bank, through its multi-country AIDS program (MAP), the Global Fund to Fight AIDS, Tuberculosis and Malaria (GFATM), the U.S. President's Emergency Plan for AIDS Relief (PEPFAR), and major donors and foundations. How relevant is the concept of exceptionalism today; indeed how relevant has it ever been?

## How Important Is HIV?

Table 7.1 presents the application of the revised estimates for HIV deaths (UNAIDS 2008a) to data from the Global Burden of Disease Estimates for the main causes of death (WHO 2001; World Bank 2006a). Globally, HIV accounts for 3 percent of all deaths (Figure 7.1), overshadowed by deaths from cardiovascular diseases, cancers, accidents and injuries, respiratory infections, respiratory diseases, and below diarrheal diseases, perinatal conditions, and digestive diseases.

In lower and middle income countries (LMICs) where, with the intense publicity given to HIV it might be expected that it contributes a greater proportion of deaths, in fact the situation is little changed. HIV accounts for 3.4 percent of all deaths in LMICs which display a similar pattern to global deaths (Figure 7.2).

Table 7.1 Main Causes of Death

| | Deaths '000 in 2001 | | | | | | | |
| --- | --- | --- | --- | --- | --- | --- | --- | --- |
| | Global | % | LMICs | % | AFRO | % | AFRO-5 | % |
| Total deaths | 55,388[1] | | 47,399[2] | | 9,784[3] | | 9,784[3] | |
| Selected causes | | | | | | | | |
| TB | 1,644 | 2.97 | 1,590 | 3.35 | 335 | 3.42 | 262 | 3.42 |
| HIV[4] | 1,700 | 3.07 | 1,600 | 3.38 | 1,300 | 13.29 | 590 | 7.71 |
| Diarrheal diseases | 2,001 | 3.61 | 1,777 | 3.75 | 703 | 7.19 | 550 | 7.19 |
| Childhood cluster Measles Tetanus | 1,318 | 2.38 | 1,362 | 2.87 | 695 | 7.10 | 544 | 7.10 |
| Malaria | 1,124 | 2.03 | 1,207 | 2.55 | 963 | 9.84 | 753 | 9.84 |
| Respiratory infections | 3,947 | 7.13 | 3,481 | 7.34 | 1,039 | 10.62 | 813 | 10.62 |
| Maternal conditions | 509 | 0.92 | 507 | 1.07 | 240 | 2.45 | 188 | 2.45 |
| Perinatal conditions Low birthweight | 2,503 | 4.52 | 2,489 | 5.25 | 576 | 5.89 | 450 | 5.89 |
| Cancers | 7,115 | 12.85 | 4,955 | 10.45 | 544 | 5.56 | 425 | 5.56 |
| Diabetes mellitus | 895 | 1.62 | 757 | 1.60 | 54 | 0.55 | 42 | 0.55 |
| Neuropsychiatric | 1,023 | 1.85 | 701 | 1.48 | 80 | 0.82 | 63 | 0.82 |
| Cardiovascular diseases Ischemic heart disease Cerebrovascular | 16,585 | 29.94 | 13,354 | 28.17 | 985 | 10.07 | 770 | 10.07 |

| Respiratory diseases COPD | 3,560 | 6.43 | 3,125 | 6.59 | 234 | 2.39 | 183 | 2.39 |
|---|---|---|---|---|---|---|---|---|
| Digestive diseases | 1,987 | 3.59 | 1,600 | 3.38 | 200 | 2.04 | 156 | 2.04 |
| Congenital abnormalities | 507 | 0.92 | 477 | 1.01 | 67 | 0.68 | 52 | 0.68 |
| Unintentional injuries Road traffic | 3,508 | 6.33 | 3,214 | 6.78 | 469 | 4.79 | 367 | 4.79 |
| Intentional injuries | 1,594 | 2.88 | 1,501 | 3.17 | 267 | 2.73 | 209 | 2.73 |

1–3  Derived by deducting recent revisions in HIV deaths from total deaths in 2001

1  56,553,860−(2,865,804−1,7000,000) gbdwhoregionmortality2001
   SOURCE: http://www.who.int/healthinfo/statistics/bodgbd2001/en/index.html

2  48,351−(2,552−1,600) Disease Control Priorities Project
   SOURCE: http://www.dcp2.org/pubs/GBD/3/Table/3.B1

3  10,680,871−(2,196,956−1,300,000) gbdwhoregionmortality2001
   SOURCE: http://www.who.int/healthinfo/statistics/bodgbd2001/en/index.html

4  Source for global and AFRO: 2008 report on the global AIDS epidemic. UNAIDS/WHO, July 2008
   Source for LMICs: Author's estimate

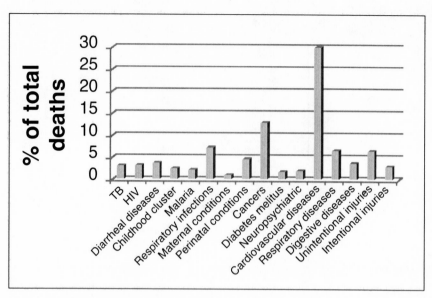

*Figure 7.1* Causes of Death Globally, 2001
SOURCE: Data from Table 7.1

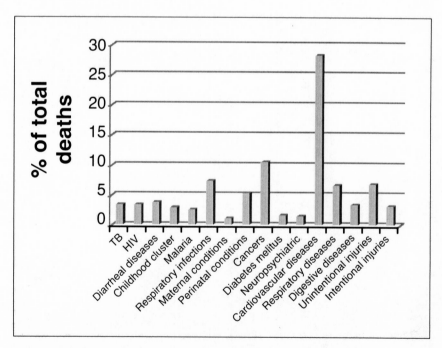

*Figure 7.2* Causes of Death in Lower and Middle Income Countries, 2001
SOURCE: Data from Table 7.1

In Africa the situation is different, with HIV accounting for 13.3 percent of deaths, ahead of respiratory infections at 10.6 percent and cardiovascular diseases at 10.1 percent (Figure 7.3). Within Africa, however, HIV is very unevenly distributed, disproportionately affecting some southern African countries. The Republic of South Africa alone accounts for some 23.33 percent of HIV deaths (2007).

Excluding the five countries with the highest number of deaths from HIV, HIV for the rest of Africa accounts for around 7.7 percent of deaths, below malaria, respiratory infections, cardiovascular diseases, maternal and perinatal conditions, and accidents and injuries, and roughly similar to diarrheal diseases, and childhood cluster (Figure 7.4). HIV may be "the biggest killer in Africa," but it is not the biggest killer in most of Africa's 53 countries.

To put the number of HIV deaths in perspective globally, HIV deaths in Africa are equivalent to: 65 percent of under five deaths in India alone from all causes; or 43 percent of child deaths from pneumonia globally; or the number of "missing girls" in China and India (combined) from infanticide and feticide.

Is HIV increasing more rapidly than other diseases in Africa? It seems not. Indeed, as shown in Figure 7.5, incidence peaked in the mid-to-late 1990s (Shelton, Halperin, and Wilson 2006). What are rising rapidly are deaths from noncommunicable diseases and accidents and injuries. Within the next decade, noncommunicable diseases, accidents, and injuries will constitute almost 85 percent of the burden of disease in developing countries (Boutayeb and Boutayeb 2005). In Zambia, for example, road accidents alone are reported as already the third leading cause of death (*Times of Zambia* 2005).

Figure 7.6 shows WHO projections for causes of death, suggesting that as deaths from HIV in low-income countries halve by 2030, deaths from cardiovascular disease and cancers will double.

So while HIV has had devastating effects in some southern African countries, this is not the story everywhere. There are other important disease priorities, and surely we must question why HIV is still singled out and promoted as "exceptional" by UNAIDS and others. Globally, for every human being who dies of HIV, five human beings die before they reach five years old, most of them from diseases that are relatively easily prevented or treated. That surely is exceptional.

How Much Money Are We Spending on HIV, and How Are We Spending It?

The amount of aid for HIV compared with other needs has been questioned for some time (England 2006, 2007; Shiffman 2006). Although HIV accounts for 13 percent of deaths in Africa, it received over 40 percent of health aid in 2006, probably 50 percent now. In some countries aid for HIV exceeds the government health budget for the whole sector. Two examples are shown in Figure 7.7a.

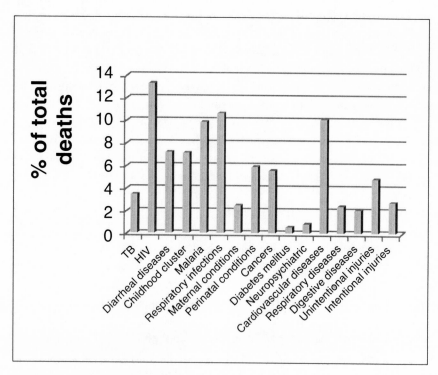

*Figure 7.3* Causes of Death in Africa, 2001
SOURCE: Data from Table 7.1

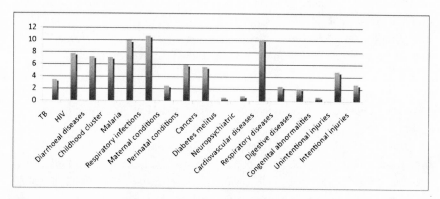

*Figure 7.4* Causes of Death in Africa, 2001 (excluding five countries)
SOURCE: Data from Table 7.1

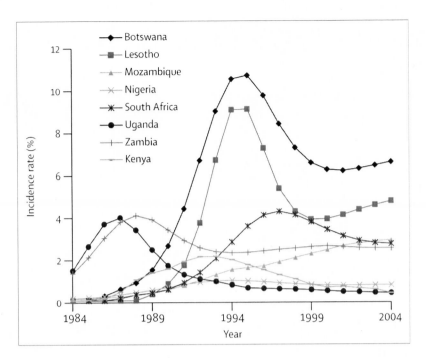

*Figure 7.5*　HIV incidence in adults (15–49 years) in high prevalence countries in Africa, 1984–2004

SOURCE: Shelton, Halperin, and Wilson (2006), Figure 2, p. 1121. Reprinted with permission from *The Lancet.*

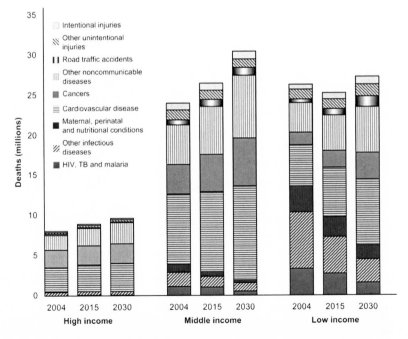

*Figure 7.6*　WHO projected deaths by cause

SOURCE: WHO (2008e), p.29. Reprinted with permission from the World Health Organization.

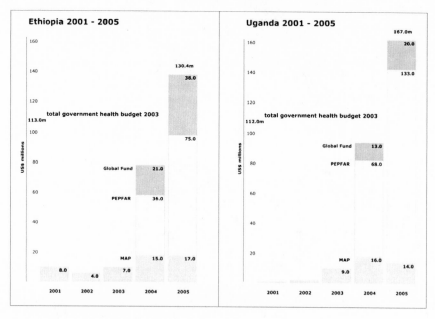

*Figure 7.7a*    Aid for HIV in Ethiopia and Uganda 2001–2005
SOURCE: Based on Center for Global Development (2007a).

HIV-dedicated funding constitutes the majority share of health aid for many countries as shown in Figure 7.7b.

Based on recent OECD DAC and WHO data, Figure 7.8 shows HIV aid against HIV as a percentage of burden of disease for aid-receiving countries. Countries above the line (i.e, almost all of them) are receiving more HIV aid than is justified by the contribution of HIV to the national burden of disease.

In fact, the proper share of health aid allocated to HIV should be decided not only by the contribution HIV makes to the burden of disease, but also by the relative cost effectiveness of available interventions compared with those for other diseases. HIV could justify more funding than its share of the burden of disease if its interventions were more cost effective than those for other diseases. But HIV interventions are not very cost effective compared with those for other diseases, HIV treatment least of all. Costs per Disabilty-Adjusted Life Years (DALYs) averted are lower for immunizations, malaria, traffic accidents, childhood illnesses, and tuberculosis (TB), for example (Jamison et al. 2006; Laxminarayan et al. 2006; WHO CHOICE). For the cost of every life prolonged by antiretroviral therapy (ART), many more lives could be saved by spending that money elsewhere.

Combined aid and domestic expenditure on HIV in relevant countries is over US$10 billion a year. What is this being spent on, and with what results? We know remarkably little. It is by no means clear precisely how much is spent on

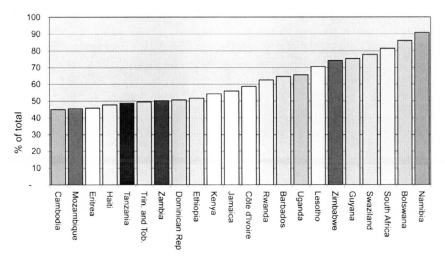

*Figure 7.7b*    Percentage of donor support for health and population dedicated for HIV, 2002–06
SOURCE: Data from OECD DAC CRS online from Pearson (2008).

prevention or what it is spent on, but we do know that billions are being wasted on ineffectual multi-sectoral projects (World Bank 2005), including disbursements to line ministries that they are unable to use (Center for Global Development 2008a), and on badly targeted prevention (Chin 2008). Chin shows that UNAIDS has grossly overestimated HIV prevalence, exaggerated the potential for HIV epidemics in general populations, and encouraged huge spending aimed at preventing general epidemics that were never going to happen.

We do not know exactly how much is being spent on treatment and what the components of those expenditures are, and, equally worrying, we know little about the benefit incidence: which income groups are getting free treatment, and who is being subsidized? The Demographic and Health Surveys show clearly that in Africa the middle classes and more educated now have the highest HIV rates (Shelton, Cassell, and Adetunji 2005; Mishra et al. 2007a). We may expect then that much of the massive global subsidy for HIV treatment is being consumed by the middle classes, the more so since it is those who live in urban conurbations and near main roads who have access to testing and free treatment, rather than the rural poor.

We know little about how much is spent on transaction costs in maintaining a whole HIV industry, including funding western NGOs providing HIV services in countries, research grants in vaguely related and ineffectual studies, and HIV components of UN projects (a recent UNDP study of hurricane preparedness on a Caribbean island included looking at whether shelters are making provision for people living with HIV), for example. UNAIDS itself costs almost US$0.5 billion

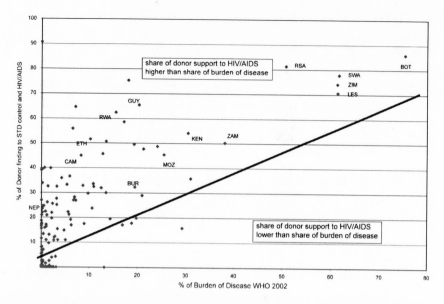

*Figure 7.8*   Percentage of aid for HIV in relation to HIV as percentage of BOD
SOURCE: Data from OECD (1–4) from Pearson (2008).

a year (UNAIDS 2008c), and transaction costs for PEPFAR may be 30–40 percent of total allocations.

## What Effects Is This Level of Expenditure Having?

Those lobbying for more money for HIV, led by UNAIDS, argue that it is not a problem that a disproportionate amount of health aid is being spent on HIV because HIV aid has been additional to health sector aid, and the success of HIV funding is bringing pressure for increased aid for health. Additionally, it is argued, HIV aid benefits health services as a whole (Rapid Responses to England 2008). How true are these claims? A discussion of each of these claims follows.

## Is HIV Aid Additional to Health Aid?

Figure 7.9 shows health aid as a percentage of total development aid, and how much of that health aid has been for HIV. With the exception of a dip in 1999, the health share of total aid has increased steadily, stabilizing at around 8 percent before increasing sharply in 2006 (the latest year for which detailed data are available). Starting in the late 1990s, however, HIV has taken an increasing share of what has been available, and non-HIV/STD health aid has declined as a percentage of total aid, picking up again only in 2006 but still not restoring even levels of 1996–98.

Although aid for health has increased as a share of total development assistance and absolutely, aid for non-HIV/STI has been less than it would have been if it had continued at trend. In 1998, non-HIV aid was 7.7 percent of all development aid. Table 7.2 shows what non-HIV/STI aid would have been if it had continued at this share up to 2006, and what it actually was.

In no year has non-HIV aid reached the trend level, and the total loss of non-HIV aid over the eight years has been US$10.3 billion. During this time, HIV aid has increased dramatically, from US$216 million to US$4.6 billion a year (OECD 2, 4). While some HIV aid may have been truly additional aid, it is hard to avoid the conclusion that much of it has been at the expense of non-HIV aid as donors have shifted their funding.

One example of this is family planning programs, vital for women to have control over their fertility and health. Given that half of all births are unwanted or unplanned, universally available family planning could prevent up to a quarter of a million maternal deaths a year and perhaps 150,000 children borne with HIV. But funding for family planning has been decimated in recent years, falling from 55 percent of all population activities to 9 percent over the decade to 2004, while funding for HIV prevention and treatment rose from 9 percent to 54 percent (UN Economic and Social Council 2005).

The U.S. President's funding request for HIV programs in the 15 PEPFAR countries increased 125 percent in just two years over the 2006 allocated level, while that for family planning and reproductive health fell by 11 percent. At just $67.5 million requested for 2008, aid for family planning and reproduction health is less than 2 percent of HIV aid at $3.6 billion (Figure 7.10).

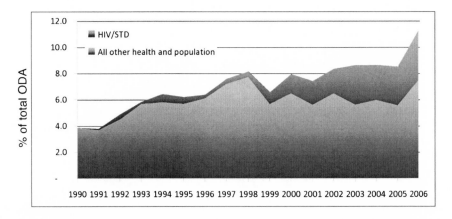

*Figure 7.9*    Health aid as a percentage of total Official Development Assistance
SOURCE: Data from OECD (1–4) from Pearson (2008).

Table 7.2 Non-HIV aid at 7.7 percent of all aid versus actual non-HIV aid 1998–2006

| Non-HIV Health AID | 1998 | 1999 | 2000 | 2001 | 2002 | 2003 | 2004 | 2005 | 2006 | Total |
|---|---|---|---|---|---|---|---|---|---|---|
| Trend | 3.8 | 4.3 | 4.3 | 4.3 | 5 | 7 | 7.6 | 9.4 | 9.3 | 54.9 |
| Actual | 3.8 | 3.2 | 3.7 | 3.1 | 4.2 | 5.1 | 5.9 | 6.8 | 9 | 44.6 |
| Shortfall | | 1.1 | 0.7 | 1.2 | 0.8 | 1.9 | 1.7 | 2.6 | 0.3 | 10.3 |

SOURCE: From Figure 7.9, with data from (OECD 1–4), taken from Pearson (2008).

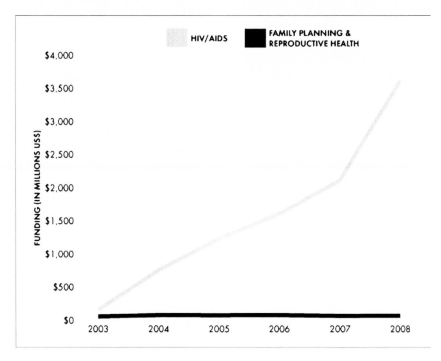

*Figure 7.10*    FP/RH and HIV Funding for PEPFAR Countries, Allocated 2003–08, Requested 2007–08
SOURCE: Population Action International (2008).

## Does HIV Aid Benefit Health Services as a Whole?

There is anecdotal and circumstantial evidence for and against HIV aid improving general health services (e.g., Box 1). Proponents point to new public health laboratories built with HIV money. Opponents point out that the only work going on in them is for HIV, because there is no money for other staff, equipment, or reagents or, worse, that the higher pay for HIV staff has attracted them away from non-HIV work. While PMTCT (preventing mother-to-child transmission) money has obvious opportunities to strengthen maternal and child health (MCH) on which its effective delivery so clearly depends, it has not done so very much (Druce and Nolan 2007). PMTCT programs have been focused on narrow PMTCT interventions, often delivered in parallel with those for MCH.

Box 1: A personal account

What I saw in a public district hospital in Zambia illustrates this point. The few available district nurses are sent to training one after the other: to improve their skills to test, treat and council AIDS patients. They appreciate this, because it enhances their knowledge and they have the opportunity to meet new colleagues. In their hospital they are now able to provide drugs for free to AIDS patients, they can spend time to council patients (30 min, much more than they were used to spending on any patient), the AIDS clinic is nicely painted, the lab is functioning, and they receive extra allowances to top up their meagre salaries. They feel rewarded and their job satisfaction has increased: they are now able to properly treat patients who they could previously not. The AIDS patients feel encouraged. They get a sense of their right to proper treatment and they start to demand these rights. It seems that this disease specific programme is strengthening the local system.

The other patients are waiting in a longer queue, for staff that has less time available because of the additional tasks, and the time spent per patient is very short. They still have to pay for the drugs they are prescribed. The ward is not painted. The nurses are not paid incentives for these 'regular' clinics and they treat the patients less friendly. They realise this, and feel guilty about it. But they feel exhausted. AIDS treatment coverage is going up, while vaccination rates are going down. The woman in child labour, the child with pneumonia, the AIDS patient with a broken leg: they don't get the care they are entitled to. In fact, they are worse off as there is less time available and they are now seen as second class patients. And the situation is getting worse, as AIDS organisations are recruiting staff from the public sector and from the private for-profit sector, to run the AIDS clinics outside of the public sector. They find the staff, because they pay higher salaries and offer better working conditions, leaving the public sector behind.

—*Ellen Verheul, Wemos (NGO), Netherlands* (pers.comm.)

In Africa, relatively excessive HIV money has resulted in a loss of skilled staff to HIV NGOs offering higher salary scales. In Ethiopia, a driver for a U.S. bilateral agency earns more than a professor in a medical school and a public health specialist four to five times a counterpart in government services. HIV money is used for HIV-dedicated training in VCT (voluntary counseling and testing) and treatment, distorting work patterns of those workers in government service who earn more from allowances at the workshops than from salaries (Davey, Fekade, and Parry 2006). Studies from Mozambique, Uganda, and Zambia indicate how HIV funding has built HIV-specific systems and processes distinct from those for other health programs (Center for Global Development 2008b). Similar stories are heard from Cambodia, Vietnam, and Kenya with health workers switching to HIV programs. In Rwanda, doctors working for NGOs are earning six times more than their public sector equivalents (Republic of Rwanda 2006).

Stories abound from Africa of "two tier" health services in which HIV patients can benefit from upgraded separate space in health facilities, separate medical records, specialist staff, and high quality protocols, whilst non-HIV patients suffer the lack of these things. Dedicated VCT services (bloods, counseling, laboratory work and equipment, training, etc.) are working to high standards, but shortages and low quality work are seen in non-HIV services (see Box 2). For HIV, there are well-designed and enforced treatment protocols, for example, but prescribing chaos exists in pneumonia treatment. Also, blood safety procedures are practiced in HIV clinics, but this is not the rule in hospital wards.

The ultimate inequity here is that the HIV patients receive their treatment free of charge while, typically, non-HIV patients must pay for their care.

---

### Box 2: Double standards

HIV money encourages higher quality services for ART rollout than for non-HIV services. Examples below are taken from Tanzania.

*Dedicated Care and Treatment (C&T) Clinics or
general health facilities providing ART have:*

- space for registration of HIV patients
- space for consultation/examination (confidentiality)
- HIV patient flow plan
- C&T coordinator
- separate HIV clinics, on separate days (losing all synergies and doubling up on travel problems for attendees)
- dedicated C&T team or individuals (medical/clinical, nurse, VCT counsellor, laboratory, pharmacy, data entry)
- dedicated C&T forms to complete
- dedicated C&T training

*Typically, VCT, PMTCT and home based care (HBC) services will provide:*

- dedicated training (compulsory 6-week course for VCT in Tanzania)
- dedicated guidelines – PMTCT, VCT, HBC, drugs, lab work

- dedicated reporting – clinical HIV surveillance forms, ART patient numbers, computerization for HIV data, all separate from the National Health Management Information System (HMIS)/Monitoring and Evaluation (M&E)
- HBC programs in training, support, and supplies for HIV, but little else
- dedicated "PMTCT plus" clinics
- dedicated PMTCT workers in MCH

*Source:* Author's work in Tanzania, unpublished.

So not only has the big increase in HIV funding been partly at the expense of non-HIV funding, but the operation of HIV services using that funding can further deplete non-HIV services by usurping components of the health delivery system, particularly staff and staff time. As the expansion of HIV treatment moves into "task shifting" (WHO 2008d), we can expect it to usurp more of the time of almost all groups of workers down to community health workers.

Even where there are examples of HIV aid improving an aspect of general services, the obvious question remains whether this is an efficient way of improving general services and achieving maximum health gain for available funding? If the latter is the objective, which it should be, then aid should be focused on achieving it. Poorer countries that have made good progress in mortality reduction are those that have selectively introduced cheap and effective interventions achieving extensive coverage of immunization, vitamin A supplementation, oral rehydration solution use, and family planning; before moving on to improving attended delivery rates, introducing management of pneumonia and short-course TB treatment by community health workers etc.; and before aiming at extending curative case management capacity (Rohde et al. 2008). It is not clear how dedicated HIV money can help countries along this path. In fact, the new funding for HIV was never intended to improve general health services or to be aligned to country priorities. It was intended for HIV and specifically for ART. It has not been delivered through country sector financing mechanisms (see below), because countries might not have chosen to spend so much on HIV given their other priorities, but that is how donors and their lobby groups have wanted it spent.

UNAIDS and others argue that the problem is not that of relatively too much money being spent on HIV, but that total health aid must be hugely increased (Rapid Responses to England 2008). Until recently, UNAIDS was calling for global HIV spending alone to rise from US$9 billion in 2006 to US$42 billion by 2010, later moderated to US$25 billion, most of which would have to come from aid (UNAIDS 2009b). What would total health aid have to be to justify that increase? Such large sums for aid are not realistic, and even if they materialized, they would likely result in macroeconomic distortions, including inflation as more money competes for limited national resources. This would disproportionately affect the poor. These effects can be reduced with careful planning and if used mostly for goods and services that cannot be produced nationally (Pearson 2009). But whatever the total health aid budget, it is important that it is used for maximum health gain, not disproportionately usurped for one disease.

## How Aid Is Delivered Is Also Important

Although it may be possible, theoretically, for HIV aid to improve all health care—to strengthen all laboratory services, not just those for HIV; to raise capacity for drugs and supplies procurement across the board, not just for HIV supplies; to strengthen MCH services, not just PMTCT services; and to improve sector-wide information and M&E systems, not just those for HIV—in practice, the HIV money arrives in ways that largely prevent this. The largest source of HIV aid comes from PEPFAR, GFATM, and World Bank. This aid bypasses country planning and budgeting systems. It is off-budget, administered by Project Management Units (PMUs), National AIDS Commissions (NACs), and others and does not conform to balanced country priorities. It is earmarked for specific HIV activities, such as creating sophisticated HIV M&E systems even when countries have no basic health management systems, for ART, for VCT, and for associated training and supplies. It is specifically budgeted for HIV purposes and accounted for in terms of how it is spent for those purposes, so it cannot be used for anything else. It leads to high transactional costs for countries in dealing with donors' project approval and appraisal systems, responding to donor information demands including separate data needs and M&E requirements. The GFATM grant application process, for example, treats health systems strengthening as an add-on to disease-specific investment, demanding convoluted and artificial applications showing how money for systems strengthening will benefit HIV (or TB or malaria) (GFATM 2008). It results in dedicated drugs, test kits, and supplies procurement and distribution (by PMUs, NACs, or directly by donors) outside national systems and thus does not improve them.

It is hard to see how HIV aid can benefit general health services unless we change the way it is delivered. Not only is the big HIV aid disproportionate to burden of disease (Figure 7.8), it is out of line with countries' own plans and priorities. Zambia has a One Sector Strategic Plan, Joint Sector Reviews, a SWAp (Sector-Wide Approach), and a Basket Funding mechanism that allows for flexible funding and a focus on national and local priorities. But in 2007, 90 percent of health aid ignored this admirable progress and was disease dedicated (mostly to HIV) with only 10 percent available for strengthening the health care system (IHP+2008a).

In Cambodia over the past five years, aid flows have been far out of alignment with the national health priorities and burden of disease. Although the National Strategic Development Plan (the Cambodian equivalent of a Poverty Reduction Strategy) sets out the intention of spending the majority of resources on primary health care (including expansion of the Minimum Package of Activities), over the period 2003–5, about 60 percent of donor funding went to HIV and other infectious diseases (Figure 7.11). This misalignment is likely to have increased since, in view of GFATM approvals amounting to over $85m in grants since late 2005. This blatant disregard by donors of countries' needs and rational planning, providing instead funding for donors' own favorite diseases, is little short of shocking.

The Cambodian Draft Health Strategic Plan 2008–2015 comments, "the predominant attention given to disease control programmes has further led to distortions in spending priorities, and effectively undermines MoH [Ministry of Health] stewardship of the sector." The disease-dedicated funding of the Global Health Partnerships (GHPs) has reinforced these distortions, in particular as far as HIV, TB, malaria, and childhood immunization are concerned.

A recent study from Cambodia comments:

> Vertical funding channels are undermining the SWiM (SWAp) thus hindering the long term development of a good aid relationship. The failure of the GHPs (alongside other donors) to harmonize and align has discouraged the development of the basic building blocks for an effective SWAp process. . . . The GHPs have also introduced major transaction costs – partly a reflection of Cambodia's success in attracting GHP funding. However, the Global Fund in particular appears to be more transaction cost intensive than other forms of donor support. . . . Future GHP allocations should not be allowed to further exacerbate the misalignment between available resources and priorities. This would serve only to further displace the fiscal space the Government needs to implement the major priorities set out in the Health Strategic Plan 2008–2015 (Pearson, Buse, and Pun 2008).

In Rwanda, government manages only 14 percent of its health aid and a review of sector financing highlights a "gross misallocation" of resources in relation to disease priorities. In 2005, Rwanda received over US$47 million earmarked for HIV (it has an adult HIV prevalence rate of 3 percent), and only US$1 million for childhood illnesses (Republic of Rwanda 2006).

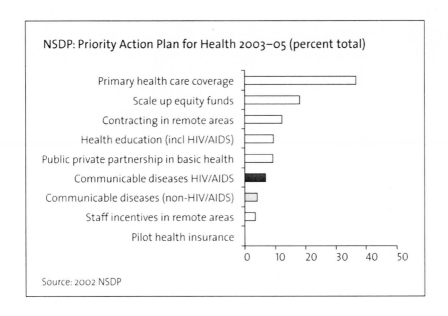

NSDP: Priority Action Plan for Health 2003–05 (percent total)

Source: 2002 NSDP

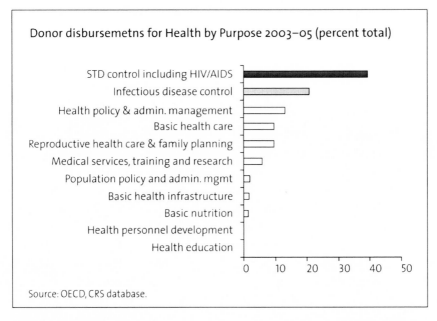

Donor disbursemetns for Health by Purpose 2003–05 (percent total)

Source: OECD, CRS database.

*Figure 7.11* Cambodia national health priorities and donor disbursements for health, 2003–2005
SOURCE: Cambodia National Strategic Development Plan 2002 and OECD CRS database, presented in WHO (2007), Fig. 6, p. 21. Reprinted by permission from the World Health Organization.

## Conclusions

It is hard to escape the conclusion that too much aid is dedicated to HIV, given other needs. Much HIV aid is not aligned to the needs and stated priorities of countries, even where countries have worked these out well and have good plans for meeting them. Furthermore, the relative imbalance in HIV aid has been dictated by donors and the agencies they fund rather than the needs and wishes of countries, a situation not helped by the existence of UNAIDS as a powerful one-disease advocacy body.

In practice, it is very difficult to use HIV for effective health systems strengthening. The way in which HIV aid is delivered is weakening country planning and budgeting mechanisms, and constraining the development of general health services and sector management capacity.

Preparatory work for the Accra High Level Forum highlights the fragmentation of health aid, with more than two-thirds of aid commitments under US$0.5 million, and with very little aid delivered through country planning and budgeting mechanisms (WHO 2008a). HIV aid may not have created all these problems but, undoubtedly, it is making them much worse.

Although, at the service delivery level, HIV funding may be used to leverage small improvements in general health services (WHO 2008c), HIV aid delivery mechanisms are undermining rather than building population health and primary care systems. The narrow obsession with HIV has resulted in missed opportunities for synergies even with tuberculosis and reproductive health services. This situation is now improving, but it would not have occurred in the first place if funding had been used to strengthen general health services (within which, *inter alia*, ART could have been delivered more cost effectively than it has been; although this does not mean that a more rational allocation of aid would have spent so much on ART given other needs and intervention cost effectiveness). Indeed because HIV funding is largely outside of government systems, there appears to be little effective coordination even within and between HIV services (Global HIV/AIDS Initiative Network 2008). And, if HIV is to continue to dictate the allocation of so much health aid, this will disadvantage most of west and central Africa where HIV rates are low, but mortality and morbidity from malnutrition, respiratory, and diarrheal diseases are very high (Halperin 2008).

## The Way Forward Now: Priorities for Change in the Aid Environment

Donor-driven HIV-dedicated aid should be replaced by general health sector aid allowing countries to decide their real priorities and act on them. This will not stop all HIV funding: donors must continue to provide for the costs of ART for example, since it is not possible to withdraw this for those who have started treatment. The (first-line) drugs costs for the three million on treatment amount to no more than US$450 million a year, and the total costs for a basic delivery package including drugs, some laboratory support, and patient care are two to three times this estimate. Significant questions arise, however, about additional spending on HIV treatment when so many other priorities exist and when many more lives could be saved by spending the next available dollar per capita on preventing and treating other causes of mortality.

Health aid should work to build country health service delivery platforms able to maximize health outcomes for all. Poorer African countries need a reliable, predictable, and flexible line of grant funding to be able to do this. It should be provided to countries through national budgeting and spending mechanisms so that countries can plan and allocate to meet national priorities. Strengthening these mechanisms must be a top priority. There will not be a structure that fits all countries, but SWAp-type arrangements still offer a large potential to coordinate external funding, combine it with domestic funding, and spend it according to agreed plans. Institutionalizing the SWAp arrangements may be one way forward, with external funders sitting as "shareholders" on national boards to ensure transparency, objective evaluation, and results. Social insurance schemes like those of Ghana and Senegal, with insurance funds as knowledgeable purchasers driving quality improvements in both public and private providers, also offer good prospects for more effective aid delivery and could be good vehicles for reaching the poor with subsidies (England 2008a).

There is growing recognition that emphasis must shift from disease-specific funding and technical support to the strengthening of country sector funding and service delivery mechanisms. Reich and others point out the potential for the G8 role in consolidating a commitment to this shift and backing it with money (Reich and Takemi 2009). A key gap is that of appropriate international institutions able to disburse the funding in ways that avoid the problems discussed in this paper and to provide the technical guidance needed for strengthening health systems. Serious reforms are needed of the roles, structures, capacities, and relationships of global health institutions and, given the instincts and consummate skills for self-preservation of UN agencies, it is likely that this can only come from a G8 initiative using a "task force" outside of the existing global institutions. The High Level Forum on Aid Effectiveness held in Accra in September 2008, calls for many of the right things: more use of country systems, more predictable aid, and more coordination to reduce fragmentation of aid and aid management costs (OECD 2008; WHO 2008a). Individual agencies are taking some steps to improve their aid harmonization performance. Global Alliance for Vaccines and Immunisation (GAVI) is moving from using its own proposal and reporting mechanisms based on its own business cycle to those of countries, starting with using the International Health Partnership and related initiatives (IHP+) processes (IHP+2008b). GFATM is moving towards replacing "rounds based" funding with "single stream" funding which will make funding more predictable and less burdensome for recipients. Progress is being made but not fast enough.

One obvious step towards creating more momentum is for the GFATM to be transformed from a three-diseases fund into a global health fund. New methods are required to finance the fund, allowing long-term commitments to countries that include more recurrent budget support not just investment, so that health workers can be paid performance incentives, for example, or independent providers be contracted to provide public services. Funding should be delivered in ways that help strengthen the coordination of aid and its alignment to country plans and poverty reduction strategies—not weaken them as GFATM funding does currently by demanding separate planning and accounting practices. Although GFATM has been making some moves towards funding health system strengthening (it claims that 20 percent of Round 7 resources were for system-related activities), these are being achieved by stealth rather than re-engineering of the organization; potential grantees must still demonstrate what any planned systems strengthening activities will do for one of the three diseases (GFATM 2008). Transformation of the GFATM along these lines would create instant pressure for reforms of technical agencies, with GFATM having to insist on coordinated, evidence-based planning and technical advice for disbursements.

Rationalization of UN technical agencies should start with the closure of UNAIDS. Its one-disease advocacy is distorting public and political understanding of the true importance of HIV in relation to other greater health care needs. The structure of the Programme Coordinating Board that governs UNAIDS comprises the HIV representatives of its cosponsoring agencies and ensures that the advice the organization provides to the UN Director General is self-serving. Its functions of strategic information, monitoring and evaluation, and projecting funding requirements should be integrated within other organizations, primarily WHO (which undertakes most of them anyway), where they may be balanced with those for all causes of mortality and morbidity. A UN Economic and Social Council inquiry into UNAIDS is needed now, developing into a task force to review health aid institutions and rationalize the UN technical structure.

Research priorities should also shift—and will do if funding shifts first. Countries must have convincing, evidence-based sector plans with which to negotiate with donors if health aid is to be aligned to real needs, priorities, and opportunities. There is much to understand about how to make health systems work and what elements of health systems are resulting in cost-effective performance and better health outcomes. This includes understanding more about whole sector funding and services, not only the traditional public sector. To be really useful, much of this must be country specific, but cross-country comparisons may provide insight, if not universally applicable answers. If we are to argue for significantly more aid for health, we must be able to show that it will be spent cost effectively and without causing adverse macroeconomic effects. On this latter issue alone, there is much practical research to be done.

Finally, there is a need to improve the performance of donors and technical agencies and to hold them to account by measuring publicly good and bad practices. This must be independent of UN institutions, possibly along the lines of the work of Transparency International and its annual country performance tables for corruption (Transparency International).

## Footnote and Update

A great deal has happened since this paper was prepared in mid-2008. There is now a much wider appreciation of the problems, as well as the benefits of disease-specific funding, and of the need to support the strengthening of health systems across the board (Pearson et al. 2009; Case and Paxson 2009; Grepin, 2009).

The issue is shifting towards "how to do it." The progress being made by IHP+ is based on recognition of the faults in the traditional aid model as outlined in this paper. In preliminary reports, the two Working Groups established to advise the Taskforce on Innovative International Financing for Health Systems recognize the imbalance in health aid and identify the need to shift the emphasis to health systems (Taskforce on Innovative International Financing for Health Systems 2009).

As a result of this, GAVI, the Global Fund, and the World Bank are collaborating in joint programming work to achieve more funding and more coordination in support for health systems strengthening. It remains to be seen what will come out of these important initiatives, and there will yet be much opposition from vested interests, but they offer the best chance yet of supporting countries with systems strengthening across the board, and perhaps of creating a permanent global health fund to continue doing so (Health System Strengthening Workshop 2009).

# CHAPTER 8

✕✕✕✕✕✕

Prevention Failure: The Ballooning Entitlement Burden of
U.S. Global AIDS Treatment Spending and What to Do About It

*Mead Over*[1]

## I. Introduction: Build on PEPFAR

Although it was unknown as recently as the 1980s, AIDS is now the most notorious disease in the world. In the United States, children study the HIV/AIDS epidemic in primary school and learn HIV prevention methods in high school. Among some poor, illiterate populations in the severely affected countries of Africa, more people correctly identify sex as a means of HIV transmission than know that mosquitoes transmit malaria, the ancient scourge that kills almost as many Africans.

The notoriety of the AIDS epidemic is due to many factors. The fact that it first came to attention as a disease that primarily affected gay men in the U.S. and other rich countries is certainly one important reason: gay men proved to be extraordinarily articulate in publicizing the ravages of the disease and in lobbying for public resources to study and treat it. The long incubation period of the virus allowed persons living with AIDS to speak and write about their suffering for years—possibilities which were less available to sufferers from more quickly fatal illnesses.

The appearance in these personal narratives of both sex and death contributed to their fascination. HIV-infected blood supplies spread the disease to many transfusion recipients in rich countries and led to scandals and more publicity. The creation of a specialized international agency called first the Special Programme on AIDS, then the Global Programme on AIDS, and currently UNAIDS provided salaried positions for people whose job it was to publicize this sole disease. The novel challenges of research on the causative agent, one of a class of little understood pathogens called "retroviruses," engendered enthusiasm in the medical and biological research communities. Based on this rapidly evolving research, multinational pharmaceutical firms discovered new drugs to combat the disease and profited from selling those drugs in rich countries and sometimes in poor ones.[2] And last, but not least, the fact is that the virus and its consequences spread in many parts of the world, despite what seemed like the best efforts to control it.

Although the AIDS epidemic is no longer a growing public health problem in the U.S. or other rich countries, UNAIDS estimates that over 33 million people are infected, and over 2 million deaths occur every year (UNAIDS 2007b). While the robust economic growth of heavily affected countries like Botswana and South Africa suggests that AIDS does not have immediately catastrophic impacts on economic growth,[3] the fact that it can reduce life expectancy by decades is, by definition, a catastrophic impact on economic well-being and development. AIDS is decimating the professional classes of the worst affected countries (Hamoudi and Birdsall 2004). Furthermore, the long-term impact of lower life expectancy and high rates of orphanhood are still unknown. One study has suggested that by the year 2080, orphanhood in South Africa might reduce its income per capita to less than half of its current level (Bell, Devarajan, and Gersbach 2004). Growing awareness of these impacts of AIDS may have contributed to President Bush's decision to propose an initiative to combat AIDS in poor countries in the same 2003 State of the Union address in which he announced his intention to invade Iraq.[4]

In response to a proposal from the White House, U.S. Congress launched the U.S. Global AIDS Initiative by passing the United States Leadership against HIV/AIDS, Tuberculosis and Malaria Act of 2003 on May 27, 2003 (United States Leadership 2003).[5] The act required the President to establish the position of Global AIDS Coordinator within the Department of State, rather than in USAID where previous U.S.-funded AIDS assistance had been managed. The Coordinator, Ambassador Randall Tobias, fulfilled his mandate to present to Congress the U.S. Five-Year Global AIDS Strategy on February 23, 2004. He gave the strategy the title: "The President's Emergency Plan for AIDS Relief" (PEPFAR) which today remains the name of the program (OGAC 2004). The strategy established the following three objectives:

1) "To encourage bold leadership at every level to fight HIV/AIDS
2) "To apply best practices within US bilateral HIV/AIDS prevention, treatment and care programs . . .
3) "To encourage partners . . . to coordinate . . . [in order] to ensure the most effective and efficient use of resources" (OGAC 2004).

The strategy defined 15 "focus countries" for US HIV/AIDS assistance, which are listed in Table 8.1.

As a result of PEPFAR, the United States was the largest single contributor to the struggle to control the international AIDS epidemic in 2006 and 2007 (Kates,

*Table 8.1* Selected Economic and Health-Related Indicators of the PEPFAR Focus Countries

| Country | Population | Income Status | GDP per capita (US$) | Life Expectancy | Adult HIV/AIDS Prevalence (ages 15–49) | | Number of physicians in 2003/4 |
|---|---|---|---|---|---|---|---|
| | | | | | *Point Estimate* | *Range* | |
| Botswana | 1,765,000 | Upper middle | 8,920 | 35 | 24.1 | 23.0–32.0 | 715 |
| Côte d'Ivoire | 18,154,000 | Low | 1,390 | 47 | 7.1 | 4.3–9.7 | 2,081 |
| Ethiopia | 77,431,000 | Low | 810 | 48 | | 0.9–3.5 | 1,936 |
| Guyana | 751,000 | Lower middle | 4,110 | 63 | 2.4 | 1.0–4.9 | 366 |
| Haiti | 8,528,000 | Low | 1,680 | 52 | 3.8 | 2.2–5.4 | 1,949 |
| Kenya | 34,256,000 | Low | 1,050 | 47 | 6.1 | 5.2–7.0 | 4,506 |
| Mozambique | 19,792,000 | Low | 1,160 | 42 | 16.1 | 12.5–20.0 | 514 |
| Namibia | 2,031,000 | Lower middle | 6,960 | 46 | 19.6 | 8.6–31.7 | 598 |
| Nigeria | 131,530,000 | Low | 930 | 44 | 3.9 | 2.3–5.6 | 34,923 |
| Rwanda | 9,038,000 | Low | 1,300 | 44 | 3.1 | 2.9–3.2 | 401 |
| South Africa | 47,432,000 | Upper middle | 10,960 | 52 | 18.8 | 16.8–20.7 | 34,829 |
| Tanzania | 38,329,000 | Low | 660 | 44 | 6.5 | 5.8–7.2 | 822 |
| Uganda | 28,816,000 | Low | 1,520 | 48 | 6.7 | 5.7–7.6 | 2,209 |
| Vietnam | 84,238,000 | Low | 2,700 | 72 | 0.5 | 0.3–0.9 | 42,327 |
| Zambia | 11,668,000 | Low | 890 | 37 | 17 | 15.9–18.1 | 1,264 |

NOTE: GDP = gross domestic product.
SOURCE: Based on data from Institute of Medicine (2007), Tables 2-3, 2-4, pp. 59–61.

Izazola, and Lief 2007). In 2006, the U.S. committed $2.6 billion for AIDS, which was 47 percent of the $5.6 billion total from all donors, with the Netherlands in second place at 17 percent (9). As illustrated in Figure 8.1, the U.S. accounted for 41 percent of the $3.9 billion that was actually disbursed (with the UK in second place at 20 percent) (10). Most of this money was channeled through the U.S. President's Emergency Plan for AIDS Relief (PEPFAR), which can properly be described as the "largest global health initiative directed at a single disease that any nation has ever undertaken" (U.S. Government 2007). For comparison, in inflation-adjusted dollars, the U.S. is spending more than 100 times as much per year now on AIDS in poor countries as it spent between 1967 and 1979 on the eradication of smallpox.[6]

The most remarkable achievement of the PEPFAR program has been its contribution to the provision of AIDS treatment to over 1.3 million patients in its 15 focus countries by September of 2007.[7] Furthermore, as Figure 8.2 shows, PEPFAR was able to accelerate constantly until March 2007, adding more patients to its rolls each six-month period than it had the previous six months. However, it is sobering to note that the number of new infections in this period in these

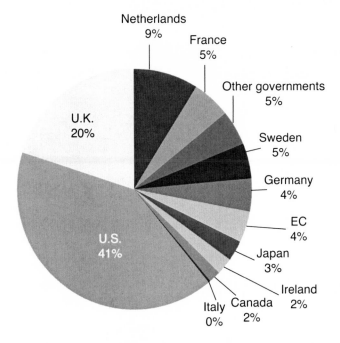

*Figure 8.1*    Shares of national donor disbursements to combating AIDS, 2006
SOURCE: Kates, Izazola, and Lief (2007, 10). This information was reprinted with permission from the Henry J. Kaiser Family Foundation. The Kaiser Family Foundation is a non-profit private operating foundation, based in Menlo Park, California, dedicated to producing and communicating the best possible analysis and information on health issues.

countries averaged about 1.4 million in every year, about three times the number of people who started therapy in the last year of the data.

The U.S. foreign assistance program is also the biggest single funder of the Global Fund to Fight AIDS, Tuberculosis, and Malaria and the second biggest (after the United Kingdom) of the World Bank, the two most important multilateral sources of AIDS financing. Also, U.S. tax laws favoring the creation and operation of philanthropic foundations have enabled U.S. foundations to dominate the world of foundation giving to fight AIDS.

Thus, U.S. AIDS policy under President Bush established a record of success on AIDS treatment, to which the actions of future U.S. Presidents will inevitably be compared. Presidential candidates choose to ignore AIDS policy at their peril. They can quietly continue the country on its present course. They can withdraw support from AIDS patients, risking a backlash of cynicism and skepticism regarding the country's ability to respect its commitments. Or, they can address the weaknesses of existing U.S. AIDS policy and, in so doing, strengthen the U.S. reputation for contributing to the solution of global problems.

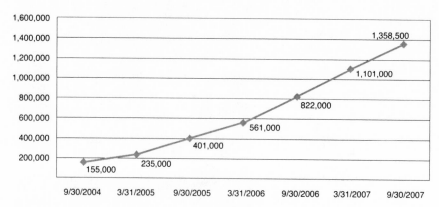

*Figure 8.2*   Number receiving U.S.-supported AIDS treatment in the 15 PEPFAR focus countries
SOURCE: OGAC (2007).

## II. Successes of PEPFAR—But Not On Prevention

The U.S.'s generous increase in AIDS funding under the PEPFAR program has achieved substantial success in two areas. The program has not only placed hundreds of thousands on treatment, but the treatment has been successful, at least initially, for most patients in keeping these patients alive. The result has been millions of years of life saved, and because most of the patients are parents, millions of years of orphanhood averted. These are tremendous achievements and justify some degree of pride.

### A. Years of life and of orphanhood saved

By placing over 800,000 patients on antiretroviral therapy (ART), PEPFAR has postponed death for most of these people by at least a year. This is already a substantial achievement. Under assumptions about the success of treatment and the continuation of PEPFAR funding, the annual report estimates the number of years of life that PEPFAR will have added through 2009 (U.S. Government 2007, Figure 4). According to their estimates, the program purchased 870, 340 years of life by mid-2007 and will purchase an additional 2.5 million life years through 2009 (Figure 8.3). And, there will be spillover benefits for others in these societies. For example, assuming the average patient has two children under 15 years of age and will have no new children while on ART, each of these extra years of life averts about two years of orphanhood.[8] That would be about 7,000,000 years of orphanhood averted through 2009, a laudable achievement.

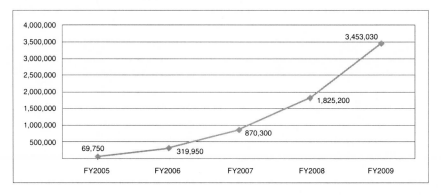

*Figure 8.3*   Estimated cumulated years of life saved through FY2009 due to PEPFAR support in 15 focus countries
SOURCE: OGAC (2007).

## B. U.S. is contributing its fair share on AIDS—if not elsewhere

U.S. citizens should be proud that their government has been the international leader in the altruistic effort to expand the availability of AIDS treatment. In view of the Bush administration's unwillingness to shoulder its share of the responsibility to prevent global warming, AIDS policy stands out as an area where the U.S. has taken the lead in assuming responsibility for a global problem—if not always in the way other countries would have preferred.[9]

The three panels of Figure 8.4 present three views of the magnitude of the U.S.'s effort to combat the international AIDS pandemic. Panel A shows that the U.S. is second among OECD countries in the percentage of its total ODA budget that it devotes to AIDS. Panel B shows that the U.S. contributes 45 percent of all OECD aid on AIDS, which is the same as its share of OECD GDP, but almost twice its 24 percent share of total aid from OECD countries.

Panel C presents the data from the previous two panels against a "Fairness Frontier." A country on the frontier is giving a share of total OECD development assistance which is in proportion to its share of total OECD income or GDP. Such a country could be viewed as giving its "fair share." Countries above the frontier are more generous relative to other OECD countries, and countries below it are stingier. The base of each arrow shows the fairness of each country's total aid contributions, and the arrow point shows its fairness for AIDS. Panel C shows that, despite its large contributions, the U.S. is less generous than most countries on total aid and exactly on the Fairness Frontier" in its AIDS contributions.[10] On at least this measure, the U.S. is performing better on AIDS than on overall foreign assistance—even if it compares less well on other dimensions of assistance.[11,12]

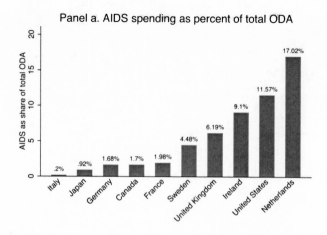

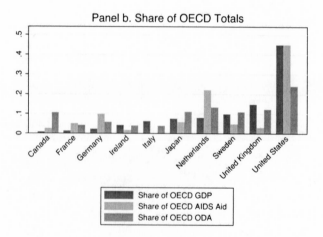

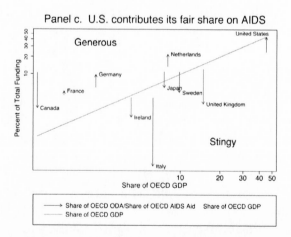

*Figure 8.4*   The U.S. has devoted a larger share of its assistance funding to AIDS than all but one of the other OECD countries. Panel A. AIDS spending as a percent of total ODA. Panel B. Share of OECD totals. Panel C. U.S. contributes its fair share on AIDS.
SOURCE: Data from Kates, Izazola, and Lief (2007) and OECD(5).

## C. U.S. assistance has made little measurable progress on prevention

Each prevented HIV infection saves many years of life in the protected individual and also has spillover benefits for all of society. It has been estimated that each dollar that Thailand invested in its HIV prevention program saved $43 dollars in avoided future treatment costs (Over et al. 2007; Revenga et al. 2006). By preventing these infections, Thailand also avoided millions of painful adult deaths and infected or orphaned children.

Despite the recognized priority of prevention in any disease control program, PEPFAR's enabling legislation first suggested, and then required, the agency to spend only 20 percent of its resources preventing future cases (Oomman, Bernstein, and Rosenzweig 2007b). Furthermore, PEPFAR was first asked, and then constrained, to spend two-thirds of those prevention resources on the A (abstinence) and B (be faithful) strategies, leaving only a third of the 20 percent, or less than 6 percent of overall funding, for use in reducing the riskiness of ongoing risky behavior (the "C" or condom-based strategy).

Since the 20 percent share for prevention was originally only a suggestion, PEPFAR actually spent more than 30 percent on prevention in its first year of operation. But as Figure 8.5 shows, in each subsequent year the share spent on prevention declined, until in 2006 the share reached the mandated 20 percent. Part of the reduction in prevention's share was due to the scaling up of expenditures on treatment. But Figure 8.6 shows that the reduction in prevention share was accompanied by a reduction in the magnitude of prevention spending in nine of 15 countries.[13]

According to law, PEPFAR's objective has been to save 7 million HIV infections by 2010 in the 15 focus countries. Over the five years of PEPFAR implementation, that would be 1.4 million infections per year. But the total number of infections per year in these countries is estimated by UNAIDS to be about 1.8 million a year. The contrast between the objective of achieving universal coverage for AIDS treatment and preventing only two out of three new HIV infections is stark. President Obama has an opportunity to push beyond PEPFAR by putting prevention on at least an equal footing with treatment. We suggest he declare a specific prevention goal as a *proportion* of total HIV infections rather than as an absolute number of infections averted. For example, he might propose that 90 percent of all HIV infections be prevented in the focus countries by 2016.

In order to provide evidence to Congress of the attainment of the percentage prevention goal, U.S. program staff would first have to work with other donors and the national government in each country to greatly improve existing estimates of the number of annual HIV infections. This effort would serve as the impetus for gathering the epidemiological data to discern where and among

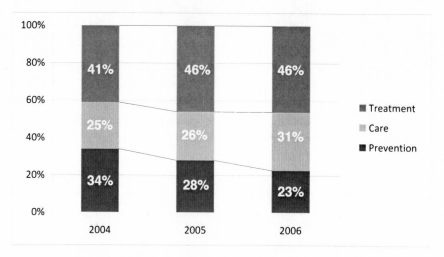

*Figure 8.5*  Prevention has declined from 33 percent to 23 percent of PEPFAR funding

whom HIV infections are spreading most rapidly, which is the first step of any successful prevention campaign.

PEPFAR's third report to Congress features its success at expanding three other prevention activities, prevention of transmission from mother to children, blood safety, and clean injections. However, since sexual transmission accounts for 80 to 90 percent of all infections in Africa, these seem like Pyrrhic victories (Institute of Medicine 2007, 137).

## III. Meeting Our Existing Commitments

If the U.S. is to maintain and enhance its reputation as an international leader in the area of AIDS funding, it must first keep up with the growing need for treatment and then consider strengthening its AIDS assistance program. Continuing to lead will require greatly increased expenditure and recognition that AIDS treatment expenditures will increasingly be viewed as an "international entitlement."

The term "entitlement" applies to a government expenditure program which engenders the expectation that current beneficiaries will continue to receive funding in future years. The expectation is created partly by the language of the authorizing legislation, which typically endows beneficiaries with the "right" to a continued flow of payments, and partly by the perception that the beneficiaries are vitally dependent on continuation of the funding. The domestic U.S. program that is most commonly described as an "entitlement" program is Social Security, any reduction of which entails a grave reputational and political risk

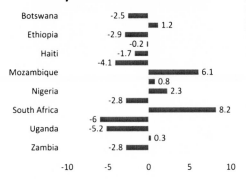

## Difference in PEPFAR Prevention Obligations, 2005/2006 current dollars

Botswana      -2.5
       1.2
Ethiopia      -2.9
    -0.2
Haiti      -1.7
    -4.1
Mozambique      6.1
    0.8
Nigeria      2.3
    -2.8
South Africa      8.2
    -6
Uganda      -5.2
    0.3
Zambia      -2.8

-10      -5      0      5      10

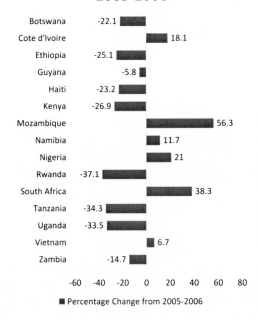

## Percentage Change from 2005-2006

Botswana      -22.1
Cote d'Ivoire      18.1
Ethiopia      -25.1
Guyana      -5.8
Haiti      -23.2
Kenya      -26.9
Mozambique      56.3
Namibia      11.7
Nigeria      21
Rwanda      -37.1
South Africa      38.3
Tanzania      -34.3
Uganda      -33.5
Vietnam      6.7
Zambia      -14.7

-60    -40    -20    0    20    40    60    80

■ Percentage Change from 2005-2006

*Figure 8.6*    PEPFAR spending on prevention declined in absolute terms in nine of 15 countries

SOURCE: Author's estimates based on data from the Center for Public Integrity described in (Oomman, Bernstein, and Rosenzweig 2007b). See Note 13.

for the politicians who propose it. Since the beneficiaries of PEPFAR's treatment component are foreign nationals, they are endowed legally with neither the right to continued funding nor the right to vote against U.S. politicians who would reduce their benefits. Nevertheless, because these beneficiaries are vitally dependent on continued receipt of AIDS treatment and linked to an international network of articulate AIDS treatment advocates, any withdrawal of treatment funding which threatens their lives will expose the governments of the U.S. and other donor countries to reputational risk at home and abroad and may threaten U.S. politicians at the ballot box.

To the extent that the U.S. is providing less than the entirety of AIDS treatment support in each of the 15 countries, the responsibility for any perceived entitlement might be shared with the other donors, reducing the reputation risk to the U.S. Figure 8.7 breaks out total external 2005 AIDS funding in the 15 PEPFAR focus countries between PEPFAR and all other donors. Across all 15 countries PEPFAR provided 77 percent of declared external AIDS funding in 2005.[14] While we do not know how this figure has evolved in all countries since 2005, in-depth study of three of these countries shows that PEPFAR's share has increased rather than decreased. According to Oomman et al., "The large majority of increases [in AIDS funding] since 2004, when spending began to rise most rapidly, can be attributed to PEPFAR alone. By 2006, PEPFAR money constituted 62 percent of HIV/AIDS resources in Zambia, 78 percent in Uganda and 78 percent in Mozambique" (Oomman, Bernstein, and Rosenzweig 2007a). In general, by carrying an average of more than three-quarters of the total external AIDS funding burden, and presumably at least as large a share of treatment spending, these AIDS treatment entitlements are incumbent upon the U.S. more than on any other donor or group of donors.

### A. The number of new HIV cases is growing faster than the number of people on treatment

The PEPFAR countries achieved extraordinary progress in increasing the numbers on treatment from a few hundred to 800,000 by 2006. On average these countries were able to roll out treatment to almost one-fifth of those who needed treatment in those countries each year. Figure 8.8 shows the projected future growth of people on treatment in the 15 PEPFAR countries under two scale-up assumptions, continued expansion at the historical rate of about 18 percent of unmet need each year and an acceleration to cover 95 percent of unmet need each year.[15] The left panel in the figure shows that even if the historical rate of increase continues, the number with unmet need for treatment in these countries, represented by the dotted line, continues to increase until about 2012. At that point, given the assumption that the rate of new cases of HIV infection declines steadily at 5 percent a year, unmet need would finally begin to fall. Under this scenario of historical expansion, the number on AIDS treatment in the focus countries will go from about 1.7 million at the beginning of President Obama's term to about 3.5 million by the time of the next presidential election. And by 2016, at the end of a possible second term, the number on treatment would be up to 5.4 million.[16]

But suppose that PEPFAR meets the demand to expand access much more rapidly, covering 95 percent of all unmet need in each future year. The right panel in the figure shows that this rate of expansion would dramatically reduce the unmet need for treatment (the dotted green line turns down and approaches the horizontal axis). Of course, the number on treatment rises much more rapidly, and many more premature deaths would be averted. Under the same assumption regarding new HIV infections, the PEPFAR countries will have about 4.6 million people under treatment in November 2008, rising to 10 million in 2012, and 15 million in 2016. In these 15 countries, most of these people will be able to thank the U.S. for their survival—or blame it, if the program falters.

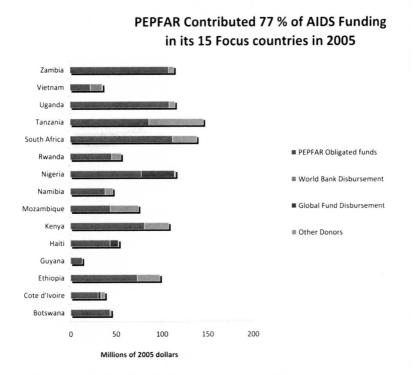

**PEPFAR Contributed 77 % of AIDS Funding in its 15 Focus countries in 2005**

*Figure 8.7*   2005 AIDS assistance received by 15 PEPFAR countries by donor (countries ranked by amount of PEPFAR 2005 spending)

SOURCE: Author's calculations based on data received from the three major donors and from the OECD database.

### B. Costs will rise dramatically, especially if PEPFAR expands to meet most of the unmet need for AIDS treatment

Growth in U.S.-funded treatment implies growth in costs. Figure 8.9 shows the cost expansion associated with the two scenarios depicted in the previous figure. The solid line represents the expanding cost of the treatment component of the PEPFAR program, which rises in the left panel from about $1.1 billion (2006 dollars) a year in 2008 to $2.4 billion in 2012 and $4.5 billion in 2016. The entire U.S. budget for overseas development assistance was $23 billion in 2006. So, if treatment is scaled up in these 15 countries at this historical rate, by 2016 the U.S. will have either increased its total overseas development assistance by 20 percent in order to sustain the AIDS treatment entitlement, or it will have reallocated about one-fifth of its budget to that use.[17]

Under this historical rate of expansion, the extra money that would be required to treat unmet need in any year, called the "funding gap" in the figure, rises from $1.8 billion in 2008 to $2.1 billion in 2012 and then falls to $1.9 billion in 2016. By this measure, the U.S. will only be funding about 40 percent of the need for ART treatment in 2008, rising to 70 percent by 2016. The dashed line shows the portion of total costs which must be spent on the small number of people on second-line therapy. Because the cost per patient is larger for those on second-line, and they steadily accumulate over time, total cost of second-line treatment grows faster than does the number of people on treatment.

The lower panel of Figure 8.9 shows how much faster AIDS spending will increase if President Obama accelerates U.S. support to cover 95 percent of unmet need each year. From $2.5 billion (2006 dollars) a year in 2008, expenditure would rise to $6 billion in 2012 and then to $11.6 billion in 2016. Thus, to achieve this faster scale-up of treatment through 2016, the country must either increase its total foreign assistance by roughly 50 percent, or it must reallocate half its assistance budget to AIDS spending. In this rapid scale-up scenario, AIDS treatment entitlements will consume somewhere between one-third and one-half of all development assistance.[18]

### C. Successfully treated patients accumulate over time and have an entitlement to more treatment

Although called an "emergency plan," PEPFAR will endure longer than most emergency programs and, unless the U.S. either abandons or hands over its patients to other funders, is likely to persist longer than most foreign assistance projects. As *The Economist* has pointed out,

> The problem with AIDS is that the more successful you are at treating it, the more you end up paying. That is because, unlike malaria and tuberculosis

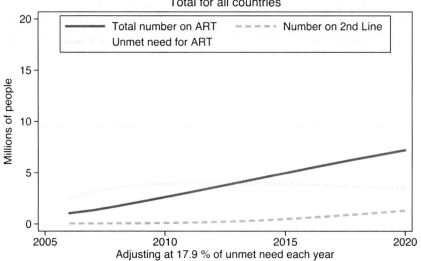

AIDS Treatment: Projected use and unmet need
Total for all countries

Adjusting at 17.9 % of unmet need each year

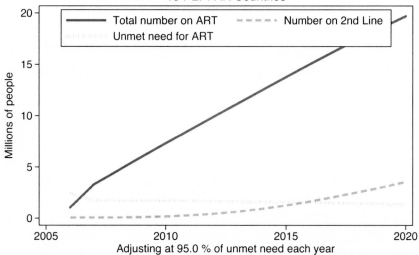

AIDS Treatment: Projected use and unmet need
15 PEPFAR Countries

Adjusting at 95.0 % of unmet need each year

*Figure 8.8*   The number of people on treatment grows much faster if access to treatment is accelerated. Panel A. Historical uptake at 17.9 percent of unmet need each year. Panel B. Aggressive uptake at 95 percent of unmet need each year.
SOURCE: Author's estimates.

(TB), it is incurable. Once someone is infected with HIV, the virus that causes it, they will end up requiring treatment for life. Good news for drug-makers, but bad news for both the poor who make up the overwhelming majority of the 40m people infected and for the taxpayers of the rich world who will be expected to find much of the money (*Economist* 2007).

Those people whose lives currently are sustained by donor funding of their AIDS treatment may feel that they are entitled to continuation of that treatment, that their donor has entered into an implicit contract to provide life-sustaining drugs in exchange for their conscientious adherence. Furthermore, international and domestic opinion will hold donors responsible for maintaining treatment subsidies to individuals who have already started treatment. As the largest national donor, the U.S. will be seen as particularly accountable for sustaining this life-giving therapy, especially in the 15 PEPFAR countries.

Discretionary spending is whatever is left in a budget after entitlements are funded. From the donors' perspective, the downside of growing entitlements—in the absence of a very large increase in the total aid budget—is that the proportion of discretionary spending in donors' AIDS budgets will decline as donors place more and more patients on treatment. From the recipients' side, the downside of entitlements is dependency. Those who receive entitlements typically become dependent on them and never more starkly than in the case of expensive life-giving drugs. There may be medium- and long-term negative repercussions from the extreme form of aid dependency that AIDS treatment represents.

Figure 8.10 projects the proportion of annual AIDS treatment expenditure that will be considered "entitlement" as coverage expands in both the historical and the ambitious expansion scenarios. In both scenarios, the percentage of total expenditure needed by continuing patients grows inexorably over time. That percentage starts lower in the more ambitious expansion scenario, because continuing patients represent a smaller portion of total expenditure.[19]

Because support for AIDS treatment converts foreign assistance from discretionary to entitlement spending, past treatment expenditure has already locked the U.S. and the rest of the donor countries into a new aid paradigm. Advocates point to the unmet need for care and call for ever increasing funding levels.[20] To the extent that the international community heeds the advocates' call for more resources, entitlement spending will greatly increase in the next few years. The increase will be both absolute and, unless total assistance expands at the same phenomenal rate, relative to total assistance.

Are voting taxpayers of the U.S. and other OECD countries ready for this new entitlement paradigm? Growing funding for AIDS treatment suggests this possibility. But there is reason for concern. Historically, when budgets expand less quickly than planned, growing entitlements often squeeze out discretionary programs. In

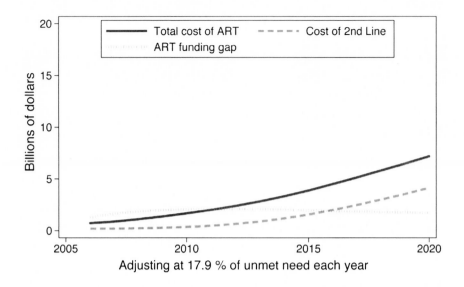

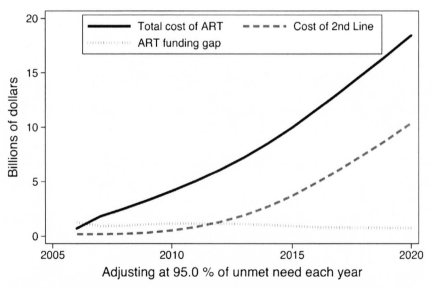

*Figure 8.9* The cost of AIDS treatment grows even faster than the number of treated especially if access to treatment is accelerated. Panel A. Historical uptake at 17.9 percent of unmet need each year. Panel B. Aggressive uptake at 95 percent of unmet need each year.

SOURCE: Author's estimates.

comparison to the moral imperative to continue funding AIDS treatment, HIV prevention *and* all other assistance programs will appear to be discretionary. So if the requested additional AIDS funds are not forthcoming, the discretionary assistance will be squeezed out. By one calculation, the $50 billion a year requested by UNAIDS from all donors to meet "universal access" objectives for treatment and prevention could squeeze out spending on all eight of the United Nations Millennium Development Goals.[21]

## IV. Reputation Risks Lie Ahead

Although reneging on entitlements would certainly be a reputation risk for the United States, maintaining AIDS treatment entitlements, or even scaling them up at current rates of increase, difficult and expensive as that will be, will not suffice to avoid such risks.

### A. Scaling up requires extending high quality treatment to less accessible populations

The cost projections in Figure 8.9 above assume constant average costs. This may seem to be a pessimistic assumption in view of the rapid decreases in drug costs that have occurred during the last decade. However, any future decreases in drug cost may be offset by the increased cost per patient necessary to scale up to reach full coverage targets. If the smallpox eradication program is a guide, reaching the last people with AIDS treatment may cost hundreds of times more per patient-year of extended life than reaching the first 25 percent. Furthermore, these cost projections do not consider the future demand for third-line and so-called "salvage" medications by those who fail second-line therapy. These medications are even more costly than the second-line therapies considered here.

Additionally, as shown in Figure 8.12, disinhibition could increase costs by as much as an additional 20 percent by substantially increasing the number of new people affected by HIV. So, on balance, it seems inconsistent to assume both rapid scale-up and continued decline in unit costs.

### B. Strong treatment programs may foster complacency and resentment in recipient countries

One potential risk from the AIDS component of the U.S. foreign assistance program to the reputations of President Obama and of the United States is that the benefits in terms of freely accessible AIDS treatment will be offset by a relaxation of prevention efforts or a "disinhibition" of risky sexual behavior.[22] A more subtle but potentially more insidiously dangerous risk is that the unusually

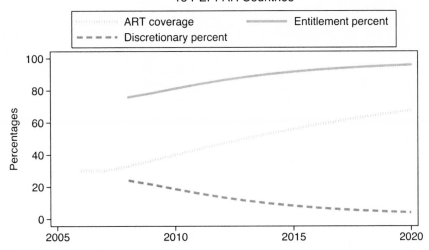

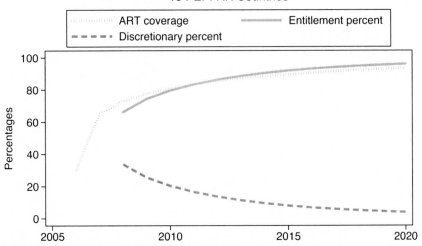

*Figure 8.10*   As coverage expands, the proportion of total expenditure that is an entitlement to existing AIDS patients also grows. Panel A. Historical uptake at 17.9 percent of unmet need each year. Panel B. Aggressive uptake at 95 percent of unmet need each year.

SOURCE: Author's estimates.

strong dependency created by U.S. funding of AIDS treatment may undermine the relationship between the U.S. and recipient countries.

## 1. COMPLACENCY IS AN UNDERSTANDABLE AND EVEN "RATIONAL" RESPONSE TO FREE AND ACCESSIBLE AIDS TREATMENT

As yet, there is little evidence of the effect of AIDS treatment on risk behavior of those at most risk of infection. There is accumulating evidence to show that treatment availability encourages people to find out their own infection status. But increased testing in response to treatment accessibility has not been convincingly shown to reduce high risk behavior among the HIV negative. Indeed, it may do the opposite depending on the knowledge and education of the individual.[23]

Visits to treatment centers in Africa turn up stories which illustrate the potentially perverse effect of free and effective AIDS treatment. For example, on a visit to a well-functioning AIDS treatment clinic in South Africa, a social worker cited the case of a woman who had asked for him to reveal which of the men were HIV positive—so that she could get infected from one of them and share in the disability payments and free food available to HIV-infected people in South Africa. Until more data is collected and analyzed, it is hard to know if such stories are representative of broader trends or are only rare and isolated, regrettable cases.[24] However, Figure 8.11 shows disturbing data from a cohort of Nairobi sex workers collected for more than a decade by a research team including researchers from the University of Manitoba. Is it only a coincidence that efforts to promote condom use suffered severe setbacks each time the press announced a supposed "cure" for AIDS? In the absence of more information, causality is hard to determine. But if news of a false cure, though expensive and hard to obtain, could persuade prostitutes to reduce condom use by almost 20 percent, what impact will a widely accessible and highly effective treatment have on risk behavior?[25]

Panels A and B of Figure 8.12 repeat the projections of Panels A and B of Figure 8.9 with one difference. Instead of declining at 5 percent a year, the annual rate of new infections (or, in epidemiologists' parlance, the incidence rate), increases by 15 percent each year. With historical uptake, the ART funding gap never turns down as it did in Panel A of Figure 8.6. With aggressive uptake, total expenditure reaches $25 billion a year instead of $18 billion a year at the end of the period.

## 2. ENTITLEMENTS MIGHT ENGENDER COMPLACENCY AND RESENTMENT

To the extent that AIDS treatment is viewed as an entitlement by all parties to the transaction—the donor governments and their citizens on the one hand, and the recipient governments and their patients on the other—the recipient governments and individuals might have diminished incentives to prevent HIV infection or to use efficiently the externally provided resources. Furthermore, it is human nature for people who are dependent on others to resent the dependency relationship.

In the extreme, it is possible that a strong AIDS program in these 15 countries will create a kind of postmodern colonial relationship between the U.S. and these countries, undermining the quality of these bilateral relationships. To take just one example, suppose the U.S. wishes a country to relinquish its rights under the WTO Trade-Related Aspects of Intellectual Property Rights (TRIPS) agreement. If millions of that country's citizens are dependent on the U.S. to fund their life-sustaining AIDS treatment, this will increase the U.S. bargaining power on this bilateral trade negotiation—and engender resentment among the government officials and the citizens of the recipient country.

### C. Individual HIV testing may aggravate the epidemic

Originally, HIV testing policies in developing countries were guided and circumscribed by the overriding ethical imperative to protect the emotional well-being and the confidentiality of tested individuals, leading to the policy of voluntary counseling and testing (VCT). This approach made sense in rich countries where prevalence rates in the general population were under 1 percent, and HIV infected people were likely to be stigmatized either as homosexuals or drug users. The epidemic's danger to public health was small, and the potential danger to the individual from stigmatization was large. However, in the worst affected countries today, the situation is reversed. With up to 30 percent of the population infected,

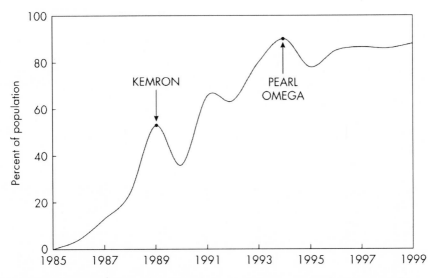

*Figure 8.11*   The announcement of false "cures" for AIDS in 1989 and 1994 apparently caused substantial reductions in condom use in a cohort of Nairobi prostitutes.
SOURCE: Adapted from Jha and Mills (2002), as cited in Over et al. (2004). Used with permission of WHO.

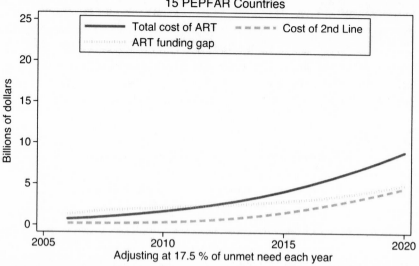

### AIDS Treatment: Projected cost & funding gap
#### 15 PEPFAR Countries

Adjusting at 17.5 % of unmet need each year

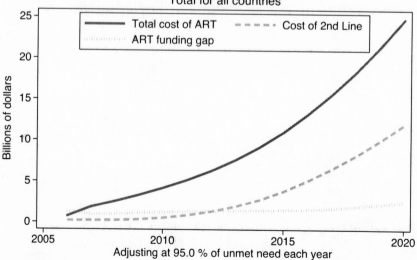

### AIDS Treatment: Projected cost & funding gap
#### Total for all countries

Adjusting at 95.0 % of unmet need each year

*Figure 8.12* If AIDS treatment disinhibits risk behavior, costs will grow even more rapidly. Panel A. Historical uptake at 17.5 percent of unmet need each year. Panel B. Aggressive uptake at 95 percent of unmet need each year.
SOURCE: Author's estimates.

the danger to the public health is astronomical. At the same time the danger of stigmatization, while still present, is receding day by day. And many of those who test positive can immediately be offered effective treatment in PEPFAR's focus countries. In response to this changed perception of costs and benefits, first Botswana and then other countries have shifted from the human rights-guided policy of individual-initiated "voluntary" counseling and testing for HIV to a public health-guided policy called "provider initiated testing," with little or no counseling for the majority who are HIV negative. This change seems to be supported by the Batswana public (Weiser et al. 2006).[26] Table 8.2 shows that this policy change has now occurred in most of the PEPFAR countries.

There is widespread and convincing anecdotal evidence that the shift to provider-initiated (or "opt-out") testing has speeded the recruitment into AIDS treatment of patients who might otherwise have waited too long before seeking treatment on their own. This policy shift is therefore almost certainly contributing to treatment success.

However, evidence is accumulating that expanded *individual* HIV testing is an imperfect prevention intervention. Many individuals who learn their HIV status seem to react by maintaining or even increasing their risk behavior.[27] For example, a review of 50 studies conducted in 1991 found mixed effects of voluntary counseling and testing (Higgins et al. 1991). Recent studies in the Rakai region of Uganda have found "no impact of VCT on subsequent risk behaviors or incidence" (Matovu et al. 2005).

Furthermore, those who have received multiple negative HIV tests (such as occurs with provider-initiated testing at every visit to a health center) were more likely to have more than two sexual partners and to use condoms inconsistently (Matovu et al. 2007). If this finding is replicated elsewhere, the expansion of provider-initiated testing driven by the availability of AIDS treatment might have the perverse effect of accelerating the epidemic.[28] Thus, it appears that a further more dramatic policy shift may be required, such as introducing and expanding couples testing. This policy option is discussed below.

### D. Expanding AIDS treatment may crowd out other health care

The extraordinary expansion of AIDS treatment currently underway in the worst affected countries is putting pressure on the supplies of all the factors of health care production, from nurses and doctors to health care facilities. There is currently a debate between those who believe that such pressures will undermine the health systems in these countries and those who maintain that improving AIDS care will have beneficial spillover effects on the rest of health care in these countries.

How much pressure will the worst affected countries actually experience? In order to understand the pressure that AIDS treatment will bring to bear on a country, it is necessary to relate the total amount of care needed to the supply of health care resources.[29] One easy way to do that is to construct a ratio between the two. Figure 8.13 presents the distribution of this ratio of need per physician for all the AIDS-affected countries in the world.

The distribution has three peaks and thus allows grouping the countries into three groups, according to the needed expenditure per physician in U.S. dollars. The group of countries on the right of the distribution, with need per physician larger than $1,778, will experience the most pressure. This is the part of the distribution which is inhabited by most of the 15 PEPFAR countries.

Figure 8.14 displays estimated current expenditure for the 15 PEPFAR countries plotted against the number of doctors in each country. Diagonal lines are drawn for equal burdens per physician of $100,000 (the upper line and $10,000 (the lower line). Botswana's health system must absorb the largest burden per physician as shown by its position to the northwest of the upper diagonal. Figure 8.15 superimposes the estimated need for AIDS expenditures on top of the estimated current expenditure. The arrow connecting the two is longer when need is a large multiple of current treatment. Note that if Mozambique and Tanzania

Table 8.2  Date of Adoption of Provider-initiated HIV Testing in 15 PEPFAR Focus Countries

| Country | Date of policy adoption |
| --- | --- |
| Botswana | 2003 |
| Côte d'Ivoire | — |
| Ethiopia | — |
| Guyana | 2006[1] |
| Haiti | — |
| Kenya | 2004 |
| Mozambique | — |
| Namibia | 2004[2] |
| Nigeria | — |
| Rwanda | 2006 |
| South Africa | — |
| Tanzania | 2006 |
| Uganda | 2005 |
| Vietnam | 2006 |
| Zambia | 2005[3] |

[1] Guyana's provider-initiated testing policy is for labor and delivery wards only.
[2] Namibia's provider-initiated testing policy is for PMTCT, antenatal clinics (ANC), and TB only and includes provision for non-laboratory personnel including community counselors to perform rapid HIV testing.
[3] Zambia adopted a PMTCT-specific provider-initiated testing policy in 2004.
SOURCE: Table 7 of OGAC (2007)

succeed in making ART available to all, their health systems must join Botswana's in absorbing more than $100,000 per physician.

If the PEPFAR program succeeds in expanding treatment to meet the need, each country will move up its arrow in Figure 8.15, and each of the physicians working in AIDS will have to manage the very large amounts of health care resources represented by the those arrows. Without changes in technology, this calculation suggests extreme stress on the health care systems of the worst affected countries. Some of the symptoms of this stress could be expected to be: physicians and nurses pulled out of non-AIDS care to focus exclusively on AIDS, reduced quality of care as individual physicians spread themselves too thinly, poor absorptive capacity of the health systems as doctors are unable to supervise such large quantities of resources, and increased leakage in the form of waste or corruption. All of these possibilities pose reputation risks for the donors viewed to be "at fault" (Piller and Smith 2007).

However, the situation is complicated by our inability to predict the future progression of the number of physicians in each country or the extent to which physicians will increase their "span of control" by supervising larger numbers of intermediate level health care personnel. Will the excess demand for the labor of health care specialists pull more of the country's brightest students into AIDS treatment (Clemens and Bazzi 2008)? If so, the dots representing the countries in Figure 8.12 will migrate towards the right as well as upward, and the burden per

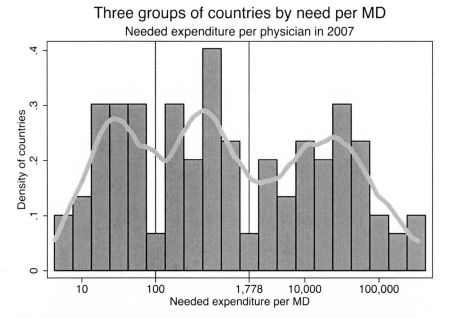

*Figure 8.13*    Distribution of needed AIDS treatment expenditure per physician
SOURCE: Author's estimates.

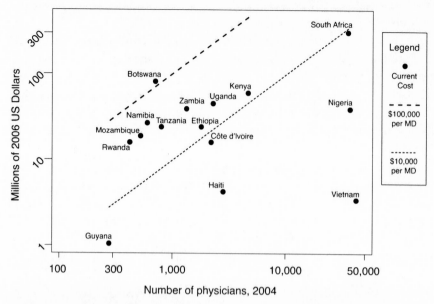

*Figure 8.14*   Estimated current AIDS expenditure is more than $10,000 per physician for 9 of the 15 PEPFAR countries

SOURCE: Author's estimates with WHO data on numbers of physicians in 2004, the latest year available.

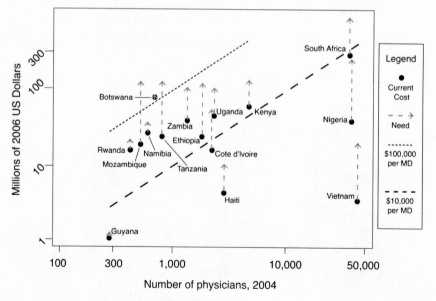

*Figure 8.15*   Needed AIDS expenditure is more than $100,000 per physician in Mozambique, Botswana, and Tanzania

SOURCE: Author's estimates with WHO data on numbers of physicians in 2004, the latest year available.

physician will be smaller. Will AIDS funding be accompanied with funding for the rest of the health care system so that patients with other health problems also benefit (Price et al. 2007)? If so, then the extraordinary increase of disease-specific funding will have few pernicious effects on the health system.

On the other hand, if health care personnel leave these countries in search of better wages faster than more can be trained, then the burden will be larger (Bärnighausen, Bloom, and Humair 2007). More research is needed to understand how severely these countries are burdened by the effort to treat all AIDS patients while maintaining their services to other patients.

## V. From an Emergency Plan to a Sustainable Policy

Foreign assistance can be classified into four types, which have different objectives and different justifications. Emergency relief and redistributive welfare programs are intended to extend a helping hand to our unfortunate neighbors out of empathy, because "there but for the grace of God go I." Military assistance is offered sometimes out of empathy for the plight of another people but more often to bolster the national security and further the strategic interests of the donor country. Development programs and projects constitute the fourth category which is intended to stimulate the economic growth of the recipient country on the grounds that, "it is better to teach a man to fish than to give him a fish every day."

While there is a growing literature on the investment benefits of programs to combat AIDS, there is only weak support for the proposition that subsidized AIDS treatment for the poorest AIDS patients will stimulate national growth—except in the health sector where it is rumored to have substantially augmented doctors' incomes. The attempts to expand U.S. support for AIDS treatment during the Clinton administration were justified on national security grounds. An innovation of the Bush presidency was to largely eschew national security as a justification for the PEPFAR program. Instead, the Bush administration used the AIDS program as the prime international exhibit for its vaunted philosophy of "compassionate conservatism." As its name signifies, PEPFAR was originally justified primarily as an emergency plan. However, the fact that it is creating entitlements which most recipient countries could not shoulder and is hard to justify on investment grounds suggests that it is really an international transfer program, comparable perhaps to U.S. food assistance.[30] Programs to redistribute resources from the U.S. taxpayers to the poor in developing countries constitute state-supported international welfare programs.

Our recommendations are grouped under three headings: manage the AIDS treatment entitlement, prevent the future need for treatment, and assure the "AIDS transition."

## A. Manage the AIDS treatment entitlement

In order to make space in the AIDS budget for HIV prevention spending, which is the only existing technology for reducing the need for treatment, and to avoid the reputation risk of failed support for AIDS treatment, the president must wisely manage the treatment entitlements that he inherited from the Bush administration.

### 1. MAXIMIZE SUCCESS OF ONGOING TREATMENT

As an assistance program expands and matures, it can become encumbered by leakages and inefficiencies. In the case of AIDS treatment, these problems would mean loss of patient life, increased resort to second-line therapies, and the consequent expense and increased transmission of drug-resistant strains of HIV. To prevent U.S.-funded AIDS treatment in the focus countries from suffering this fate, the U.S. must assure the effective supervision of AIDS treatment personnel and supplies in the 15 countries. Furthermore, the U.S. should provide small start-up funds for the formation of patient-managed adherence support organizations.[31] Such groups would help slow the development of drug resistance not only for antiretroviral medications but for medications against malaria and TB and even for antibiotics. Such demand-side mechanisms can help assure quality treatment in the private sector, where command and control supervision does not reach.

### 2. REDUCE UNIT COSTS OF TREATMENT

While the continuing drive to extend treatment to almost all who need it will drive up unit costs, U.S. support for AIDS interventions should work to bring down unit costs in other ways. President Obama should actively collaborate with the WHO's program to certify generic versions of antiretrovirals for use in PEPFAR countries and should cooperate with the Clinton Foundation's efforts to lower drug prices through long-term contracts for large quantities. As a last resort, when patent holders fail to "sufficiently" reduce their prices for poor countries, the U.S. should support compulsory licensing of AIDS drugs by poor countries and by third-party countries such as Canada which can then export to poor countries. The U.S. should cease using bilateral trade agreements to constrain the use of compulsory licenses for treating diseases that are specific to poor countries (Fink and Elliot 2007).

### 3. LIMIT THE EXPANSION OF AIDS TREATMENT ENTITLEMENTS

In view of the reputational risk to the U.S. of AIDS treatment entitlements, the new president should moderate the expansion of treatment entitlements to new beneficiaries while at the same time he upholds and even strengthens existing ones. Several strategies for limiting the imprudent expansion of entitlements are available. First, the president should resist the pressure to expand the number of focus countries targeted by PEPFAR. This group of countries already accounts for almost half of existing AIDS cases and more than half of new cases worldwide. The U.S. should concentrate on doing a good job in these countries at least through the next two presidential terms, leaving the rest of the donor countries, the Global Fund, and other mechanisms to deal with the other countries.[32] If the U.S. does a good job in these countries, spillovers to the other countries will benefit the rest of the world, whereas poor performance in the focus countries will cast a shadow on treatment efforts in other countries. Examples of benefits that would spill over from focus countries to their neighbors include low generic drug prices, lessons about what works in treatment and prevention, reduced stigma for AIDS patients, and safer norms of sexual behavior.

Limiting expansion of AIDS treatment in the 15 countries to the rate of increase that PEPFAR has achieved up to now would require the AIDS treatment budget to grow as in Panel A of Figure 8.16, to about $5 billion per year in 2016 and $7 billion per year in 2020. This rate of expansion saves $7 billion a year in 2016 to $10 billion per year in 2020, compared to the aggressive uptake scenario in Panel B—money which can be spent on urgently needed HIV prevention and on strengthening the health care systems of the recipient countries.[33]

A second strategy open to the president for limiting the growth of U.S. entitlements is to increase the proportion of U.S.-financed AIDS funding that passes through multilateral institutions, including the Global Fund and the World Bank. Not only does this strategy shift the entitlement from the U.S. government to the multilateral institutions, but it can benefit the recipient nations and patients by stimulating competition on the ground among alternative AIDS treatment and prevention institutions. The HIV/AIDS Monitor project (Center for Global Development 2007b), which compares the performance of the three largest AIDS funders in three countries, already shows how recipient countries benefit when the evaluators can compare the funders to one another.

Figure 8.17 shows the percentage of AIDS financing that passes through the Global Fund for each of the OECD donors. The U.S. is ranked sixth in the group, passing only about 17 percent of its resources through the Global Fund. There is room for substantial expansion here.

### 4. SUPPORT THE CREATION OF A GLOBAL HEALTH CORPS

As the U.S. continues to extend AIDS care in the 15 PEPFAR countries, the burden on the existing health care systems will grow more and more onerous. From the current levels of more than $10,000 per physician, expansion will soon require expenditures of up to $100,000 per physician each year (see Figure 8.15). This additional burden on top of the existing health care needs threatens to divert

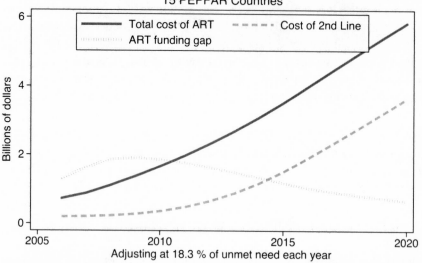

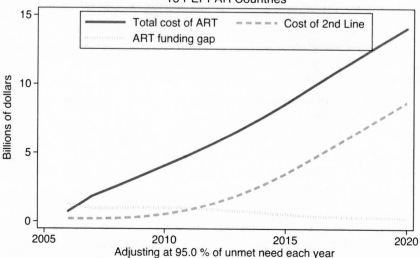

*Figure 8.16* The cost of AIDS treatment grows even faster than the number of treated especially if access to treatment is accelerated. Panel A. Historical uptake at 18 percent of unmet need each year. Panel B. Aggressive uptake at 95 percent of unmet need each year. SOURCE: Author's estimates.

resources away from patients suffering from other health problems (Piller and Smith 2007).

While one obvious answer to this problem is for the U.S. to support general health system strengthening like that documented in Rwanda (Price et al. 2007), more is needed. The president should support the creation and deployment of a global Health Corps (Levine 2008). A key feature of this Corps is its offer to fill the most serious gaps in the health care needs of the host country, not just contribute to AIDS treatment. By responding to requests to send American health care personnel to PEPFAR countries and by bringing selected members of those countries' medical professionals to the U.S. for a year of study, the president will be demonstrating the country's willingness to engage its most valuable resource—its own people—in the struggle against the health problems of the PEPFAR countries.

## B. Prevent the future need for treatment

The old proverb that an ounce of prevention is worth a pound of cure has never been truer than it is now with the AIDS epidemic.[34] The president should propose a dramatic new objective: *prevention of 90 percent of new infections in the focus countries by the year 2012.* Since the current number of new infections each year in the 15 focus countries is about 1.4 million, this goal would commit the U.S. to reducing this number to about 140,000 by the year 2016. Establishment of such a goal recognizes the superior cost-effectiveness of prevention in

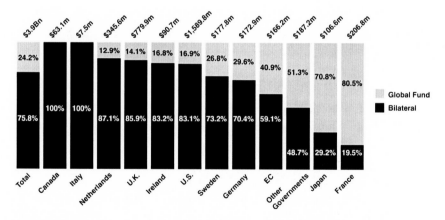

*Figure 8.17* The U.S. should channel more than the current 17 percent of AIDS resources through the Global Fund

SOURCE: Kates, Izazola, and Lief (2007). This information was reprinted with permission from the Henry J. Kaiser Family Foundation. The Kaiser Family Foundation is a non-profit private operating foundation, based in Menlo Park, California, dedicated to producing and communicating the best possible analysis and information on health issues.

the long run and commits the country to developing and applying interventions and measurement tools which will advance the prevention agenda and measure its progress.[35]

### 1. PREVENTION WILL EVENTUALLY SAVE MONEY

Because every new HIV infection adds to the AIDS treatment burden five to ten years later, it is becoming a fiscal imperative to slow the progress of HIV infections. Figure 8.9 above showed how the treatment burden would grow if HIV infection rates decline by only 5 percent each successive year. Figure 8.18 shows the effects of a more dramatic decline of 90 percent each year. If the U.S. is able to help the 15 focus countries to slow the growth of HIV by this much starting in 2008, and the rate of treatment uptake is maintained at 18 percent of unmet need each year, by 2020 the cost of treatment will be smaller by about $1.4 billion a year, releasing resources for discretionary foreign assistance objectives.[36]

The imperative to strengthen HIV prevention programs is reinforced not only by the cost of treatment, but also by the possibility that access to treatment may itself speed infection. As pointed out above, free access to widely available and demonstrably effective treatment can engender complacency leading to the disinhibition of risk behavior. Following the Hippocratic injunction to "first, do no harm," the U.S. must strengthen prevention programs at least in focus countries.

A possible unintended consequence of the rapid and effective rollout of ART in PEPFAR focus countries may be to attract immigration from neighboring countries where AIDS treatment is less accessible. Because successful prevention in those neighboring countries will eventually slow that influx of AIDS patients to PEPFAR countries, PEPFAR should also contribute to prevention programs in countries bordering with PEPFAR countries.

### 2. SUPPORT PROMISING PREVENTION OPPORTUNITIES

Much has been published about prevention strategies, and this is not the place to review all the options. It is depressing and even scandalous that after more than 20 years of donor-funded prevention efforts, so few prevention interventions have been rigorously evaluated (Wegbreit et al. 2006). Five neglected prevention strategies that seem both technically and politically feasible, based on current knowledge, deserve particular attention in PEPFAR countries: (i) improved targeting of prevention efforts in places frequented by those at most risk of contracting and transmitting the infection; (ii) the mobilization for HIV prevention of the people who receive U.S.-funded AIDS treatment; (iii) the expansion of access to male circumcision; (iv) the integration of family planning services with HIV testing and AIDS treatment; and (v) the reorientation of HIV testing toward in-home services for couples, rather than facility-based testing of individuals.

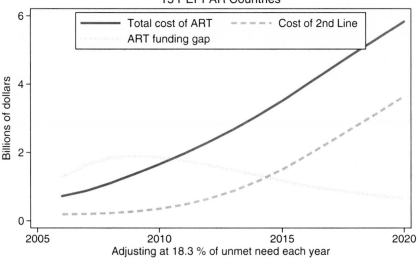

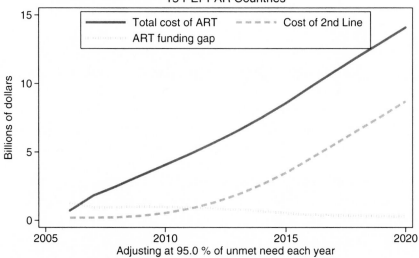

*Figure 8.18* Cost projection of AIDS treatment in 15 PEPFAR countries if rate of new infections decreases by 90 percent a year. Panel A. Historical uptake. Panel B. Aggressive uptake.

SOURCE: Author's estimates.

a. Target HIV prevention efforts to hot spots

The first step in a successful prevention campaign is to gather the epidemiological data to discern where and among whom HIV infections are spreading most rapidly. As the Institute of Medicine (IOM) points out in its recent assessment of PEPFAR's implementation, PEPFAR has never done the basic survey work that would be required to monitor its own progress on prevention (Institute of Medicine 2007). In the words of the IOM report,

> PEPFAR and other U.S. government-funded programs before it have supported the collection, analysis and appropriate application of both sentinel and behavioral surveillance data in many of the focus countries. . . .However, only a few of the countries have conducted behavioral surveys focused specifically on high risk populations. Without behavioral data on these populations it is difficult for countries and donors to know what specific factors are driving each epidemic and what particular interventions would be the most successful for each country in preventing further spread of HIV (Institute of Medicine 2007, 133).

There are a variety of techniques for reaching high risk populations with the needed interventions which promote and distribute condoms and train people in their effective use. Unfortunately, few of these techniques benefit from the rigorous impact evaluation that has been exercised on biomedical prevention techniques or treatment interventions (Wegbreit et al. 2006; Lagakos and Gable 2008). The great success of the 100 percent condom program in Thailand in the 1980s was predicated on the existence of brothels which were active and easily identifiable foci for an effective prevention campaign (Ainsworth and Over 1997). A technique called the "PLACE Method" was developed in the last ten years to achieve the same objective in African epidemiological contexts (Weir et al. 2002; Weir et al. 2003; Weir et al. 2004). The method uses interviewers' contacts with taxi drivers, market women, and other people in the street to identify the so-called "hot spots" in the town where people gather to look for a date. Although the formative research to develop this technique and field test it in a dozen African cities was funded by USAID, neither that agency nor PEPFAR has attempted to evaluate the method using rigorous impact evaluation methods or scale up its implementation in order to saturate all or any region of any African country with prevention messages and condoms.

b. Mobilize AIDS patients for HIV prevention

It is easy to misunderstand the intent of this suggestion. Doctors will tell you that they are already counseling their patients in safe sex and suggest that more effort like this is the kind of mobilization that is needed. A study on ART patients in Côte d'Ivoire showed no increase in self-reported risk behavior among ART patients who were counseled to maintain safe behavior (Katzenstein, Laga, and Moatti 2003). However, we know from biological studies that patients who are effectively adhering to antiretroviral medication are in any case less likely to transmit infection during unprotected sex. The challenge lies elsewhere.

Patients who, thanks to their precise adherence to their medication regime, are in good health can be an important channel for reaching out to the much larger population of people whose risk behavior places them in danger of infection. With proper training, motivation, and monitoring, patients can work to assure that AIDS treatment does not engender complacency and disinhibition among non-patients, but instead encourages reductions in their risk behavior.

One way to use such patients would be to build on the adherence support organizations mentioned above. When multiple adherence support organizations exist in a community, they can be judged against one another not only by their success at maintaining adherence among their members, but also on their efforts to reach out to non-members with HIV prevention interventions. Organizations which do well only on adherence would not lose their funding; reducing their funding might disrupt the treatment of their members. But neither would such poor performers receive funding to enroll additional members. Organizations which excel at both adherence support and outreach prevention would, on the other hand, be rewarded with funding for additional members. In this way, through a process of muted competition among treatment support organizations, treatment subsidies would also be leveraging prevention efforts in the places that need both.

### c. Expand access to male circumcision

The evidence that male circumcision (MC) protects men from HIV infection has accumulated now from both observational and experimental studies. The first observational study was the cross-country regression by Bongaarts and co-authors in 1989 (Bongaarts et al. 1989), and showed a remarkable association between MC prevalence and HIV prevalence. Skeptics expressed doubt regarding the causal link since MC prevalence was correlated with religious affiliation, which might be directly responsible for differences in HIV prevalence because of religious differences in sexual mores. For example, one cross-section study of HIV prevalence found that prevalence of MC was statistically insignificant, when percent-Muslim and seven other socioeconomic variables were controlled for (Over 1998).[37] However, in the last few years, randomized controlled trials in Uganda (Gray et al. 2007), South Africa (Auvert et al. 2006), and Kenya (Bailey et al. 2007) have confirmed that the association between MC and HIV is indeed causal. For example, the ethical review process halted the Kenyan trial after observing that 22 of the 1,391 circumcised men became HIV infected compared to 47 among the 1,393 in the uncircumcised group. Since the risk of becoming infected during the trial period was 53 percent smaller for the circumcised, the researchers concluded that MC is comparable to a 50 percent effective vaccination. Circumcision seemed to be equally protective in Uganda (51 percent reduction in risk) and perhaps more so in South Africa (60 percent reduction in risk).[38] Furthermore, none of the studies was able to find evidence that circumcised men might be "disinhibited," increasing their risky behavior and thereby offsetting some of the advantage of the circumcision.

As the encouraging results on MC have accumulated, researchers have increasingly turned from the question of efficacy to that of feasibility. Small scale nonrandom studies have generally supported the feasibility of scaling up MC access to the general population in Africa.[39] Building on these research results, PEPFAR should now allocate a substantial portion of its discretionary resources to making clean and safe circumcision at least as easily accessible to men as antiretroviral therapy in all the PEPFAR countries.

### d. Integrate family planning with AIDS treatment

Another key strategy to prevent infections, which has not been sufficiently deployed, is family planning. While programs to prevent mother-to-child transmission (PMTCT) of HIV are having increased success, they are still difficult and complicated. Every child that is infected, despite PMTCT efforts, will be costly to treat for his or her entire life. Furthermore, such children stand a greater than average chance of becoming orphans, despite the efficacy and increased availability of AIDS treatment.

In view of the private and social cost incurred for each HIV-infected child, AIDS treatment programs and family planning programs should join forces to assure that every HIV-positive woman has free and easy access to the birth control method of her choice, without fear of stigmatization. Unfortunately, due to the lack of integration of family planning and AIDS treatment, there appears to be substantial unmet need for contraception among HIV-positive women. As early as 1993, a study found that 60 percent of HIV-positive women would prefer not to have more children (Allen et al. 1993). Medical intervention to prevent mother-to-child transmission of HIV once pregnancy has occurred has been found to be less than or equally cost-effective as family planning in several studies (Reynolds et al. 2006; Stover et al. 2003; Sweat et al. 2004). In a letter to the editor of *Sexually Transmitted Infections*, three of the authors of these studies point out that the existing low levels of contraception in sub-Saharan Africa have probably prevented 173,000 HIV-infected births each recent year, and that provision of family planning services to the those with unmet need can avert an additional 160,000 HIV-positive births every year (Reynolds, Steiner, and Cates 2005).[40]

e. Reorient HIV testing toward couples

As a supplement to provider-initiated testing, PEPFAR should evaluate the feasibility and effectiveness of widescale couple counseling in the home. While couple counseling has been found to be effective with discordant couples (where one is HIV infected) (Allen et al. 1992a; Allen et al. 1992b; Allen et al. 1993; Padian et al. 1993; Roth et al. 2001), it has an even more promising role for concordant-negative couples, in which neither person is yet infected. Furthermore, a few studies suggest that people are more likely to accept couple counseling in their home than at health care facilities (Farquhar et al. 2004; Matovu et al. 2002; Were et al. 2003). When couples learn each others' HIV status as well as their own and receive counseling about the dangers of unprotected sex outside the couple, such knowledge might not only increase condom use with other partners but also reduce the frequency of such partners. Thus, couple counseling, especially couple counseling in a couple's home, might be the intervention that would achieve Helen Epstein's elusive "invisible cure," by discouraging the practice of multiple concurrent partnerships thought to be a major contributor to the epidemic (Epstein 2007; Halperin and Epstein 2004; Morris and Kretzschmar 1997).

## C. Ensure the AIDS Transition

Just as there have been demographic transitions and epidemiologic transitions which have occurred in the past, the world can aspire to accomplish an "AIDS Transition" in the next few decades.[41] What would an AIDS transition encompass?

First, in the epidemiological dimension, an AIDS transition would see the growth of the number of people infected with HIV decrease below the growth of the number of people on treatment. Even with the enormous progress in the last few years, the number of people placed on treatment worldwide in 2007 was only about one-fourth the number of new HIV infections that year. So to accomplish the AIDS Transition, we will need to both accelerate treatment access *and* greatly reduce the rate of new infections.

As outlined above, for the PEPFAR program the AIDS Transition can mean the program's gradual transformation from a predominately bilateral program to a more multilateral one. If the prevention part of the AIDS Transition is to succeed in PEPFAR countries, the millions of people receiving AIDS treatment must be used as a force for the dramatic expansion and improved effectiveness of prevention programs.

*More generally the AIDS Transition must mean a refocusing of the rhetoric, goal-setting, and results orientation that is gaining force in AIDS treatment to target also AIDS prevention.* The U.S. president should assure that the successor to WHO's unsuccessful "3 by 5" program to expand treatment to three million by 2005 and its current program "Towards Universal Access by 2010" will be a program aimed at *preventing 90 percent of current annual infections by 2012*. Such a program should use all means available—including schools, adherence support groups, and local governments. Measures of success must use biological markers of risk behavior like pregnancy, HIV infection, or infection with another sexually transmitted infection, not just self-reports.

The most forward looking part of the AIDS Transition will be to broaden U.S. research funding on AIDS. Because NIH's mandate is to focus on biomedical research, the critical questions of how to scale up treatment programs and how to improve the effectiveness and reach of prevention programs are underresearched (Institute of Medicine 2007; Klag 2007). The next U.S. president should ask Congress to channel 10 percent of all AIDS research funding to health services research on the effective delivery of HIV/AIDS prevention and treatment services in a manner that complements, rather than undermines, other locally needed health care services.

President Bush's "emergency" AIDS assistance program to 15 of the countries affected by the epidemic is in the best, generous traditions of American foreign assistance. PEPFAR has already prolonged the lives of more than a million people, provided care and support for orphans and other vulnerable children, and prevented many cases of HIV infection. Although the evidence is not yet in on the program's effects on the health care systems of all recipients, some countries' systems seem to have benefited from positive spillover effects from PEPFAR. Together with the Millennium Challenge Account, PEPFAR is arguably the Bush administration's most notable foreign policy success.

However, the research and analysis presented in this chapter suggest that the potential for several serious failures lies hidden within this apparent success. If the U.S. is seen to renege on its implied commitment to existing AIDS patients, or if it is thought to have allowed treatment quality to degrade over time, failed to prevent new cases of HIV infection from swelling the ranks of those needing treatment, harmed the health care of patients who do not have AIDS, or facilitated the emergence and spread of drug-resistant forms of HIV, President Bush's initial success will metamorphose before our eyes into a deadly and shameful example of overreaching American incompetence—to be blamed inevitably on President Obama. We argue that the president can build on PEPFAR in such a way as to prevent these worst-case scenarios. If, in the existing 15 PEPFAR focus countries, the next government can effectively manage the current AIDS treatment entitlement, prevent future need for treatment, and help ensure the AIDS transition to the point that the disease becomes a manageable, chronic condition, then President Obama will deserve a full measure of credit for the long-run benefits of PEPFAR, credit equal to or greater than that due to President Bush for launching the program. This chapter has suggested some of the specific ways that President

Obama and his successors can avoid the worst-case scenarios and assure this desirable outcome.

## Annex A. A model for projecting future AIDS treatment costs

Parameters of the projection model for predicting future AIDS treatment expenditures

| | | |
|---|---|---|
| Proportion of HIV+ newly eligible for ART | erate | .11 |
| ART Death Rate during first year on 1st line | adrate1 | .13 |
| ART Death Rate during subsequent years on 1st line | adrate2 | .04 |
| ART Death Rate of AIDS patients on 2nd line | bdrate | .01 |
| Non-ART Death Rate of AIDS patients | ndrate | .3 |
| Starting coverage rate for 2nd line ART[42] | strtcov2 | .05 |
| Target coverage rate for 2nd line ART | trgtcov2 | .95 |
| 2nd line ART to reach target in year | trgtyr | 2016 |

Scale-up of 1st line modeled as constant proportion
(1 - lambda) of unmet need, where lambda is constant
across all countries and equal to:

| | | |
|---|---|---|
| Historical scale up | lambda = | .82 |
| Rapid scale up | lambda = | .05 |
| Annual cost per patient of first-line drugs[43] | | $227 |
| Annual cost per patient of second-line drugs | | $2,681 |
| Annual cost per patient of clinic time | | $278 |

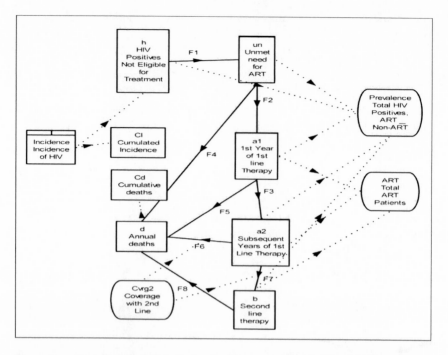

*Figure 8.19*    Flow diagram for predicting the future growth of AIDS treatment costs
SOURCE: Author's construction using ModelMaker software. See White (2007) for discussion of appropriate parameter values for the model and the Spectrum projection model for an alternative modeling platform: http://www.futuresinstitute.org/. On cost assumptions, see Bollinger, Stover, and UNAIDS (2007)

# Annex B

*Table 8.A.1*  Projected annual cost of treating AIDS patients in 15 focus countries by uptake and prevention scenarios (Thousands of 2006 U.S. dollars).

| | Costs of AIDS treatment at historical uptake & 90% reduction in incidence each year | | | | Costs of AIDS treatment at historical uptake & 5% reduction in incidence each year | | |
|---|---|---|---|---|---|---|---|
| | 1st line | 2nd line | Total cost | | 1st line | 2nd line | Total cost |
| 2006 | 529,785 | 191,727 | 721,512 | 2006 | 529,785 | 191,727 | 721,512 |
| 2007 | 673,329 | 201,623 | 874,952 | 2007 | 673,329 | 201,623 | 874,952 |
| 2008 | 874,949 | 227,439 | 1,102,388 | 2008 | 874,949 | 227,439 | 1,102,388 |
| 2009 | 1,093,394 | 274,306 | 1,367,700 | 2009 | 1,093,394 | 274,306 | 1,367,700 |
| 2010 | 1,303,451 | 353,146 | 1,656,597 | 2010 | 1,316,705 | 353,146 | 1,669,851 |
| 2011 | 1,493,607 | 474,165 | 1,967,772 | 2011 | 1,537,707 | 474,165 | 2,011,872 |
| 2012 | 1,659,169 | 645,144 | 2,304,313 | 2012 | 1,752,010 | 646,776 | 2,398,786 |
| 2013 | 1,799,050 | 871,376 | 2,670,426 | 2013 | 1,956,904 | 879,399 | 2,836,303 |
| 2014 | 1,914,054 | 1,155,985 | 3,070,039 | 2014 | 2,150,721 | 1,179,388 | 3,330,109 |
| 2015 | 2,005,932 | 1,500,249 | 3,506,181 | 2015 | 2,332,462 | 1,553,030 | 3,885,492 |
| 2016 | 2,076,820 | 1,903,999 | 3,980,819 | 2016 | 2,501,578 | 2,005,589 | 4,507,167 |
| 2017 | 2,128,992 | 2,324,288 | 4,453,280 | 2017 | 2,657,823 | 2,493,208 | 5,151,031 |
| 2018 | 2,164,638 | 2,756,281 | 4,920,919 | 2018 | 2,801,161 | 3,012,715 | 5,813,876 |
| 2019 | 2,185,840 | 3,195,719 | 5,381,559 | 2019 | 2,931,717 | 3,560,905 | 6,492,622 |
| 2020 | 2,194,497 | 3,638,869 | 5,833,366 | 2020 | 3,049,732 | 4,134,636 | 7,184,368 |
| | | | Least costly | | | | |
| Total | 24,097,507 | 19,714,316 | 43,811,823 | Total | 28,159,977 | 21,188,052 | 49,348,029 |
| By presidential term | | | | | | | |
| '09-'12 | 5,549,621 | 1,746,761 | 7,296,382 | | 5,699,816 | 1,748,393 | 7,448,209 |
| '13-'16 | 7,795,856 | 5,431,609 | 13,227,465 | | 8,941,665 | 5,617,406 | 14,559,071 |

*(continued)*

*Table 8.A.1*  Projected annual cost of treating AIDS patients in 15 focus countries by uptake and prevention scenarios (Thousands of 2006 US dollars). (continued)

| | Costs of AIDS treatment at rapid uptake & 90% reduction in incidence each year | | | | Costs of AIDS treatment at rapid uptake & 5% reduction in incidence each year | | |
| --- | --- | --- | --- | --- | --- | --- | --- |
| | 1st line | 2nd line | Total cost | | 1st line | 2nd line | Total cost |
| 2006 | 529,785 | 191,727 | 721,512 | 2006 | 529,785 | 191,727 | 721,512 |
| 2007 | 1,635,364 | 201,623 | 1,836,987 | 2007 | 1,635,364 | 201,623 | 1,836,987 |
| 2008 | 2,307,005 | 227,439 | 2,534,444 | 2008 | 2,307,005 | 227,439 | 2,534,444 |
| 2009 | 2,970,273 | 335,242 | 3,305,515 | 2009 | 2,970,273 | 335,242 | 3,305,515 |
| 2010 | 3,528,288 | 537,685 | 4,065,973 | 2010 | 3,604,610 | 537,685 | 4,142,295 |
| 2011 | 3,989,774 | 857,925 | 4,847,699 | 2011 | 4,206,920 | 857,925 | 5,064,845 |
| 2012 | 4,366,528 | 1,308,550 | 5,675,078 | 2012 | 4,775,381 | 1,317,404 | 6,092,785 |
| 2013 | 4,669,214 | 1,896,367 | 6,565,581 | 2013 | 5,308,801 | 1,935,101 | 7,243,902 |
| 2014 | 4,907,290 | 2,624,207 | 7,531,497 | 2014 | 5,806,506 | 2,727,520 | 8,534,026 |
| 2015 | 5,089,106 | 3,491,710 | 8,580,816 | 2015 | 6,268,233 | 3,708,719 | 9,976,952 |
| 2016 | 5,222,058 | 4,496,040 | 9,718,098 | 2016 | 6,694,088 | 4,890,296 | 11,584,384 |
| 2017 | 5,312,678 | 5,530,143 | 10,842,821 | 2017 | 7,084,481 | 6,156,945 | 13,241,426 |
| 2018 | 5,366,727 | 6,583,190 | 11,949,917 | 2018 | 7,440,050 | 7,500,065 | 14,940,115 |
| 2019 | 5,389,291 | 7,645,843 | 13,035,134 | 2019 | 7,761,645 | 8,911,297 | 16,672,942 |
| 2020 | 5,384,857 | 8,710,115 | 14,094,972 | 2020 | 8,050,268 | 10,382,518 | 18,432,786 |
| | | | | | | | Most costly |
| Total | 60,668,238 | 44,637,806 | 105,306,044 | Total | 74,443,410 | 49,881,506 | 124,324,916 |
| By presidential term | | | | | | | |
| '09–'12 | 14,854,863 | 3,039,402 | 17,894,265 | | 15,557,184 | 3,048,256 | 18,605,440 |
| '13–'16 | 19,887,668 | 12,508,324 | 32,395,992 | | 24,077,628 | 13,261,636 | 37,339,264 |

SOURCE: Author's calculations based on assumptions in Annex A.

## Notes

1. Mead Over is a senior fellow at the Center for Global Development (CGD). The author is grateful for the comments by Martha Ainsworth, Michael Bernstein, Nancy Birdsall, Jimmy Kolker, Ruth Levine, Michael Merson, Phil Musgrove, Nandini Oomman, John Stover, Steve Radelet, and Steve Rosenzweig; for the editorial suggestions of Lawrence MacDonald and Pearl Subramanian; and for the expert research assistance of Martina Tonizzo and Owen McCarthy. The views expressed in this chapter—and any remaining errors—are those of the author. This paper was made possible in part by financial support that the Bill and Melinda Gates Foundation provides to CGD's Global Health Policy Research Network.

2. See Note 11.

3. For a recent contrary view on the economic benefits of AIDS treatment, see Ventelou et al. (2008).

4. See Radelet (2003) for a discussion of the shifting politics of Bush's foreign aid policy.

5. This paragraph draws on page 24 of the IOM report (Institute of Medicine 2007).

6. The U.S. is estimated to have contributed about $25 million over the 12 years of the smallpox eradication campaign or an average of about $2.5 million per year (Levine 2004). In current dollars this would be about $5 million per year which is less than one percent of the U.S.'s 2006 expenditures on AIDS.

7. Of the 1.4 million individuals receiving treatment, PEPFAR provided treatment directly to about one million and provided indirect support to the treatment of an additional 350,000 (OGAC 2008).

8. Unfortunately people on ART have trouble getting access to family planning methods and so may not be able to prevent additional births even if they want to, as many do. Expansion of family planning services in conjunction with antiretroviral therapy is an urgent need. See Section V.B for discussion of priority prevention programs.

9. For example, Pedro Chequer, the director of Brazil's AIDS program explained his country's refusal to accept U.S. requirements to condemn prostitutes and promote abstinence-only prevention programs, with the following remark: "'Obviously abstinence is the safest way to avoid AIDS,' Dr. Chequer said. 'But it's not viable in an operational sense unless you are proposing that mankind be castrated or genetically altered, and then you would end up with something that is not human but something else altogether.'" (Rohter 2005).

10. One country's AIDS generosity can, by this measure, make another look stingy. For example, if the United Kingdom were to double its AIDS funding, total AIDS funding would be increased, so the U.S. would be providing a smaller share of the total, and the point of its arrow would be pushed below the "Fairness Frontier."

11. The direction of the arrow in Panel C of Figure 8.3 shows how the individual OECD country funds AIDS in comparison to its other international contributions. The U.S. joins the Netherlands and Germany in revealing a preference for AIDS assistance over other types of ODA, as indicated by the upward directions of their arrows in the figure. Despite France's rhetorical promotion of assistance for AIDS treatment (http://www.ambafrance-uk.org/2nd-International-AIDS-Society.html; http://www.africa.upenn.edu/Urgent_Action/apic_11 098.html), the shortness of its upward arrow in Panel C reveals that it gives only slight preference to AIDS in comparison to other types of ODA. The other OECD countries contribute smaller, sometimes much smaller, shares of AIDS assistance than of other types of aid

12. For instance, on the environmental dimension, the Center for Global Development has ranked the U.S. in last place for 2007: (http://www.cgdev.org/content/publications/detail/14716).

13. Data released by the Office of the U.S. Global AIDS Coordinator (OGAC) to the Center for Public Integrity includes no information on 2006 funding that had not yet been obligated at the end of 2006. However, the data do allow us to estimate the proportion of late obligations for funding years 2004 (15.8 percent) and 2005 (9 percent). In order to construct Figure 8.6, which compares 2005 and 2006 funding, we have excluded the 2005 funding of 9 percent which was not obligated in 2005. With this exclusion, the data show a reduction in the absolute amount of prevention spending in eight of 15 focus countries. Assuming that the percentage of unobligated funding at the end of 2006 was not much larger than the 9 percent that had been achieved in 2005, this conclusion is robust to the inclusion of that data.

14. Among the 15 PEPFAR countries, South Africa is the only one to fund a sizable share of the costs of its AIDS interventions from its own budget.

15. For more information on the projections used in this chapter, see McCarthy and Over (2009).

16. See Annex A for details on the model used to make these projections and Annex B for the numerical projections for Figures 8.9 and 8.12. Model assumptions are based on White (2007).

17. Calculated as $4.5 billion divided by $23 billion.

18. These projections rely on many assumptions, most of which are detailed in Annex A. Among these is the assumption that unit costs remain constant over time. A brief discussion on this point is presented in paragraph IV.A.

19. Whether expansion to the new patients is considered "discretionary," as it is termed in the graph's legend, is ultimately a political decision. The suggestion is that the moral imperative to treat will be particularly strong for existing patients who will be deemed to have an "entitlement," whereas new patients might, at least in theory, find other sources of support.

20. On September 26, 2007, UNAIDS published "Financial Resources Required to Achieve Universal Access to HIV Prevention, Treatment, Care and Support" to request $50 billion a year in AIDS funding, up from the current level of about $10 billion a year.

21. A 2002 World Bank study (Devarajan, Miller, and Swanson 2002) in support of the UN-mandated Millennium Development Goals estimated that the cost of achieving all eight of the goals by the year 2015 would be between $40 and $60 billion a year.

22. One of the first uses of the term "disinhibition" was in two publications reporting a modeling study of the impact of AIDS treatment on India (Over et al. 2006; Over et al. 2004). Also, see Cassell et al. (2006).

23. See Section IV.C of this paper.

24. Preliminary analysis of cross-section survey results from Burkina-Faso and Ghana, done jointly with Damien de Walque and Harounan Kazianga of the World Bank, suggests that knowledge of the availability and effectiveness of AIDS treatment leads to extramarital sex for married individuals but also leads to more condom use on these contacts. If these findings are borne out by detailed analysis, the question will arise whether the net effect of these two offsetting influences is to increase or decrease HIV transmission.

25. In an op-ed piece in the *Baltimore Sun*, Michael Klag, the dean of the Johns Hopkins School of Public Health calls for PEPFAR to fund "research to investigate the effect of PEP-FAR's HIV therapy on the spread of HIV and on drug resistance" (Klag 2007).

26. Although the case for this policy is not as strong in the U.S., the Center for Disease Control has recommended a shift to "opt-out" testing domestically as well (Holtgrave 2007).

27. This result was predicted by economists based on the observation that confidential individual testing increases the asymmetry of information between the tested person and everyone else (Over 1999; Philipson and Posner 1993). People tend to take advantage of privileged information in their business transactions (e.g., insider trading scandals on Wall Street). If a similar tendency in sexual transactions is not completely restrained by altruism, people who learn they are HIV positive may increase their risk behavior on the grounds that they have nothing to lose. On the other hand, people who have previously taken risks and learn they are HIV negative may falsely conclude that they are immune to infection and hence take even more risks (Thornton 2005).

28. Suppose that adults at risk of HIV infection are not all equally motivated by a desire to protect their sexual partners from infection, but all are equally motivated by a self-interested drive to avoid their own deaths from AIDS. Those who are most altruistic would have been motivated to learn their own infection status even in the absence of effective AIDS treatment. As news spreads of the accessibility of effective treatment, a surge in demand for testing will come disproportionately from those who would not have sought testing only to protect others. If condom use is even slightly inconvenient or unpleasant, more self-interested people will respond to the information that they are HIV positive by reducing their condom use rather than increasing it. Under this set of plausible conditions, accessible AIDS treatment accelerates HIV testing by differentially recruiting those who

are most likely to use the knowledge they are infected in a socially irresponsible way. Thus it is inescapably plausible that the expansion of AIDS testing in the presence of effective AIDS treatment will accelerate the spread of HIV.

29. An alternative approach would be to relate the cost of treating AIDS patients to total national health expenditure. However, this approach amounts to assuming that the total consumption of care is a good index of the available supply, an unreasonable assumption when physicians are overworked in some countries and unemployed in others.

30. The U.S. constituency for U.S. food aid is a coalition between supporters of altruistic aid to hungry people in developing countries and U.S. farmers who benefit when the U.S. buys the food to be donated overseas. The U.S. constituency for the PEPFAR program has analogously consisted of a coalition between supporters of altruistic treatment for AIDS patients and U.S. multinational pharmaceutical manufacturers who benefit when the U.S. buys their products for donation overseas. The recent shift of U.S. policy towards approval of the purchase of generic drugs from non-American sources weakens but does not completely vitiate this analogy.

31. Such organizations can include tuberculosis patients, because HIV positive patients more easily contract TB and can spread it to people regardless of their HIV status; adherence to TB medication is an important public health issue whether or not one has AIDS and inclusion of TB patients in the group might reduce the stigma on AIDS patients. To the author's knowledge, no such group has been subjected to rigorous impact evaluation, which is urgently needed. The potential cost-effectiveness of such groups has been estimated for Thailand (Over et al. 2007).

32. Since Congress has authorized an increase in the annual funding level of PEPFAR to $50 billion over the next five years, there is discussion of whether to expand the number of focus countries. Proponents of expansion argue that the absorptive capacity of the original 15 countries is limited and may not accommodate such a large increase in funding, while substantial expansion of treatment coverage can be achieved more easily in other countries not currently included, such as Malawi or Lesotho. However, while the goals of universal treatment access and reduced incidence of new cases are far from met in the original 15 countries, the U.S. will better manage its entitlements by channeling any funds not usable in those countries through the multilateral AIDS funding agencies, especially the Global Fund.

33. The right two panels in the Annex table present the numerical projections under historical and rapid uptake, assuming incidence declines at 5 percent per year. Over the five-year period of the proposed PEPFAR reauthorization, 200910-134, this table predicts that AIDS treatment expenditures will total up to $25.8 billion. Congress has recently authorized that 80 percent of $50 billion, or $40 billion, be spent on AIDS of which more than 20 percent ($8 billion) should be spent on HIV prevention and another substantial portion on care and support for patients and their orphaned children. Furthermore, a large, but unknown proportion of the $40 billion would flow to the Global Fund for AIDS, Tuberculosis and Malaria. Thus $25.8 billion represents up to 25 percent more AIDS treatment expenditure than has yet been authorized. These projections include estimates of the variable cost per patient in each country but do not include any fixed cost per country or per treatment site.

34. This proverb suggests that the benefit to cost ratio of prevention might be 16 to 1, but the Thailand calculations cited earlier suggest a ratio of 43 to 1. In the AIDS epidemic, an ounce of prevention is worth two and a half pounds of cure.

35. This goal is consistent with the president's call to avert 5,000,000 new infections over the next five years. However, calculating averted infections requires estimating the number of infections there would be in the absence of U.S. effort. This is a tricky exercise

partly because of the well-known difficulties of attributing changes in national indicators to the contributions of any one partner, and partly because the same person's infection can be multiplied repeatedly, month after month, year after year. The latter problem means that any estimate of cumulated infections averted exaggerates the number of people helped and can obscure lack of progress in reducing the *rate* of infection. A preferable approach is to set a target for the maximum absolute number of annual new infections which is 90 percent lower than the estimated current level. Note that women, who now bear a dispro-portionate share of the burden of the epidemic, will reap most of the benefits of a vigorous prevention campaign. Thus there is no need to establish separate objectives regarding pre-vention among women.

36. This figure is the difference between \$7.18 billion and \$5.83 billion, the figures for 2020 "Total Cost" in the top two panels of Annex B. At rapid uptake the saving in 2020 would be \$4.34 billion, more than twice as large. This figure is the difference between the 2020 "Total Cost" in the bottom two panels of the Annex B.

37. A more recent cross-section analysis found a statistically significant impact of male circumcision but did not control for socioeconomic variables (Drain et al. 2006).

38. However, the confidence intervals overlap.

39. Whether this would be true in South Asia, where the foreskin is a distinction of Hindu men, is a separate and potentially more difficult question.

40. Her estimate rests on the assumption that the proportion of unwanted pregnancies is similar between HIV-positive and HIV-negative women. This assumption finds support in a recent working paper on Lesotho in which the author found no statistically significant difference in desire for children with respect to known HIV status (Adair 2007).

41. See Over (2004) for discussion of the implications of an AIDS transition.

42. The model embodies the assumption that, for those people who fail first-line ART, access to second-line ART expands along a logistic curve from about 5 percent of all patients needing it now to 95 percent of all patients needing it in 2016.

43. Drug costs are assumed to vary across countries with the 2006 GDP per capita of the country according to the patterns observed by WHO in that year and then to remain constant in any given country over time. While the costs of drugs may be reduced as markets for antiretroviral drugs become more contestable, the unit costs of achieving high ART uptake and strong adherence may increase at the same rate, leaving average costs per patient unchanged.

# CHAPTER 9

⋈⋈⋈⋈⋈

HIV Prevention in Africa: What Has Been Learned?

*Peter Glick*

## 1. Introduction

In an era of massive scale-up of antiretroviral therapy (ART) for HIV-positive individuals in Africa, prevention remains at the heart of efforts to turn back the epidemic. Presently, new infections are outpacing the expansion of ART treatment. Even if all who are in need were to be covered, the costs of providing ART will escalate cumulatively, and possibly, prohibitively, if new infections are not reduced (Over 2010). Vaccine trials have so far proved disappointing, and by any measure, an effective vaccine against HIV is many years from being available. Effective prevention is thus indispensible to strategies for dealing with HIV/AIDS in Africa.

Nevertheless, resources for prevention in Africa, which have grown much more slowly in recent years than have resources for treatment, are inadequate to the task (Bertozzi et al. 2008; Piot et al. 2008; Horton and Das 2008). A range of reasons might explain this shortfall. For donors and governments alike, funding treatment may be more attractive than funding prevention. Treatment produces clear benefits and does so in the short term. It is less controversial to treat the sick than to publicly discuss and promote change in sexual behavior and attitudes. Further, there is usually not a mass political demand for prevention measures (Piot et al. 2008).

Another important factor, however, is that there is legitimate confusion over which prevention interventions will be effective and in which contexts. This chapter grapples with this question by surveying what is known (and what remains to be learned) about the effectiveness of HIV-prevention interventions in Africa. Following the standard typology of policies (Global HIV Prevention Working Group 2008), I consider evidence for three kinds of interventions: biomedical interventions that attempt to block infection or decrease infectiousness; behavioral interventions that attempt to get people to reduce HIV risk behaviors; and broader structural interventions that try to change the underlying social and economic contexts that condition risk behaviors, including factors such as gender relations and social norms.

These distinctions are not as hard and fast as such a categorization might suggest, because almost all interventions, and not just explicitly behavioral interventions such as HIV testing and counseling or promotion of sexual fidelity, will depend on behavioral responses to be effective. For example, interventions such as microbicides and male circumcision potentially reduce transmission of the virus in the biomedical sense (for the latter, this effect has been established clinically). But both will depend on behavior to have strong prevention impacts: women must apply microbicides as needed, and circumcised men must refrain from "compensating" increases in sexual risk behaviors. The dominant role of behavior—and the need for behavioral modification for effective prevention—is a recurrent theme in what follows.

The focus here will be on HIV prevention in the context of concentrated epidemics, in which infections are occurring throughout the adult population rather than being concentrated within specific high-risk groups such as sex workers and intravenous drug users.[1] Virtually all countries of sub-Saharan Africa have generalized epidemics so defined, but there is a great deal of regional variation. Prevalence is generally stable and relatively low (under 5 percent but over 1 percent) in West Africa and stable or declining in much of East Africa but at higher rates (over 6 percent in Uganda, Kenya, and Tanzania). In most countries of southern Africa, prevalence is extremely high—over 15 percent in Botswana, Lesotho, Mozambique, Namibia, South Africa, Swaziland, and Zimbabwe—and generally is only now beginning to peak. Prevention approaches will need to be quite different—and typically, more complex—in such environments, compared to settings with concentrated epidemics where it is possible to have major impacts by targeting programs to a few well-defined high-risk groups. Also, the focus in this chapter will be on prevention of infection in adults. Hence, I do not discuss the use of antiretroviral drugs to reduce mother-to-child transmission of HIV, which happens to be one of the few clearly successful prevention interventions in the region.

The remainder of this paper is organized as follows. The next section sets the stage by considering the extent of changes in HIV risk behaviors in Africa in recent years. This is followed in Section 3 with a brief discussion of how the effectiveness of prevention policies and interventions can be assessed, making the distinction between focused impact evaluations and the broader country-level assessments of HIV policy that are needed to relate population-level changes in behavior to policy. Sections 4, 5, and 6 consider the evidence for biomedical, behavioral, and structural interventions, respectively. Section 7 draws several broad conclusions from the evidence.

## 2. Is Behavior Changing?

Both the public and behavioral responses to the epidemic in Africa were for many years tragically inadequate (Caldwell 2000). However, there were early exceptions to this pattern, notably in Uganda and Senegal. In recent years there is evidence of more widespread increases in HIV-prevention knowledge and reductions in risk behaviors. Information on both comes largely from Demographic and Health Surveys (DHS), which are nationally representative surveys conducted at regular (usually five-year) intervals in many countries in Africa and in other regions. Since behavior is self-reported, there is inevitably the possibility of bias. If increasing exposure to HIV messages raises awareness of what behavior is deemed "appropriate," respondents in later surveys may tend to understate (or understate more) their levels of risk behavior (e.g., number of current sexual partners), leading to overestimates of reductions in risk. There is inferential evidence of such "social desirability bias" in surveys (Zaba et al. 2004; Gersovitz 2005; Glick and Sahn 2008). One, therefore, has to be cautious about inferring changes in behavior from such sources, though to some extent they can be confirmed via epidemiological modeling, as discussed below. Note that this concern applies equally to program evaluations when outcomes are self-reported behaviors, as opposed to objectively measured biomarkers.

In Uganda, DHS data from 1989 and 1995 point to large behavior changes over this interval—in particular, a 60 percent reduction in the share of men reporting having casual or non-regular partners, as well as modest increases among young people in age at sexual debut (Stoneburner and Low-Beer 2004)—although there is some concern over the comparability of the surveys over time (Gray et al. 2006). This period corresponds to the timing of the country's major decline in prevalence, and more relevantly, incidence (inferred from trends in infection among younger cohorts). Based on these declines in prevalence and in risk behaviors, Uganda has widely been hailed as a rare African success in turning back the epidemic through behavior change. There is emerging evidence, however, of more recent (after 2000) increases in multiple partnerships and some other risk behaviors in Uganda as well as rising, or at least no longer falling, HIV prevalence (Shafer et al. 2008; Green et al. 2006).[2]

Reductions in self-reported sexual risk behaviors have also been observed in several other African countries, again corresponding to declines in HIV prevalence or incidence. In Zimbabwe, where a general population cohort was followed from 1998–2003 in Manicaland province, prevalence declined slightly, mirroring antenatal site trends for the country overall showing declines in 2000–2004 (Gregson et al. 2006). Sexually experienced men and women reported reductions in casual sex of 49 percent and 22 percent, respectively, over this period, and younger cohorts reported delayed sexual debut. DHS data present a similar picture of behavior change for Zimbabwe overall, with a substantial increase in condom use with non-regular partners and an increase in fidelity. For Zambia, DHS surveys present a more mixed picture, showing declines in several risk behaviors to 1996, especially strong in the capital, but less movement afterwards. The changes in behavior are thought to explain declining incidence in the 1990s in Zambia (Fylkesnes et al. 2001). In Kenya, antenatal sentinel surveillance data indicate a decline in national HIV prevalence from 10 percent in the late 1990s to 7 percent in 2004. DHS surveys from the same period show increases in age at first sex and in condom use and a falling share of adults with multiple partners (Cheluget et al. 2006).

Glick and Sahn (2008), attempting a more comprehensive look, consider recent changes in self-reported risk behaviors (number of partners, condom use at last sex, and age at first sex, using comparable DHS surveys in nine African countries. Overall, the picture is one of reductions in risk behaviors over recent 4–6-year periods, most consistently for condom use among single men and women, which increased in almost all countries. In three of five countries where strictly comparable information on number of partners was available (Benin, Kenya, and Zambia), proportional reductions were observed that appear to be roughly comparable to that noted above for Uganda. Cleland and Ali (2006), considering DHS evidence for condom use among young people in a larger number of countries (18), find changes on an annual basis comparable to those reported in Glick and Sahn.

Whether the changes in (self-reported) risk behaviors measured in some countries are sufficiently large to impact the course of the epidemic is not immediately clear. This is the case even where HIV prevalence is declining at the same time, because change in prevalence can be driven purely by epidemiological factors (especially, death rates among the infected), and because unlike incidence, prevalence should respond to behavior change only with a lag. To answer this question requires epidemiological modeling. One approach is to simulate the natural course of the epidemic, and see how closely the observed pattern in prevalence over time corresponds to the model predictions. Where there is a divergence such that prevalence is falling faster than predicted, it can be inferred that behavioral changes have also been at work, altering the natural course of the epidemic.

Hallet et al. (2006) apply this approach to several African countries (see, also, UNAIDS 2005b). The simulations indicate that behavior change in Uganda, Zimbabwe, and urban Kenya contributed to reduction in HIV prevalence beyond that caused by the natural dynamics of the disease—that is, beyond the changes in mortality and incidence that would occur as the disease progresses. In each of these countries, significant behavior change was in fact measured in surveys.

Elsewhere (Côte d'Ivoire, Malawi, Rwanda, and Ethiopia), the model explains patterns in prevalence without behavior change. It should be emphasized that in countries where it appears that behavior change has brought down HIV prevalence, this means only that the epidemic has been diminished, which is far different from eliminating it. The need for continued and effective prevention policy is hardly "over" in such cases.

Finally, to the extent that behavior did change and in turn had epidemiological impacts, how much of the former was driven by policy (not to mention, which policies) is not clear. Changes in behavior may reflect endogenous population responses to the devastation caused by epidemic, rather than (only) the impacts of public awareness campaigns and other interventions (UNAIDS 2005b; Caldwell 2000). However, the unfavorable experiences of very high-prevalence countries such as Botswana and South Africa, and earlier, differences between Uganda and similarly afflicted counties in the region, make clear that endogenous behavioral responses to AIDS mortality are not the whole story: policy and possibly also cultural differences and practices (notably, male circumcision) are important. Examination of specific country experiences provides insights into the role of policies and the nature of successful approaches to prevention, though as discussed below, this evidence is never unambiguous. The other major approach to assessing policy impacts—more rigorous but more narrow—is efficacy studies of specific interventions.

## 3. Assessing the Impacts of Policies

A growing number of behavioral HIV interventions in Africa—and traditionally, most biomedical ones—have been investigated using randomized controlled trials (RCTs). In RCTs, individuals (or communities or other groups) are randomly assigned to treatment or control group status by the researchers. Randomization permits truly causal inference of the effect of a treatment on the study population—what is known as "internal validity." For logistical, cost, or ethical reasons, however, randomization is not always feasible. A range of methods is used to evaluate the effects of interventions in the absence of random assignment—that is, using non-experimental data. Each uses a different approach to generate an appropriate control or comparison group. A common approach in the evaluation of HIV interventions is to simply compare outcomes for program participants before and after treatment; here the participants serve as their own control group. This approach has the serious shortcoming that it does not control for factors other than the intervention that may have influenced outcomes over the period. More reliable are designs that select a comparison group and record outcomes for both it and treatment groups at baseline (i.e., prior to treatment) and follow-up (post-treatment). Comparing changes over the interval for the two groups controls for common trends as well as differences in characteristics, both observed and unobserved, in the two groups that may affect the outcomes. It does make the assumption that in the absence of the intervention, trends in outcomes would have been the same for the two groups. An alternative (or complementary) approach is to match treatment individuals or communities to appropriate controls based on observed characteristics: the assumption here is that unobservable factors do not differ for the two groups in such a way as to affect the outcomes of interest.

These alternatives to RCTs each must impose certain assumptions to generate a valid control group, unlike a true randomized design. For this reason, RCTs are considered the ideal approach for evaluating efficacy. However, both RCTs and other approaches, when used on small study populations or to evaluate pilot programs, have important limitations. First, there is the problem of scale up. Efficacy trials, whether of drugs or behavioral interventions, essentially show whether an intervention has impacts under ideal conditions. Outcomes under routine conditions once an intervention is scaled up to cover the target population nationally may be significantly less favorable. The agencies implementing the larger program—typically, the health ministry—may have less competent or enthusiastic personnel than were used to carry out a trial. Resource shortfalls (of personnel, drugs, and health infrastructure) may seriously impinge once a program is taken to scale, reducing quality; this is especially pertinent in resource-strapped countries. Study participants themselves may also be more motivated to comply with protocols (or to change their behavior in the desired direction) in a pilot study of a new program.

These problems mean that while efficacy studies can establish the potential value of an intervention, they may be limited in what they can say about the society-wide impacts of a scaled up program on behavioral or other outcomes, and ultimately, HIV incidence and prevalence. One can instead turn to broader observational evidence, by considering at the national level how major changes in policy correlate with changes in behavior (measured, for example, in nationally representative surveys such as the DHS) and in epidemiological outcomes. Countries with similar initial conditions, but without the policy or with different policies, may serve as rough controls. Much of the literature discussed below takes this approach. However, while such associations may be suggestive of causal impacts of policy, causality cannot be established. Many factors cannot be accounted for that may have also led to the observed changes, including changes in economic conditions, the natural course of the epidemic, and the population's endogenous (non-policy determined) behavioral responses to the epidemic.[3] This leaves room for uncertainty and debate over true policy impacts.

Another limitation of efficacy studies is that they almost always consider interventions in isolation. It is possible that behavior change on a national scale requires multiple complementary prevention strategies. Although RCTs can accommodate complementarities through study designs with multiple treatment arms (for say, two interventions separately and combined), this is rarely done in practice because of the increased complexity and sample size required for such designs. Country case study evidence discussed below also suggests that factors such as national leadership and aggressive society-wide mobilization are key determinants of success in behavior change. There may be complementarities between these broad factors and specific behavior change interventions; for example, people may be more willing to respond to the local availability of HIV testing when their national leaders have been strongly promoting openness about HIV and attempting to end the stigmatization of people living with AIDS. If this is the case, testing the efficacy of an intervention in isolation from these complementary policy efforts will provide a misleading picture of the potential role of the intervention in prevention.

These issues pose a real dilemma for research and policy. Researchers can test individual interventions well enough via RCTs or other rigorous means, but complementarities among multiple interventions, and between individual or community interventions and national-level mobilization, will be missed. Again, it is necessary to broaden one's perspective and consider national-level evidence and cross-country comparisons of policy and behavioral and epidemiological outcomes. This comes at the expense of formality and the ability to assign causal impacts to policies—and in the presence of multiple interventions, to specific policies. The debate over what happened and why in Uganda in the 1990s, discussed below, illustrates well the uncertainty that arises from this situation. It is clear that rigorous efficacy studies of interventions and broader observational analysis both have an important role to play in understanding how policy may impact the epidemic.

## 4. Biomedical Prevention Interventions

### 4.1 Control of other sexually transmitted infections

Africa has high rates of untreated non-HIV sexually transmitted infections (STIs) that are cofactors for HIV infection. STIs such as syphilis and herpes increase susceptibility to HIV via genital ulceration, which increases the likelihood of blood transmission during intercourse (Kapiga and Aitken 2003). Further, STI infection in HIV-positive men is associated with greater viral load of HIV, which increases the likelihood of transmission to the partner (Cohen et al. 1997). Oster (2005) develops an epidemiological model incorporating plausible sexual behavior parameters for Africa and the U.S. that attempts to decompose the growth of HIV prevalence into behavior and transmission rate determinants. In line with earlier theorizing about HIV and STIs in Africa, her simulations suggest that a great deal of the vast differences in U.S. and African prevalence rates are due to differences in the transmission rates of the virus, which would largely be a reflection of the high levels of untreated STIs in Africa.

Given these considerations, there were initially high expectations that comprehensive prevention or control of STIs would have significant positive HIV prevention impacts. There have been three large community randomized trials of comprehensive STI programs in Africa: in Rakai and Masaka, Uganda, and Mwanza, Tanzania, all in rural areas (Grosskurth et al. 1995; Wawer et al. 1999; Kamali et al. 2003). Disappointingly, while STI incidence fell in each case, outcomes for HIV incidence were less favorable. Only in the Tanzania case was there also a reduction in new HIV infections. Together these three studies suggest that STI control will yield HIV prevention benefits when (as in Tanzania) the epidemic remains relatively concentrated, that is, when transmission is still occurring primarily in specific high-risk groups, and when STI rates themselves are high (Korenromp et al. 2005). In other contexts, population-level impacts on HIV infection may be limited.

### 4.2 Male circumcision

Another important cofactor for HIV infection is male circumcision, or more precisely, not having been circumcised. In East and Southern Africa, the regions in Africa with the highest HIV prevalence, most men are not circumcised; in West Africa, where HIV rates are lowest, most men are. Non-circumcision may raise susceptibility to HIV infection directly[4] as well as indirectly by increasing susceptibility to cofactor STIs. A review of observational studies for Africa indicates that male circumcision is associated with a significantly reduced risk of HIV infection among men, with an adjusted relative risk of 0.42 (Weiss et al. 2000). These comparisons cannot account for all cultural and behavioral differences that distinguish circumcised and uncircumcised male populations, but recent experimental evidence confirms that circumcision substantially reduces transmission risk. In the first such study, the French National Agency for Research on AIDS (ANRS) randomized trial in South Africa, incidence was about 60 percent lower in the group of men getting the procedure relative to controls (Auvert et al. 2006). Following on the heels of this study were two more RCTs of male circumcision, in Rakai, Uganda, and Kisumu, Kenya (Gray et al. 2007; Bailey et al. 2007), which found approximately the same level of protection from infection. These trials therefore suggest very significant prevention benefits to men (and by extension, to women) from getting circumcised—almost certainly larger than most behavioral interventions. Further, surveys consistently show that acceptability of the procedure among African men is high (Westercamp and Bailey 2007).

However, there is concern that male circumcision will lead to adverse behavioral responses via "risk compensation" (Cassell et al. 2006). It is hard to convey the concept of partial protection, which is what circumcision provides, so men may feel freer to engage in riskier behavior than before. This can result in a net increase in their infection risk. In the case of the ANRS study, the estimate of the protective effect of circumcision was not sensitive to adjustment for participants' self-reported sexual behaviors, but it is noteworthy that most indicators of sexual risk behavior were higher in the treatment group than the controls following the start of the trial. Similarly, in the Kisumu trial on young men, several of the indicators of risk (having two or more recent partners, having had unprotected sex, inconsistent condom use) were higher at follow-up in the circumcised group than in the controls (Bailey et al. 2007). In this case, however, risk behaviors actually fell in both groups, possibly reflecting behavior modification counseling that was provided to both, but the decline was smaller in the treated group. It would be particularly useful for epidemiological models to estimate the net HIV impacts under a range of plausible scenarios for behavioral response (see Kalichman, Eaton, and Pinkerton (2007)). For policymakers, the key question is whether it is possible under conditions of routine program implementation to effectively counsel men to use condoms and follow other safe sex practices after being circumcised.

Patients also need to be counseled to avoid sexual relations while they recover from the procedure. A recent study by Wawer et al. (2009), in Rakai, Uganda (a parallel trial to the one mentioned above in Rakai), was the first RCT to investigate the effects of male circumcision on HIV risk to female partners of male patients who were HIV positive. Disappointingly, the trial did not show lower number of infections in women in the treatment group compared with controls (indeed the experiment was stopped prematurely after 24 months for this reason). This was probably due in part to couples engaging in intercourse before the male partners' surgical wounds had healed, when the probably of transmission is likely high, despite counseling to avoid relations during this period. However, despite these results for serodiscordant couples—and as the authors of this study themselves argue—male circumcision still holds substantial promise for reducing infections among both men and women.

### 4.3 Microbicides

Microbicides are substances designed to prevent or reduce the sexual transmission of HIV when applied topically, meaning, inside the vagina or rectum. They can take a number of forms, including gels, creams, suppositories, or sponges or rings that release the active ingredient over time. One attraction of microbicides is that they would offer a means of protection that is largely in the hands of women. In contrast, (male) condoms, as well as partner fidelity or relationship termination, are difficult means to employ when women lack economic or social power. Even so, like virtually all HIV-prevention methods, the effectiveness of microbicides still depend on behavior, in this case, the willingness or ability of women to routinely use the product.

Different microbicides are designed to work in different ways: *surfactants* disrupt microbial cell membranes, thereby inactivating or killing the virus; *vaginal defense enhancers* make the vagina a hostile environment for HIV by enhancing the naturally protective acidity of the vagina or by increasing the colonization of protective microorganisms; *fusion or entry inhibitors* block cellular receptors so that HIV is unable to attach to target cells. Finally, *antiretroviral (ARV)-based* microbicides prevent HIV from replicating once inside a cell and hence use the same mechanism prophylactically as the ARV drugs used for the treatment of HIV-positive individuals.

The idea of using microbicides in HIV prevention has been around for some years. However, given the years-long progression from laboratory studies through multiple-phase clinical trials to ultimate approval for widespread use, no microbicide has yet been added to the arsenal of HIV prevention. On the contrary, a significant number of compounds have been shown not to be effective and some to be possibly harmful (increasing HIV infection risk). One of the first products tested was Nonoxynol-9, a surfactant initially developed as a spermicide. Clinical trials showed that it was not effective against HIV and may increase HIV risk by irritating the vaginal surface. Similarly disappointing results came in more recent Phase III trials (in which effectiveness as well as safety are tested on large samples) of several other microbicides—Carraguard and Cullulose Sulfate (both inhibitors) and Savvy (a surfactant). A just concluded Phase IIb trial in the U.S. and several locations in Africa (Malawi, South Africa, Zambia, and Zimbabwe) showed no benefit to BufferGel (a defense enhancer) but a potential benefit to PRO 2000 (an inhibitor) which was associated with a 30 percent reduction in infection probability (NIAID 2009). The latter result was not statistically significant at conventional levels but was strong enough to warrant additional clinical trials. At this point, this is the only microbicide that has been shown to have at least the potential of eventually being an effective means of HIV prevention.

However, laboratory or clinical trials are underway or planned for a number of additional agents. Most of these involve a newer generation of more complex microbicides that fall in the fourth category above, those containing antiretroviral agents. Further, a significant number (seven at this writing) of clinical trials are underway or planned for ARVs taken orally rather than topically prior to high-risk exposures, products commonly called "pre-exposure prophylactics" (though this term could equally apply to topical microbicides containing ARV agents.) Note that the use of these compounds in effect integrates prevention and treatment—something that will appear again in a very different strategy (directed at *already infected* individuals) known as "test and treat" and described in the Section 4.4

below. Given the success of ARVs as treatment for those who are already HIV positive and in preventing mother-to-child transmission of HIV, there are reasons to expect that topical or oral pre-exposure prophylactics will be successful. It should be noted, however, that even if a clinically effective agent is found, it will be years before it is widely available. It will likely also offer only partial protection against infection. And like condoms, the product will require consistent and correct use, which is not assured even if use is under control of women. For these reasons, even a successful microbicide will not be a "magic bullet" for prevention.

### 4.4 Antiretroviral therapy

The use of antiretroviral therapy for adults, long available in the developed world, has in the last decade expanded dramatically in Africa, thanks to massive increases in donor support. Several studies confirm the life-extending benefits of antiretrovirals in low-income settings (Ferradini et al. 2006; Bussmann et al. 2008; Coetzee et al. 2004). While expansion of ART coverage has been rapid, it remains well below needs: worldwide, less than half of those in need receive ART, and the share is lower in Africa (Granich 2009). Although ARV therapy for adults was not conceived of as a prevention intervention *per se*, it nevertheless may have impacts on the spread of HIV. On the biomedical side, the drugs can reduce the presence of the virus in the bloodstream to imperceptible levels, making patients much less infectious than prior to treatment. The risk of infection may in fact be close to zero (Granich et al. 2009). This suggests a potentially strong prevention impact, but note that it requires that ARVs are given to people who are still sexually active. This group presumably excludes many or most of whom have already become sick with AIDS-related illnesses. In situations where ARVs are rationed to such highly symptomatic patients, any biomedical prevention impact may be very small since such patients were effectively no longer capable of spreading the virus. This may well be the prevailing situation in African settings, as discussed below. However, if ARVs were given to apparently healthy, sexually active HIV-positive individuals on a large enough scale, there could be significant prevention benefits. A strategy of providing the drugs to all HIV-positive persons has recently been advocated, based on epidemiological modeling of the potential impacts. It, too, will be taken up below.

On the behavioral side, there is some concern that expanded ARV coverage will lead to higher levels of risky sexual behavior in the population. Individuals who are not ill may experience "treatment optimism"—knowing that they can get treatment if they contract HIV encourages them to engage in more risky behaviors. There are also potential beneficial prevention impacts. These include reductions in AIDS stigma and a greater willingness of people to get tested if they know treatment is available (Moatti 2002). Since the evidence (discussed in Section 5.2 below) indicates that those who test positive do reduce risky behaviors, increased utilization of testing services may be a beneficial prevention side effect of ARV availability. Informal evidence (see Glick (2005)) indicates that testing surges when clinics begin offering ARVs. Still, it is not clear whether the demand for testing increases primarily among those who are already ill with AIDS (hence less likely to be sexually active and in danger of infecting others) or instead or also among the apparently healthy, including HIV-positive but asymptomatic individuals who are still sexually active and therefore at risk for spreading the virus. From a prevention perspective this distinction is important. These and the risk behavioral effects of ART provision in the general population have yet to be considered rigorously. To do so requires the use of population-based data, not just clinic-based data on individuals receiving treatment. Several studies now underway are taking this approach to examine the impacts of ARV availability on risk behaviors among non-ARV clients, including in Burkina Faso (by World Bank researchers) and in Uganda as part of the ongoing Rakai Community Cohort Study.[5]

Returning to the possibility of biomedical prevention impacts of ART, Granich et al. (2009) consider the impacts of a strategy of universal annual (voluntary) HIV testing with immediate initiation of ARV treatment for all those testing positive, even if the status of their immune systems (measured by T-cell or CD4 count or by their viral load) would not otherwise yet warrant the therapy (current WHO guidelines in resource poor settings recommend initiating therapy when the CD4 T-cell count falls below 200, while for resource-rich settings a threshold of 350 is the standard recommendation). Epidemiological modeling suggests that this "test and treat" approach could essentially end the epidemic within 10 years. This result obtains because treatment lowers infectiousness to essentially zero—and because essentially *all* HIV positive persons are treated.

This is a remarkable prediction—no such claim has been made for any existing prevention intervention. Consequently, this proposal is generating substantial interest among researchers, but also considerable skepticism. Criticisms have been leveled at key model assumptions, in particular the assumption that being on ARVs reduces an individual's infectiousness by 99 percent (Wilson 2009). The extent of actual reductions in infectiousness has not been shown clinically. Ruark et al. (2009) also question the assumptions of Granich et al. (2009) about transmission prevention, noting that even frequent testing will miss most acute infections, that is, the period within a month or so after infection during which an individual is far more infectious than later in the progression of the disease. Acute HIV infection is not usually detectable using standard HIV antibody tests, as it takes time for the immune system to produce antibodies in response to infection. However, for now, antibody tests are the only tests feasible for widespread use in resource poor settings. Therefore, the success of the strategy will depend crucially on what share of infections are transmitted during the chronic stage of the disease, during which time infectiousness is lower but which lasts a much longer time (several years at least).

There are also ethical issues arising from the recommendation that a therapy with the potential for toxic side effects and long term complications be initiated at the earliest possible moment (Dieffenbach and Fauci 2009). From a practical point of view, the Test and Treat strategy would seem to be well out of range of what is currently possible in Africa. First, the commitment of resources to supply and deliver ARVs would have to be on a much larger scale than that currently available. To many, it would seem absurd to discuss providing ARVs to all HIV-positive individuals when delivery even to the sickest in Africa falls well short of need. Modifying the approach to lower the threshold for therapy such that only individuals with CD4 counts below 350 are started on ARVs—which the results of Granich et al. (2009) suggest would still have a preventative impact but fall well short of eradication—still implies a large increase in resources. However, if the strategy did eliminate or greatly reduce HIV prevalence, aggregate costs of providing ARVs would tail off in the long run—a cost-saving investment.

A second practical issue is that universal (and regularly repeated) testing of adults in African settings would almost certainly be very hard to achieve, given current levels of testing and what these imply for the demand for testing, discussed below in Section 5.2. The promise of access to ARVs may substantially increase the demand for testing, as noted above. On the other hand, even if demand were to increase significantly, it is not clear that it would be possible to convince individuals to enroll in therapy earlier than currently medically recommended; essentially, this is asking individual patients to produce a public health externality. Once they are enrolled, ensuring adherence to the therapy among those who have not experienced AIDS illness and who feel healthy may also be difficult. In sum, the test and treat approach in African contexts must confront significant issues regarding epidemiological assumptions, feasibility, and ethics. As noted, one issue concerns the relationship between the stage of HIV infection and the transmission probability, and the effect of viral suppression via ART on infectiousness. Current randomized trials are investigating the impact on transmission to infected partners of immediate (on testing positive) as opposed to later (CD4<250) initiation of therapy, and so should provide evidence on these questions (HIV Prevention Trials Network 2009). Additionally, conducting further epidemiological modeling under different assumptions about testing coverage and frequency, as well as efficacy in preventing transmission, is an important research direction.

## 5. Behavioral Interventions

HIV prevention interventions that are explicitly designed to alter behavior include public campaigns emphasizing prevention behaviors, such as the "ABC" approach (Abstinence, Be faithful, use Condoms); voluntary testing and counseling (VCT);

provision and social marketing of condoms; and a host of education programs aimed at youth to provide HIV knowledge and encourage safe behaviors, most commonly, later sexual debut.

## 5.1 The "ABC" approach—A, B, or C?

Uganda remains the standard bearer for behavior change in high-prevalence countries, and its experience has inspired a great deal of discussion and debate. From the early 1990s to 2001, HIV prevalence in Uganda fell by two-thirds, from 15 percent to around 5 percent of the population. Much of this reduction is attributable to the natural course of the epidemic, via rising mortality as the initial group of HIV-infected persons began to succumb to AIDS; mortality also reduced incidence by removing infected individuals from sexual networks. However, it is generally agreed that large reductions in risk behaviors (described in Section 2) also played a significant role (Singh, Darroch, and Bankole 2003; Slutkin et al. 2006; Stoneburner and Low-Beer 2004).

One can consider Uganda's (and other countries') experience along two dimensions: the broad policy stance, meaning the overall nature and intensity of the efforts of government and other actors in getting prevention messages across, and the content of the messages themselves. Uganda clearly indicates the importance of the former dimension. Under the very visible leadership of President Yoweri Museveni, the government attempted to counter the epidemic earlier (starting in the mid 1980s) and far more aggressively than in other countries.[6] This involved the use of mass media and the mobilization of community and church leaders as well as NGOs in education campaigns. Many observers have noted that the frequent open public discussion about AIDS served to destigmatize the disease. This is a somewhat difficult concept to quantify empirically, but it is noteworthy that by the mid-1990s the share of individuals in DHS surveys indicating that they knew someone with AIDS or who had died of AIDS was substantially higher in Uganda than in similarly (or worse) afflicted countries where general awareness of AIDS was equally high: 91.5 percent of men and 86.4 percent of women (in 1995), compared with 68 percent to 71 percent in Zambia, Kenya, and Malawi and below 50 percent in Zimbabwe. In South Africa, the share was below 50 percent as late as 2002 (Stoneburner and Low-Beer 2004). This suggests a widespread willingness to acknowledge the disease and presumably also, the risks that it poses.[7] Along these lines, it has been argued that there were fundamental changes in Uganda in attitudes toward the disease and social norms regarding appropriate sexual behavior. This question is explored further in Section 6.

Regarding the content of the messages, debate continues over exactly which behavior change messages were successful—and which should be used now in Uganda and elsewhere. Uganda is widely said to demonstrate the power of the

"ABC" approach to prevention. However, condom promotion was not a major plank of Uganda's early national prevention strategy, and condoms were not distributed or used widely enough to have played a significant role in the decline in HIV in the early 1990s (Hogle et al. 2002). Nor did the early messages emphasize abstinence *per se*, though among the young, delayed sexual debut was encouraged (Slutkin et al. 2006). The strongest emphasis was on faithfulness to one's partner ("zero grazing"), or failing that, minimizing the number of casual partners (Epstein 2007).[8] The survey evidence cited in Section 2 indicates success in reducing the incidence of sex with non-regular partners, or more generally, of having multiple partners, as well as more modest reductions in sexual activity among youth.

"Being faithful" or partner reduction may be especially potent as a prevention behavior in the African context because of the prevalence of multiple *concurrent* long-term partnerships. With concurrent partnerships, many more people at a given point of time are linked in sexual networks than in situations where serial monogamy is predominant, as is more typical in the West and Asia, for example (Morris and Kretzschmar 1997; Halperin and Epstein 2004). These networks allow the virus to spread rapidly in the population. The effects of concurrency are exacerbated by the fact that, as noted earlier, HIV viral load, and thus infectivity, is much higher during the initial weeks or months after infection.

There are more recent cases where partner reduction may have been responsible for reductions in HIV incidence and prevalence.[9] The cases of Zimbabwe and Kenya were cited in Section 2. In Ethiopia, a cohort study of male factory workers, a high-risk group, documented reductions in risk involving primarily reductions in casual sex over a several year period in the late 1990s when prevalence was declining at the national level (Mekonnen et al. 2003). Recent evidence that policy can influence behavior with respect to casual sex and number of partners comes from the 2006 "Secret Lover" campaign in Swaziland, where the number of people reporting two or more partners in the past month was halved after an intervention aggressively focused on the dangers of infidelity to one's main partner (Halperin et al. 2006). While these country experiences are cited as further evidence of the benefits (and feasibility) of strategies focusing on partner reduction (Shelton et al. 2004), claims of specific impacts are not easy to establish. In the Zimbabwe and Kenya cases, other self-reported risk behaviors such as condom use or age at first sex also changed in the direction of greater protection. In the Ethiopia study, the sampled cohort was provided prevention education and HIV testing so changes in the behavior of the cohort was likely not representative of changes in society at large.

Unlike Uganda in the early 1990s, where condoms fairly clearly did not play a significant role, it is generally not possible in later country examples to attribute changes in prevalence or incidence to changes in specific behaviors (as noted, it is indeed not straightforward to establish what role behavior as a whole may have played). Still, while reductions in the number of sexual partners may not have been the only behavioral factor in later cases of HIV decline, they were probably essential to success. There are no cases in Africa of a generalized epidemic being significantly altered that did not coincide with substantial reductions in the average number of sexual partners.

## CONDOM PROMOTION[10]

Few would argue against the benefits of providing condoms to commercial sex workers and other typically very high-risk groups such as truck drivers and the military. Such drives, beginning with Thailand's 100 percent condom use policy for brothels and subsequently copied elsewhere in Asia, have generally been quite successful (UNAIDS 2000; WHO 2004b), both in achieving very high rates of condom use in the targeted populations and in bringing down infection rates in concentrated epidemics, where transmission was still occurring largely via these high-risk groups. However, in Africa's generalized epidemics, transmission occurs throughout the general population. Countries with generalized epidemics that have focused prevention efforts primarily on condom promotion have had rather disappointing results. Kenya (early on), Botswana, and South Africa had policies strongly promoting condoms for years, with apparent success in increasing their acceptance and use but with little to show in terms of reduced prevalence (Hearst and Chen 2004). It is hard to draw conclusions from these simple cross-country comparisons, because countries also differ in how aggressively government in general pursued its AIDS education and prevention objectives.[11] Still, these experiences suggest that it is unlikely that condom promotion in the absence of successful promotion of other risk behavior reduction, especially reduction in the number of partners, is sufficient to turn back the epidemic—there is no such "condom success story" (Green et al. 2006).

One problem is that users of condoms tend not to use them consistently (Hearst and Chen 2004). Further, it is possible that such intermittent use of condoms provides a false sense of security, so that people feel comfortable persisting in high-risk behaviors (Ahmed et al. 2001); that is, they exhibit risk disinhibition. A second problem is that people are reluctant to use condoms in long-term partnerships, as this implies a lack of trust; it is also, obviously, incompatible with the desire to have more children.[12] Unfortunately, long-term partnerships are the context in which much or most HIV transmission occurs in Africa's AIDS epidemics.

In Uganda, condoms began to be promoted more heavily in the early to mid-1990s using social marketing campaigns. This new emphasis seems to have affected the nature of prevention. Longitudinal data from Rakai province for the period 1994–2003 indicate that falling HIV prevalence was due to a combination of (primarily) rising AIDS mortality, on the one hand, and behavior change, on the other. In contrast to the reduction in casual partnerships that characterized the earlier period, behavioral adjustment took the form of increased condom use; levels of other self-reported risk behaviors did not change or even increased over the period (Wawer et al. 2005a). While in Rakai condom use may have contributed modestly to HIV decline in spite of unfavorable movements in terms of number of partners, in Uganda as a whole, a similar change with respect to multiple partnerships (increases seen in successive DHS surveys following earlier sharp declines) has coincided with an increase in HIV prevalence after 2000 (Shafer et al. 2008).[13]

The evidence discussed above on condom promotion does not come from controlled studies or evaluations of specific programs. For policies promoting condom use among the general public (as opposed to specific high-risk groups), such evaluations unfortunately are uncommon. Evidence of effectiveness of condom promotion or social marketing programs often relies on the numbers of condoms distributed or sold, and occasionally, changes in self-reported condom use. While condom promotion in Africa does appear to work in this sense (Hearst and Chen 2004; Foreit 2001; Myer et al. 2001), the effect on prevention remains unclear without information on which groups (in terms of risk levels) use them, on whether they are used consistently, and on what happens with respect to other risk behaviors—and ultimately, of course, on changes in the rate of new infections.

A rare evaluation that does attempt to gather such data is a randomized trial in Kampala, Uganda (Kajubi et al. 2005). Recruited men in one poor community participated in a workshop that taught condom skills and encouraged condom use. Men in a control community received a brief informational presentation about AIDS. All participants received coupons redeemable for free condoms from distributors in both communities and completed questionnaires at baseline and six months later. It was found that men in the intervention group redeemed significantly more condom coupons than men in the control group, but they also increased their number of sex partners by 0.31 compared with a decrease of 0.17 partners in the control group. Thus the gains from increased condom use seem to have been offset by increases in the number of sex partners. This study provides evidence of a disinhibition or "risk compensation" effect of condom use: individuals adopted one form of protective behavior and compensated by being less careful in other dimensions, possibly leading to an increase in net HIV risk (especially if condoms were not used consistently). The trends in behavior in Rakai since 1993, with respect to condom use and other prevention behaviors, are also consistent with this process. Therefore, questions remain about the overall impacts of condom promotion in generalized epidemics. Studies are needed, in particular, of the impacts of programs promoting condoms in conjunction with a strong emphasis on other risk behavior reductions. Ideally, the measured endpoints would include change in HIV incidence as well as behaviors.

Despite these concerns, it is important to point out that access to and use of condoms is essential when (as in Uganda today) half or more of new infections occur in serodiscordant couples (couples in which one partner is infected but the other is not). For many of these couples, abstinence is presumably unattractive (Merson, Dayton, and O'Reilly 2000). For single people, condoms may remain the most effective or likely to be used means of prevention.

## 5.2 HIV testing

Despite the urgency of the AIDS epidemic, Demographic and Health Surveys indicate that up to 80 percent of adults in Africa have not been tested for HIV (De Cock 2007). Many governments are attempting to change this by expanding access to testing and counseling services. Voluntary HIV Testing and Counseling typically consists of a pretest counseling session with a trained counselor, the serotest itself, and a posttest session in which individuals are counseled on behaviors to insure that they remain uninfected (if they test negative) or avoid infecting others (if positive). Those testing positive are also provided emotional support and directed to services to provide other forms of support, including medical care. For many thousands of Africans, this care, which used to be limited to palliative care, now includes antiretroviral treatment; testing is the gateway to ART.

Although VCT is often touted as a key prevention strategy, conceptually the responses to learning one's status are likely to be complex and heterogeneous. Cognitive theories of behavior change might predict that counseling will lead to reductions in risky behaviors because clients are provided with information about the levels of risk and prevention methods.[14] Economic models of behavior potentially yield different predictions. If those who test negative (the majority of cases if testing coverage is high) came to testing thinking there was a significant probability they were infected, they would enjoy an upward revision in life expectancy. Since this increases the cost of current risky behavior (more years of life are at stake), these behaviors may be curtailed. On the other hand, such individuals may also perceive themselves to be less at risk from their partners than they feared, and also will correctly see themselves as less of a risk to others (Glick 2005). Both factors could lead negative testers to increase rather than decrease their levels of risk behavior. Those who test positive, if they are altruistic, will take steps to prevent infecting others. On the other hand, simple economic models would predict greater risk behavior (if individuals are selfish), because a positive test means there is little to be personally gained from adopting safer behaviors.

There are a number of evaluations of VCT in Africa, most based on simple single group pretest and posttest designs, whereby (self-selected) clients are interviewed before they receive the testing and counseling and are followed up some time later (see Glick (2005) for a review of this research). Without similar baseline and follow-up information for a control or comparison group, it is not possible to distinguish the effects of the intervention from general trends in behavior over time. Equally important is the problem of self-selection. Given heterogeneity in the population with respect to (for example) the motivation for behavior change and risk avoidance, those who choose to use VCT may be especially responsive to the information received about their serostatus and about HIV prevention. Hence they may adjust their behavior following VCT more than would individuals in the target population in general.

For these reasons, the first randomized controlled trial of VCT in Africa, conducted in urban Kenya and Tanzania as well as Trinidad (Voluntary HIV-1 Counseling and Testing Efficacy Study Group 2000), attracted significant attention both in the research community and the popular press. Volunteers interested in testing were randomly assigned to intervention and control groups; the latter were given general information about HIV/AIDS but not VCT. [15] Relative to controls, there were reductions in unprotected sex among testing serodiscordant couples and among HIV-positive testers in general. Behavior change among those testing negative were much smaller. This is the same general pattern found in many nonexperimental studies. It suggests that the testing and counseling has some value in secondary prevention (i.e., preventing infection of the partners of those who are HIV positive), but little impact on preventing primary infection among those who are HIV negative.

The public health effectiveness of voluntary programs such as VCT depends not just on the response of those who participate, but on the extent of participation, or program coverage. For most countries in Africa, DHS surveys indicate low numbers reporting having had an HIV test, but high shares (about two-thirds) saying they would like to learn their status (Glick and Sahn 2007). In Kenya, where the government in recent years has been rapidly expanding the number of testing sites, the overall numbers tested annually have increased dramatically, from 1,100 in 2000 to over a half million in 2005 (Marum Taegtmeyer, and Chebet 2006), pointing to a strong demand for testing that had been constrained by a shortage of facilities. However, a formal analysis of the demand for HIV testing requires the use of population-based survey data collected in areas where the service is available. The findings from several such studies provide a mixed picture. In a rural Rakai, Uganda study (Nyblade et al. 2000), VCT services were offered to all individuals, who could choose to receive the service in their homes or at a nearby clinic. Despite significant outreach, demand in the initial year of the program (1995/6) was not very high—32 percent of women and 35 percent of men agreed to receive their test results. However, this jumped to 65 percent for both sexes in 1999/2000 (Matovu et al. 2002).[16] In an urban Zambia study (Fylkesnes and Siziya 2004), uptake was much lower. Even where there was similar flexibility in setting (a clinic or at home), the probability of both indicating "readiness" for testing and using the service was only about 18 percent.

Similarly, in a more recent study of rural Malawi (Thornton 2008), only about 40 percent of participants offered free testing chose to attend clinics to learn their HIV status. On the other hand, demand was very sensitive to monetary incentives: small cash payments (offered on a randomly assigned basis) were enough to double the use of the testing service.[17] This study not only randomized the testing incentive, it also used an objectively measured rather than self-reported behavioral outcome, namely, the participants' purchases of subsidized condoms. Consistent with studies of VCT outcomes discussed above, testing had no effect on condom purchases for those testing negative, but those who tested positive and had a partner purchased significantly more condoms than non-testers. However, the average number of condoms purchased was small, so the overall cost-effectiveness of VCT in this setting was low.

The evident reluctance on the part of many to get tested may reflect a number of factors: significant stigma attached to AIDS, stress, and a strong reluctance to reveal a positive test result to a partner, particularly for women who may fear domestic violence or divorce as a consequence. In view of these factors, some observers have questioned the usefulness of the VCT model for Africa (and elsewhere). The VCT approach, as the word "voluntary" implies, typically places a premium on privacy and personal choice in health care. In contrast, a policy of "mandatory"—or more accurately, "routine," "opt out" or "provider-initiated"—testing would automatically test all individuals entering the health care system. [18] Such a policy treats HIV as a public health issue in the same manner as other communicable diseases have been treated in the past in the West. Botswana and Lesotho have recently become the first African countries to initiate national policies of routine HIV testing.

Both the ethics and efficacy of mandatory testing have been hotly debated (see UNAIDS (2004b) and Holbrooke and Furman (2004) for opposing views). The impacts on risk behaviors and on coverage of testing itself remain unknown; with regard to the latter, it is possible that certain high risk or vulnerable groups will respond to a policy of automatic testing by deciding to stay away from the health system entirely. However, there is evidence from several Africa countries (Weiser et al. 2006; Perez et al. 2006; Chandisarewa et al. 2007) that routine testing has a high level of acceptability in the population. The impacts of routine testing should be amenable to formal assessment if the health authority was willing to institute routine testing in some health locations, e.g., districts, and not others in an initial rollout of the policy.

In sum, hopes that simply expanding HIV testing will have large behavioral impacts in the general population are not likely to be realized. The key problem identified from evaluations is that those who test negative—the majority—do not seem to reduce their levels of risk behavior. A second problem is that achieving very high rates of testing has proved to be difficult. Even so, testing remains an indispensable tool in prevention policy. Individuals who test positive and those in couples appear more likely to take steps to reduce risk. Given that in high-prevalence countries of Africa half or more of new infections occurs within discordant couples, this is an important benefit. Further, as noted, testing is the gateway to life-prolonging ARV treatment.

It would seem that the way to maximize the prevention impacts of testing would be to somehow attract a larger share of individuals who are (1) HIV positive but (2) also asymptomatic, that is, who continue to feel healthy. The first characteristic is important because impacts on behaviors are by and large seen only for those who test positive. The second is important because among those who are HIV positive, apparently healthy individuals are more likely to be sexually active, hence a danger to others, than those already ill with AIDS.[19] For the former group there is scope for behavior change that would reduce secondary infections, and the evidence indicates that they will alter behavior upon learning their status.

The promise of antiretroviral drugs may be a way to induce such individuals to get tested. The WHO guidelines for developing countries (WHO 2003b) recommend that individuals with a T-cell (CD4) count below 200 cells/mm$^3$ be started on ARVs, whether they display symptoms or not. Based on observational evidence of lower early mortality of patients who are started earlier on therapy, there have been calls to initiate therapy at CD4 counts of 350, again whether the patient is ill or not (see Walensky et al. (2009); Wood and Lawn (2009); When to Start Consortium (2009)). Even under the current guidelines (but more so if the threshold CD4 level were raised), individuals who do not feel ill would still have an incentive to test, since they would have the benefit of early access to therapy if they test positive. The key is the promise of getting life-prolonging treatment even before serious illness sets in. However, in practice in resource-poor settings, it is likely that treatment will be prioritized to favor those who are most ill; in any case, lack of access to sophisticated CD4-testing technology will force practitioners in many settings to wait until patients are symptomatic (Glick 2005; McGough et al. 2005). The median CD4 count of individuals put on treatment in such environments is only about 100 (Egger 2007). This suggests that rationing of therapy to the very ill may be taking place, though it could also be that, as discussed earlier, mostly individuals who are already quite ill come to these sites. But if the former (rationing) is taking place, people who are not ill may have little new incentive to seek testing, since they would be ineligible for early treatment should they test positive.

This suggests a potential tradeoff between the objectives of allocating scarce drugs only to those who need them most, on the one hand, and of increasing the demand for and prevention impacts of testing by offering drugs to individuals who are infected but not yet sick, on the other. Note this is not the same as the universal "test and treat" policy discussed above, which relies on biomedical factors, namely an ARV-caused reduction in transmission probabilities combined with near complete coverage of testing. The idea here is not necessarily to begin all HIV-positive testers on ARVs immediately, but to make it possible for individuals who are not ill to still perceive a strong benefit from testing (because if their CD4 is count below some relatively high threshold, they will be eligible for therapy), with the expectation that those testing positive will take action to reduce their chances of infecting others.

## 5.3 Programs aimed at youth

In Africa as elsewhere, many programs have sought to educate young people about HIV risk and reduce behaviors that expose them to risk: early sexual initiation, sex without condoms, or sex before marriage. Most commonly these programs operate through schools. Drawing general conclusions about efficacy from the many published program evaluations is difficult. For one thing, methodologies vary; some feature randomized designs, but most do not. While some use objective biological endpoints such as HIV infections, pregnancy, or STIs, most rely on self-reported attitudes and risk behaviors. A further complication is that the programs are heterogeneous in terms of the content of the messages and how they are communicated to young people.

A review of 11 school-based HIV education programs in Africa (Gallant and Tyndale 2004) indicates that while such interventions can be successful at improving young people's HIV awareness and attitudes, most did not produce sustained changes in behavior. A broader survey (Kirby, Laris, and Rolleri 2005), including studies from other developing regions and several additional ones from Africa, similarly finds strong improvements in knowledge while also finding that a significant share of such programs also led to (at least short term) reductions in self-reported risk behaviors. Recognizing the heterogeneous nature of school-based interventions, Kirby, Laris, and Rolleri attempt to identify the characteristics of programs that were successful. With regard to behavior change, apparently successful programs tended to be curriculum-based programs, which are more intensive and structured than non-curriculum-based interventions such as awareness-raising events or in-school counseling about sexual activity and HIV. Also, curriculum-based interventions using adults (i.e., educators) were more effective in changing behavior than those relying on peers.

As noted, most of these evaluations did not employ randomized designs, and most used self-reported behavior outcomes as endpoints rather than HIV infections or other biological endpoints such as teenage pregnancy or STIs. Given the possibility of biased self-reports of behavior, the paucity of research using biomarkers is unfortunate. However, several recent evaluations of school-based prevention programs in Africa do make use of randomized trials and in a few cases, the measured outcomes include HIV incidence or other biomarkers. These, too, have produced mixed results. In rural Tanzania, a community-randomized design was used to evaluate a project including in-school education, youth-friendly health services, and community-based condom promotion and distribution. The program led to improved knowledge, attitudes, and reduction in self-reported risk behaviors in the 10 intervention communities relative to the controls, but there was no consistent impact on biological indicators of HIV, other STIs, or pregnancy (DFID 2004). A Rakai, Uganda RCT of an extracurricular education program (Kinsman et al. 2001) found no significant impacts on teenagers' self-reported behaviors; in this case, poor implementation may be partly to blame.

A multi-arm randomized evaluation in Western Kenya (Dreyfuss et al. 2006) found that training teachers for the HIV/AIDS curriculum did not lead to any reduction in teenage pregnancy but did increase the likelihood that teenage pregnancies occur within marriage. In-class debates over condoms and opportunities to write essays on ways of protecting oneself against HIV/AIDS led to increased self-reported use of condoms without an increase in self-reported sexual activity. Reductions in the cost of schooling led to reductions both in dropout rates and teen pregnancies. As Dreyfuss et al. note, in the absence of HIV outcome measures, the implications of each of these program effects for HIV risk, while promising, are not clear. For example, an increase in teenage pregnancy within marriage, at the expense of pregnancy outside of it, may actually increase HIV risk if there is a greater tendency for the former to involve unprotected sex with older men.

On that score, a promising recent finding (Dupas 2009), from an extension of the same Kenya project, is that a program informing girls about the much higher HIV risk from older men relative to teenage boys led to a 65 percent decrease in the incidence of pregnancies by adult partners among teenage girls in the treatment group relative to the control group. Given these striking results, it would be of interest to replicate and evaluate this type of program in other contexts. Further, the fact that in at least one case (the Tanzania randomized study), self-reported risky behavior declined without any measurable impact on a range of biological HIV-related indicators shows the need for evaluations using the latter endpoints—despite the fact that such studies will generally be more complex and larger, hence more expensive.

The need for rigorous evaluation would certainly apply to "abstinence-only" programs, which are being heavily promoted in Uganda and elsewhere. There are no evaluations in Africa of this approach or comparisons of it with other programs for youth, but abstinence-only programs in the U.S. have by and large been found to be ineffective at delaying sexual initiation and reducing sexual risk-taking behaviors in the long term (Kirby 2001).[20]

The foregoing review has concerned school-based awareness and prevention programs. Evaluations of non-school interventions aimed at youth are less common.[21] Agha (2002) reports on a quasi-experimental evaluation of adolescent sexual health interventions in four African countries (Cameroon, Botswana, South Africa, and Guinea) in the mid to late 1990s. These interventions combined to varying degrees mass media (radio messages), sponsored events, peer education, and youth-friendly contraceptive services. Changes between baseline and follow-up surveys were compared for intervention towns or neighborhoods and selected comparison locales. Population impacts on perceptions and self-reported behaviors varied (and tended to be larger for young women), but one conclusion is that more intensive interventions using a variety of channels are needed to insure that a large share of adolescents is reached. This is especially relevant for Africa, where many such young people will no longer be attending school.

## 6. Structural Approaches

Frustration with the lack of success of many individual-focused interventions for behavior change has led to emphasis on changing the underlying "structural" factors that condition individual HIV risk behavior (Gupta et al. 2008; Coates, Richter, and Caceres 2008). The range of possible structural determinants is very wide, and includes political, legal, economic, and cultural factors and social norms—essentially, any social factor that is beyond the control of individuals but conditions their sexual behavior. Because they affect HIV outcomes at a remove from individual behavior, structural factors are "causally distal" or "upstream" determinants. A distinction is frequently made between "macro" and "meso" levels: the former refers to national institutions, laws, and economic conditions, as well as to cultural norms regarding gender and sexual relations, while the latter may refer to individuals' social and sexual networks, community norms, and local access to health care services.

Many structural interventions operate at the meso—typically, community—level. These include programs to change behavior by training respected community leaders to promote prevention, or by exploiting "influential networks" to transmit information. Many others operate essentially at the individual level but are considered to be structural because they address the context of risk. One important example, discussed below, is interventions to empower women, either through training in negotiating risk or by improving their economic situation. In this case, the structural factor that is addressed is women's lack of power in sexual relationships. Macro-level policies might include changes in the legal climate relevant to HIV risk (for example, regarding gender equality and creation and enforcement of laws against rape) and policies to address poverty and migration. Importantly, macro-level policy also encompasses efforts to change behavioral or gender norms via national education campaigns and social mobilization.

The distinctions between levels are important from the point of view of evaluation. Structural interventions at the community level can be assessed like any other community-level intervention, including through the use of RCTs (Bonnell et al. 2006). Measurement of outcomes at the community level (including direct participants and non-participants) will capture spillovers within the community, which are likely to be important—indeed, some interventions such as those utilizing social networks are designed precisely to operate through such externalities. Macro-level policies which affect a country as a whole cannot be analyzed so simply—there is no readily available control group in such cases. In cases of a discrete shift in policy, a natural experiment might be possible. For example, one can compare outcomes shortly before and shortly after a change in laws. In other cases, it will be very difficult to say whether changes in outcomes (behavioral or epidemiological) are related to the policy in question or to other policies or other trends, such as endogenous behavioral responses to HIV prevalence and mortality. Because of this, assessment of macro-social policy usually makes use of simple comparative analysis of trends in different (but, hopefully, similar) countries. As noted in Section 3, this approach is open to a good deal of ambiguity. On the other hand, while meso-level structural interventions may be easier to assess rigorously, it may be the case that structural interventions are only really successful, or are more successful, when they are national in scope. This issue is taken up below.

Evaluation of structural interventions is made more challenging by the fact that the links between the intervention and the intended outcomes are indirect ("casually distal") and complex. For an individual-level intervention such as HIV education in the classroom, one looks for a direct impact of the education (with appropriate control for non-random selection) on adolescents' knowledge or self-reported risk behavior, or on biomedical outcomes such as pregnancy or HIV status. Consider instead an intervention designed to reduce HIV risk by "empowering" women via microcredit, workshops on gender relations, or a combination of the two. To be successful the intervention must first lead to empowerment, however defined. Empowerment in turn must lead to other changes, such as a change in the risk behavior of one's sexual partners (getting them to use condoms or to be monogamous) or a switch to different partners or to fewer or no partners. These changes in turn may affect HIV risk. Simply finding that women were "empowered" as a result of the intervention does not establish that the intervention reduces HIV risk. For this reason, biological markers (HIV incidence) are particularly important for evaluating structural interventions. As always, this raises the necessary sample size for trials and is often not feasible.

STRUCTURAL INTERVENTIONS FOR HIV PREVENTION IN AFRICA—
MESO OR INDIVIDUAL LEVEL:

Many programs that qualify as "structural" are being carried out in Africa. A number of interventions at the meso or individual level address norms of gender inequality, partner violence, or intergenerational sex, and are tailored specifically to either female or male participants. Several of these are RCTs and include measures of HIV as outcomes.

The Stepping Stones program, which so far has been implemented in at least 40 countries, uses participatory learning to build knowledge of sexual health, awareness of risks and the consequences of risk taking and communication skills, and to provide opportunities for "facilitated self-reflection" on sexual behavior. The South African version of the program is rare in that it used a cluster (village) randomized evaluation and measured changes in HIV status (Jewkes et al. 2006b). The design of the trial was intention to treat: the sample in each treatment cluster consisted of randomly selected individuals who were offered the program, and outcomes of both participants and non-participants in the (gender segregated) sessions in these clusters were measured. Among men there were reductions in the self-reported number of current partners at 12- and 24-month follow-up in treatment relative to control clusters, as well as a greater likelihood of condom use at last sex at 12 months and reductions in transactional sex at 12 months. The proportion of men in the Stepping Stones arm who disclosed perpetrating severe intimate partner violence was lower at 12 and 24 months. These findings suggest some impact on behavior, but also that several of these were not sustained (present after one but not two years). They are, of course, also self-reported, hence may be affected by bias; for example, men may have been more ashamed to admit to abusive behavior after participating in the program and being told that such behavior is inappropriate. HIV infection rates were too low in the sample to detect any statistically significant differences among men; but among women, there were 15 percent fewer new HIV infections after two years in the Stepping Stones arm than in control clusters (Jewkes et al. 2007).[22]

Other interventions are designed to use social influence and social networks to promote behavior change. The National Institute of Mental Health Collaborative HIV/STD Prevention Trial, a multi-site community randomized study in China, India, Russia, Zimbabwe, and Peru, is testing an intervention to mobilize and train community popular opinion leaders (CPOLs) to promote change in sexual risk behavior and norms throughout a community. The study, results of which have not yet been presented, will assess both behavioral and biological (HIV infection) outcomes. An earlier, non-randomized study trained influential individuals ("Influence Network Agents") from the health, religious, non-governmental, and private sectors in Kigali, Rwanda and Lusaka, Zambia (Allen et al. 2007).

These individuals then invited couples known to them for HIV testing and counseling. The response rate to the invitations among couples was disappointingly low—14 percent in Zambia and 27 percent in Rwanda.

A related approach was used in an AIDS prevention project implemented in Muslim communities in Uganda (Kagimu et al. 1998). This intervention trained religious leaders who in turn educated their communities about AIDS. After two years, there was a significant increase in the share of residents with correct knowledge of HIV transmission, methods of preventing HIV infection, and the risks associated with ablution of the dead and unsterile circumcision. Reductions in sexual risk behaviors were also recorded. However, the simple pretest-posttest framework study design did not allow for the disentangling of intervention effects from trends in these communities or in the country as whole.

Interventions to Increase Women's Power
Women's lack of power in relationships is commonly cited as a significant source of HIV risk in African societies. Women may be unable to refuse unwanted sexual relations and may lack the power or skills to negotiate condom use with partners who they fear are HIV positive. Further, there is an association of intimate partner violence, on the one hand, and HIV infection in women and high-risk behavior on the part of their male partners, including having multiple partners and alcohol abuse, on the other (Dunkle et al. 2006; Maman et al. 2002; van der Straten et al. 2008). These patterns have led to the advocacy of programs to "empower" women as a means of reducing their vulnerability to HIV—in addition to providing direct benefits to women in the sense of giving them greater control over their lives. This is "structural," as it addresses underlying factors of female poverty and gender inequality which condition sexual behavior and risk. How can women be empowered? Although a number of earlier interventions tried to provide women with skills to negotiate safe sex, several recent programs have folded this training into microcredit programs. Such programs have become widely popular in development policy as a means both of reducing household poverty and increasing women's economic independence, though findings from a large number of studies are mixed.[23] Greater economic autonomy in turn is assumed to increase women's power in relationships, over both household decisions and sexual relations. Therefore, for microfinance combined with HIV/gender training to affect HIV risk among women, it must, as a first step, be shown to empower women. Despite popular perceptions, research does not always find that microcredit is empowering of women, measured variously through self-reported economic independence, levels of intimate partner violence, freedom of movement and association, and related indicators.[24]

Assuming that participation does empower women and, specifically, gives them more say in their sexual lives, there are several possible links to reduced HIV risk.

Risk reduction can occur if one or more the following takes place: women negotiate safer sex (condom use) with high-risk partners; insist their partners get
tested for HIV; end relationships with partners who engage in high-risk behaviors
or are or abusive (the latter as noted is often correlated with the former); are able
to alter the risk behavior of their partners (e.g., the number of outside partners
they have); or have less need to exchange sex for income or goods. While this
list suggests a range of pathways, for many women—especially those in stable
long-term partnerships— most may not be very likely. For example, it may be too
much to expect such women to demand that their partners use condoms, even if
they felt they had the power to do so; as noted earlier, evidence suggests this does
not happen unless one partner is known to be HIV positive. Some women may
use their greater independence to end high-risk partnerships, but it is unclear
how many would take this major step.[25] Women with greater bargaining power
might be able to demand that their partners reduce risk behaviors outside of the
relationship, but they cannot easily verify compliance (e.g., whether the spouse
sees other women, visits commercial sex workers, or uses condoms with other
partners). Some studies show that participation in microcredit leads to a reduction in self-reported incidence of intimate partner violence (IPV); IPV in turn is
linked to greater male HIV risk behaviors, as noted above. However, the second
association does not imply that reducing IPV will also reduce risk behaviors of
male partners outside the relationship—unless the reduction in IPV comes about
via a change in partners to less violence prone/lower risk men. Where women are
in stable relationships, this is not to be expected. These *a priori* considerations
suggest that the possibilities for empowerment to lead to reduced HIV risk may
be limited, especially among women in long term partnerships.[26]

Turning to the evidence, several integrated microfinance/HIV prevention programs have been implemented in Africa. The most rigorous evaluation is the cluster randomized trial of the Intervention with Microfinance for AIDS and Gender
Equity (IMAGE) Program conducted in rural Limpopo, South Africa, which provided women with training in gender equity, domestic violence prevention, and
HIV/AIDS prevention (Pronyk et al. 2006). Self-reported incidence of domestic
violence fell 55 percent after one year for program participants compared to controls (the latter defined below). Indicators of "empowerment" also improved (Kim
et al. 2008). Finally, young women (aged 14–35) who took part in the intervention
showed significantly higher levels (relative to controls) of HIV-related communication, were more likely to have accessed HIV testing, and were less likely to have
had unprotected sex at last intercourse with a non-spousal partner (Pronyk et al.
2008). The program also measured HIV incidence among women in intervention
and control villages (not between participants and non-participants). No differences were found.

These results suggest that combined microfinance/HIV prevention programs can reduce the prevalence of factors associated with HIV risk among poor women, but the findings need to be carefully interpreted. As stressed, improvements in empowerment indicators do not imply reduction in actual HIV risk. In view of the considerations discussed above, the findings for younger women, who are less likely to be married or in a stable partnership, may be the most promising in terms of suggesting reduced risk. On a methodological level, while the intervention was randomly assigned to communities, the comparison of outcomes for participants and non-participants, which is the core of the impact evaluation, does not benefit from randomization; instead, participants in intervention communities are matched on basic characteristics with women in control villages. Participants are a self-selected group of women who chose to apply for loans, hence may differ from randomly selected, observationally similar women in the control communities in ways that affect their responsiveness to the gender training as well as to the microfinance program. Therefore is it not clear that the "controls" so defined are an appropriate comparison group.

With respect to the finding of no impacts on HIV incidence in this study, follow-up rates were quite low (only 64 percent). Equally fundamentally, incidence was measured in random samples of women in treatment and control communities, not from program participants; this apparently was necessary because of the relatively small size of the participant sample. This part of the analysis does exploit the cluster level randomization and is a standard intention to treat analysis. However, for the evaluation to capture effects on HIV incidence at the community level, there would have to be significant spillover effects on behavior from participants to non-participants in treatment communities. This seems to set the bar quite high for finding impacts on incidence.[27]

Two other interventions in Africa combining microfinance and HIV prevention are unusual in that they are directed at young women or adolescent girls, rather than older women as in most microfinance programs. The norms that are targeted by these programs are those relating to intergenerational sex. Girls' vulnerability to HIV infection is typically much higher than for boys of the same age, because of the prevalence of relationships of with older men. Since these relationships are often characterized by the exchange of sex for gifts or income, it is possible that programs that increase the economic independence of young women will help them avoid these risky relationships. The SHAZ! (Shaping the Health of Adolescents in Zimbabwe) Program in Harare combined business training and mentoring, microcredit loans, life-skills training, and HIV prevention for out-of-school, orphaned girls, aged 16–19. A pilot study of 50 girls found that a large share of the young women were unable to pay back the loans. Some also experienced sexual exploitation from men they came into contact with while conducting their economic activities (Dunbar et al. forthcoming). The next phase of the study, involving a larger sample of girls and using a randomized assignment into the program, placed less emphasis on microcredit. Preliminary results (Kang-Dufour et al. 2009) suggest that participation led to reduced experience of partner violence as well as to lower rates of unintended pregnancy.

The second program was TRY (Tap and Reposition Youth) directed at girls aged 15–19 in slum areas of Nairobi, which again combined gender training and access to loans as well as other vocational assistance. There was some evidence that participants were more likely than members of a comparison group (matched, as in the IMAGE evaluation, on several individual and household characteristics) to demand condom use or refuse sexual relations (Erulkar and Chong 2005). However, the low follow-up rate (68 percent) raises the possibility of selection biases and may explain why the level of reported condom use actually fell in both treatment and control groups. While overall the income and asset situation of participants improved, the loan component was less successful. Repayment rates were relatively poor, similar to the pilot study in Zimbabwe.

One thing these two evaluations suggest is that although poor young women are particularly vulnerable to risky sexual relationships because of their greater economic dependency, programs to remedy this dependency by combining loans and HIV training may not work well, in part because there are multiple dimensions to their vulnerability. For example, in the Zimbabwe intervention, girls who were given the means to be economically active faced new threats in the marketplace. Further, microcredit may not be appropriate for this age group, who for the most part would not meet the criteria for loans in standard microcredit programs, as Dunbar et al. (forthcoming) point out with respect to SHAZ!. Therefore the microcredit-empowerment link does not seem promising for young women; although for more mature women, the South Africa evaluation suggests (though tentatively) that there may be risk reduction benefits. Other means to improve livelihoods may help young women in terms of empowerment and risk reduction, as the more recent SHAZ! findings imply.

One might conclude from these experiences that structural interventions to prevent HIV transmission from older men to younger women should instead, or additionally, try to alter the norms and behaviors of the men who would enter into these relationships. A more general issue, when assessing the evidence for individual- or community-level structural change interventions, is whether achieving real change in norms of behavior is a society-wide process that can only be effective if it takes place at the broader, macro-social level.

## STRUCTURAL INTERVENTIONS FOR HIV PREVENTION IN AFRICA—MACRO LEVEL

Macro-level policies that affect the structural determinants of HIV can be as diverse as those at the meso or individual level. A wide range of economic and social factors ultimately influence HIV behavior or risk. It should be pointed out that most macro-level policies that alter the context of HIV risk are not explicitly directed at the epidemic—for example, macroeconomic or trade policy that affects income levels or geographic mobility. Some are patently unrealistic as a means of combating HIV/AIDS in anything but the very long term: for example, "ending poverty." This discussion focuses specifically on macro-level structural policies explicitly designed for HIV prevention, in particular by changing social, sexual, or gender norms.

Again, Uganda takes center stage in the discussion. One could view what happened in Uganda in the 1990s from the perspective of the standard cognitive behavioral approach: public campaigns informed people and motivated them to reduce risks to their health. What distinguished Uganda from other similarly afflicted countries of the region, from this perspective, would be that these campaigns were implemented early, aggressively, and in multiple fora, and that they emphasized the most effective change in behavior for slowing the epidemic (partner reduction). However, as noted in Section 5.1, many have argued that what happened in Uganda went beyond this and represented a concerted effort to change behavior not by influencing individuals' calculus of costs and benefits of different sexual behaviors, but by changing ideas of what was and was not socially acceptable (in particular, that multiple partnerships were not acceptable behavior for men) (Shelton et al. 2004, Epstein and Kim 2007; Murphy et al. 2006). Epstein and Kim argue that this shift in norms was inextricably tied to the activities of women's groups, which traditionally have been strong in Uganda. At the national level, these groups pressed for laws guaranteeing gender equity and against rape. At the community level, women's organizations broadcast the notion that infidelity on the part of men was not acceptable and, it seems, managed to enforce a moral sanction (shame) to such behavior. Presumably, the authority of these groups at the local level was significantly enhanced, or even made possible, by what was taking place at the national level, including President Musevini's strong support for women's rights. The observational evidence for such activities and their impacts is necessarily very different from the evaluations of meso-level interventions discussed above, consisting essentially of informed observation of scholars and others.[28]

Other national scale attempts to alter social norms related to HIV have been noted. In South Africa, the Soul City project (4th series) was a multi-level program to address domestic violence (not HIV risk explicitly) using television, print media, and radio. An assessment using various means, including representative household surveys, indicated that the campaign reached a large share of the population and was associated with statistically significant changes in attitudes toward domestic abuse (Usdin et al. 2005). Usdin et al. also suggest that the campaign was instrumental in the implementation of the country's Domestic Violence Act.

Although the project was not directly concerned with HIV, and causal impacts cannot be inferred, the experience does suggest the possibility of large scale mobilization to alter norms of behavior related to gender (and likely by extension, HIV behavior). In Thailand, the aggressive campaign for 100 percent condom use among sex workers, which involved massive publicity and engagement of numerous groups in society, is also often described as having changed social norms of behavior.

The idea that social norms can be changed by macro-level policy has notable precedents in developed countries. Examples from the U.S. include large shifts in attitudes toward smoking after several decades of public health messages and changes in attitudes toward racial and gender equality. Still, the Ugandan examples and others related to HIV raise several questions. First, it is inherently hard to say whether outcomes reflect shifts in social norms or (as in the cognitive theories of behavior change) changes in knowledge and incentives for altering behavior. Presumably, both are at play to some extent. Second, the more recent backsliding in the gains made in Uganda, in terms of risk reduction (including, with respect to multiple partnerships) noted in Section 2, may lead one to question whether something as profound as a change in social norms had been achieved in a meaningful sense. It is worth noting that the changes in social attitudes and behaviors described above for the U.S. took several decades to be realized. Finally, to return to a point made at the end of the previous subsection, it is possible that community-level structural interventions of the type discussed in the previous section are more effective (or are only effective) in the presence of substantial mobilization toward the same goals at the national level. If this is the case, evaluations of isolated structural interventions where society-wide mobilization is not occurring will understate the potential value of these approaches.

## 7. Conclusions

In an earlier review of HIV prevention interventions, Potts et al. (2008) classified interventions into two groups: those that have been shown to be effective and those that appear to be ineffective or only weakly effective. This is a simple but useful exercise, though we might also add a third category for interventions whose promise has recently been touted but whose effectiveness remains unproven.

The evidence described in this chapter yields an overall picture that is far from overwhelmingly positive. Interventions that clearly belong in the "proven effective" group unfortunately remain very limited. They include, essentially, two: partner reduction campaigns (based on experiences in Uganda and several other countries) and male circumcision (based on strong findings in several controlled trials and prior observational evidence). The list of interventions that have so far shown either mixed or little effectiveness is longer: control of other STIs, HIV testing and counseling, condom promotion, programs targeting students or youth, most microbicides, and microcredit programs for women. Interventions that have been advocated but not yet widely or rigorously assessed for prevention impacts include antiretroviral-based microbicides, ARV provision, and many structural interventions.

The foregoing suggests that greater attention and resources should be focused on the two interventions in the first group than currently is the case, but it hardly suggests that there should be a wholesale shift to them. The complexities of the epidemic—especially of Africa's generalized epidemics that are no longer confined to specific vulnerable groups—and of the behavior related to it preclude an exclusive focus on one or two key interventions. Specifically, the following factors imply the need for a broad approach.

First, many of the interventions that, at least on their own, have not shown consistent effectiveness in prevention are nevertheless clearly essential to broader prevention efforts. A prevention strategy with condom promotion as the main plank seems unlikely to be successful in a generalized epidemic, but condoms are nevertheless essential for prevention of transmission within serodiscordant couples, and as protection for single, sexually active people. HIV testing and counseling overall has limited impacts on behavior but is an essential component of risk reduction for certain groups (partners of those who test positive) and is the gateway to ARV therapy. In-school HIV education may not consistently change risk behaviors among youth, but it is hard to imagine a successful national AIDS prevention program that does not seek to education young people about risks.

Second, even for interventions that have shown significant success—and all the more for those that appear promising but have not yet been well tested—expectations must be realistic. To echo a phrase that has come to be used frequently in the literature, there is no "magic bullet" for HIV prevention in Africa. Male circumcision has had very impressive results in clinical trials and holds promise as a scaled up intervention, but the possibility of compensation in risk behavior that could significantly offset the benefits is real. Circumcision also, of course, provides only partial protection against infection, and this will almost certainly be true as well of any microbicides that are found to be effective (for that matter, even an eventual vaccine will likely not offer complete protection). Partner reduction is both possible to achieve and effective against the epidemic, as Uganda and other cases show, but as Uganda also shows, these gains are hard to sustain. Structural interventions now are held out by many as the logical place to focus attention and resources, but the evidence base is still weak and there are reasons, discussed above, why the benefits may turn out to be modest.

Third, even for biomedical prevention interventions that are successful or appear promising, effectiveness will depend strongly on behavioral responses.

The example of male circumcision was just given. Others include microbicides: even if one is eventually shown clinically to be effective, it will still require that individuals be willing or able to use it consistently. Antiretroviral therapy, though not directly a prevention intervention, may lead to changes in behavior that possibly hurt (through treatment optimism) prevention efforts. These "non-behavioral" interventions need to be integrated with behavioral approaches that seek to prevent such negative or offsetting outcomes, for example, counseling men who are getting circumcised about the need to not increase other risk behaviors.

With most interventions at best only partially successful in changing behavior or in providing protection against risk, or only successful with specific groups (e.g., VCT with HIV-positive clients), it is necessary for national strategies to be multipronged, that is, feature multiple prevention approaches (McCoy, Fikree, and Padian 2009; Merson et al. 2008; Coates, Richter, and Caceres 2008). This needs to be done, of course, with due consideration to appropriateness for the context as well as feasibility and cost effectiveness (both of which are outside the scope of this chapter).

Another general conclusion—gleaned not from individual impact evaluations but from broader country-level observation—is that a high level of national commitment and leadership (not limited to providing financial resources), and a corresponding engagement with different levels of society in prevention campaigns, is essential. This happened in the very different environments of Uganda, Senegal, and Thailand.

With regard to research, there is a need for more rigorous testing of interventions, both existing and new, to improve the evidence base for choosing among policies. Many of the evaluations discussed above lacked credible treatment or control groups, or failed to control for trends affecting outcomes that were unrelated to the intervention. In most cases randomized controlled trials are the optimal method for evaluation. Compared with strictly biomedical interventions, the share of behavioral interventions evaluated in Africa using RCTs remains small but is growing. For the (many) cases where RCTs are not feasible, rigorous quasi-experimental approaches need to be routinely employed to derive appropriate treatment and control or comparison groups. Structural interventions raise particular challenges to formal evaluation, but given the increased interest in such approaches, these challenges need to be faced in future research.

It is also important to expand, where possible, the use of objective biomedical endpoints to assess outcomes, whether this is HIV infection itself or proxies for risk behaviors such as other STIs or teenage pregnancy. Given the unreliability of self reports of behavior change, this would be an important advance in providing a firmer evidence base for policies—though admittedly, it will not always, or even typically, be possible, given the costs (sample size) and potential invasiveness (testing participants) of such a design. Use of biomedical outcomes may be especially important for structural interventions, for which the pathways to behavior and risk are potentially very complex.

Finally, in view of the need for multiple interventions to achieve effective HIV prevention, more effort needs to be made to test the effectiveness of combinations of interventions. The vast majority of evaluations to date have focused on single interventions.[29] Related to this, it is also necessary to gain a better understanding of how individuals respond in terms of risk behavior to new biomedical interventions such as male circumcision or, as in the case of ARV provision, to the availability of such interventions, and to evaluate interventions that combine biomedical components with behavioral modification.

## Notes

1. UNAIDS defines a generalized epidemic as one in which adult HIV prevalence among the general adult population is at least 1 percent and transmission mostly heterosexual, and a concentrated epidemic as one in which HIV is concentrated in groups with behaviors that expose them to a high risk of HIV infection. (See http://data.unaids.org/pub/GlobalReport/2006/2006_Epi_backgrounder_on_methodology_en.pdf)

2. The evidence for recent behavior change comes from the 2000 and 2004 DHS (Green et al. 2006) and a rural cohort survey (Shafer et al. 2008); evidence for rising or leveling prevalence, from the cohort study and from antenatal surveillance sites.

3. As noted above, it is possible via epidemiological modeling to infer whether trends in national HIV prevalence reflect changes in risk behavior as opposed to the natural course of the epidemic. However, it is not possible with such methods to say what the role of policy was in producing these outcomes.

4. Among other factors, the tissue of the internal foreskin contains large concentrations of "target cells" for HIV infection. See Bailey, Plummer, and Moses (2001); Auvert et al. (2006).

5. Community randomized experiments would be the ideal approach for learning about the prevention impacts in the general population. The introduction of testing sites providing the drugs is typically staggered, reflecting resource and logistical constraints: the drugs will initially be available in certain areas and not others. The latter can form natural "late treatment" controls during the period for which ARVs are still unavailable in them. Even if it was not possible to randomize the rollout, quasi-experimental methods (difference in difference, matching, or both) can be used to control for differences in early and late treatment communities.

6. Senegal also is notable for an aggressive and early policy stance against AIDS. Unlike Uganda and most of sub-Saharan Africa, these actions were able to contain the disease before it reached generalized epidemic stage; HIV in Senegal still appears concentrated among specific high-risk groups such as sex workers (UNAIDS 2006a).

7. The responses from the DHS indicate either that people in Uganda were more likely to recognize others' illness and mortality as being caused by AIDS, or that others or their families were more likely to admit to having AIDS, or both. Since AIDS victims do not die from the HIV virus itself but from a variety of other infections that take advantage of weakened immune systems, it is easy (and very common) for families to claim that death was from some cause other than AIDS.

8. Thus "ABC," in the sense of an equal emphasis on each element, is not a totally accurate characterization of Uganda's early successful prevention campaign; indeed the phrase apparently came into use only later, in the mid-1990s (Slutkin et al. 2006).

9. Antenatal clinic surveillance data on young women provide insight into incidence, not just prevalence: given relative closeness to sexual debut, HIV-positive status in young women reflects recent infection.

10. Condoms, strictly speaking, are a biomedical intervention that blocks transmission of the virus. However, because prevention success depends so strongly on behavior (the willingness and ability to use them), it makes more sense here to consider them as a behavioral intervention.

11. Though Allen and Heald (2004) argue that policymakers in Botswana indeed pushed hard, but that the emphasis of policy—on condoms—was misdirected.

12. Condom use appears to be high within serodiscordant couples who have been tested (see below in the discussion of VCT), but with testing rates still low, the vast majority of serodiscordant couples in Africa are not aware of their HIV status.

13. Epstein (2007) describes how official prevention messages in Uganda have in recent years abandoned the strong focus on "zero grazing" or fidelity. In addition to condom promotion, abstinence has played a much larger role (including abstinence only messages for youth), encouraged by social conservatives, the U.S. government, and Ugandan First Lady Janet Museveni.

14. However, if this information is already widely known, the marginal contribution of VCT to knowledge will be diminished.

15. However, as Glick (2005) notes, this much cited study may suffer from external validity problems, since the study population consisted of volunteers for an HIV prevention study whose motivation or ability to change behavior in response to testing is not likely to be representative of the broader target population for VCT.

16. Though, it should be noted that this is conditional on having agreed in the first place to give a blood sample (78 percent of respondents).

17. This experiment is a rare example in Africa of a policy to reduce HIV risk using conditional cash transfers (giving a payment conditioned on a specific behavior). Medlin and de Walque (2008) discuss the potential for this approach to enhance HIV prevention in developing countries.

18. Under this approach, an HIV test is given by default as part of any medical care, but the patient has the option of refusing the test; hence it is an "opt out" approach to testing as opposed to the "opt in" approach of VCT.

19. Unfortunately, as noted, HIV-positive individuals are most infectious (hence pose the greatest risk to others) in the first month after contracting the virus. During this period they may experience illness that is non-AIDS symptomatic and thus may not lead them to suspect that they have been infected. Hence identifying such individuals is very difficult.

20. A related controversy is whether advising young people about condoms encourages earlier sexual activity. As noted, Dreyfuss et al. (2006) found in western Kenya that condom education increased condom use by teenagers but not rates of sexual activity (both behaviors self-reported).

21. The survey by Gallant and Maticka-Tyndale (2004), covering interventions in all developing countries published as of two years earlier, could not locate a single evaluation study of non-school based adolescent prevention programs that used as outcomes measures either self-reported condom use, number of partners, or age at first sex.

22. A related intervention (directed solely at men) is Men as Partners, implemented in several African countries including South Africa and Nigeria. This has not been subjected to rigorous evaluation using HIV endpoints, but in a pilot evaluation in Nigeria, the

intervention group had significantly higher self reported condom use, "self-efficacy for negotiation," and "power sharing" in relationships than the comparison group at three-month follow-up (Exner et al. 2009).

23. Several recent randomized trials found no impacts on household consumption (Banerjee et al. 2009; Karlan and Zinman 2009).

24. For conflicting views and evidence, see Goetz and Gupta (1995); Johnson and Rogaly (1997); Kabeer (2001); and Rahman (1999).

25. In the South African IMAGE project described below, rates of divorce or separation were not different for participating and non-participating women, even though various measures of empowerment improved among the participants.

26. Further, improved economic circumstances and mobility of women may actually increase risk by increasing access to sexual partners, as is the case for men (Hirsch et al. 2007).

27. It should also be noted with regard to this study that it is not clear whether the apparent changes in prevention behaviors came through the HIV training (a gender-based HIV prevention approach), the greater income or economic independence via the loans (i.e., a standard microfinance intervention), or their interaction. A multi-armed evaluation would be needed to assess this.

28. DHS surveys in many countries now regularly include modules on Domestic Violence and Women's Status, which could provide indications of changes in gender norms. These may prove useful for charting changes elsewhere and in the future, but they or alternatives are not available for the period of the 1990s in Uganda.

29. A rare exception is the evaluation by Williams et al. (2003) of an intensive HIV intervention started in 1998 in a mining community in South Africa that combined peer education, condom distribution, syndromic management of sexually transmitted infections, and presumptive STI treatment for sex workers. There was little evidence of significant behavior change over a two-year period (and an actual increase in the prevalence of other STIs), though it should be noted that the method was a simple pretest and posttest design without a control group. The authors suggest that the context was important in explaining the lack of response to the intervention: AIDS mortality was still low, and the South African government was not putting out broader messages about HIV risk and behavior change—in other words, a further important complementarity with national-level policy was missing.

# CHAPTER 10

Treating Ourselves to Trouble? The Impact of HIV Treatment in Africa:
Lessons from the Industrial World

*Elizabeth Pisani*

## Introduction

As the HIV epidemic approaches its fourth decade, there are many failures and
rather fewer successes to reflect on. The greatest failure is surely in the area of
prevention. This viral infection, preventable by avoiding the exchange of body
fluids between infected and uninfected individuals, has killed an estimated 27
million people since AIDS, the syndrome it causes, was identified in 1981. At the
end of 2007, between 30.6 million and 36.1 million people were believed to be
living with the virus, which remains incurable (UNAIDS 2008a). Two-thirds of
these people lived in sub-Saharan Africa; in several countries in Southern Africa,
over one adult in five is infected with a preventable disease that governments,
communities, and individuals have, collectively, failed to prevent.

Though dwarfed by failures in preventing the spread of HIV, there have been
important successes in treating the virus and delaying the onset of AIDS-defining
illnesses and death. Highly active antiretroviral therapy (HAART) became widely
available in wealthy countries in 1995. AIDS incidence and AIDS deaths both
dropped precipitously as a result (UNAIDS 1998b). One of the effects of antiretroviral drugs (ARVs) is to reduce the viral load—the amount of virus circulat-
ing freely in blood and genital fluids. The likelihood that an infected individual
will pass HIV on to another person during unprotected sex or while sharing
injecting equipment is strongly related to the infected person's viral load (Quinn
et al. 2000; Wawer et al. 2003, 2005b). This led to widespread optimism that treatment of those infected would reduce the number of new infections. Some predicted that treatment would essentially spell an end to ongoing transmission of
HIV in well-resourced settings such as the United States (Blower, Gershengorn,
and Grant 2000).

Unfortunately, that has not yet proven to be the case. Indeed the data reviewed in this paper suggest that new infections are rising among men who have sex with other men (MSM) in rich countries where access to treatment is very good. Despite this, policymakers from the World Health Organization have recently posited that a massive expansion of treatment across Africa may be the best hope for preventing the continuing spread of the virus (Granich et al. 2009).

This paper outlines the conceptual basis for HIV treatment as effective prevention. It looks at issues of infectiousness linked to virology, co-infection and health service use, as well as assumptions about sexual behavior, examining experiences in these areas to date. The vast majority of this experience comes from gay communities in wealthy countries, but the still sparse data from sub-Saharan Africa are also reviewed. The paper discusses the extent to which the experiences of the industrial world are likely to be duplicated in sub-Saharan Africa.

The conclusions are necessarily speculative. The epidemiology of HIV is very different in sub-Saharan Africa than in other parts of the world, and it varies considerably within the continent. In most of the world, including North Africa, HIV remains largely concentrated among people who inject drugs, sell sex, or buy it, as well as among men who have anal sex with other men. In parts of West Africa, these groups are also overrepresented among people infected with HIV, though prevalence among those who do not have any particularly high-risk behavior can also be high. In those parts of East and Southern Africa where concurrent sex partnerships are common, HIV has spread widely through sexual networks, affecting a significant proportion of working-age adults. The complex relationship between HIV treatment and prevention is likely to be very different in a country such as Swaziland where a third of adults are infected with HIV, than it is in Niger where prevalence is less than a tenth as high. This paper focuses largely on likely outcomes in the higher-prevalence epidemics of East and Southern Africa; these are also the sources of much of the limited treatment data available from the continent.

It is worth noting that those data that do exist come largely from well-resourced research settings in the early stages of treatment rollout. The people who have access to these programs are probably not representative of all those in need, and the quality of service delivery may not be replicable on the much larger scale required to meet existing and future treatment needs. To the limited extent possible, the paper discusses how treatment-prevention interactions may change as services are expanded over time.

## Treatment as Prevention: The Biological Basis

Early in the HIV epidemic, studies of discordant couples (in which one partner is HIV-infected and the other is uninfected) attempted to measure the infectivity of

HIV per sex act. Some estimated extremely low levels of infectivity, ranging between 1 infection per 3,000 sex acts for uninfected men in vaginal sex with infected women to 1 infection per 1,600 sex acts in receptive anal sex, but there was considerable variation in the estimates (Downs and de Vincenzi 1996; Leynaert, Downs, and de Vincenzi 1998; de Vincenzi 1994; Mastro and de Vincenzi 1996; Galvin and Cohen 2004).

It has since become clear that the likelihood of HIV transmission is strongly (though by no means exclusively) linked to the viral load of the infected partner, and that the viral load varies in a predictable way over time, peaking at very high levels within weeks of first infection, dropping rapidly to a "set point" within a few months, and continuing at low levels for periods of up to several years before rising again shortly before the appearance of AIDS-defining illness (Pilcher et al. 2004a, 2004b).

At the start of this decade, researchers in Uganda identified a strong "dose-response" relationship of plasma viral load with HIV transmission. They found no instances of seroconversion among uninfected people whose infected partners had a viral load of under 1,500 copies of HIV-1 RNA per milliliter (ml). HIV transmission rose steadily with viral load, even after controlling for other factors. For the sex partners of people whose viral load was over 50,000 copies/ml, the incidence rate was 23 seroconversions per 100 person-years of exposure (Quinn et al. 2000; Wawer et al. 2003, 2005b). This finding has been mirrored in a number of other studies in similar but also in different settings (Pedraza et al. 1999; Hisada et al. 2000; Tovanabutra et al. 2002; Buchacz et al. 2004; Castilla et al. 2005; and Brocklehurst 2002).

ARV treatment effectively reduces plasma viral load for a high proportion of people who take the medication correctly, often to levels below which detection with current tests is no longer possible, and well below the 1,500 copies/ml threshold at which transmission is rarely observed. The effect can be seen at the population level. In the U.S., Routy and colleagues found that there was a significant fall in the mean viral loads of people chronically infected with HIV from 4.3 log copies/ml in 1996 to 2.9 log copies/ml in 2000, a period during which the proportion of study participants on ARVs rose from 37 percent to 69 percent. The proportion with undetectable viral loads rose from 14 percent to 55 percent over the same period (Routy et al. 2004).

In an early study of treatment and HIV transmission in Uganda, Bunnell and colleagues reported that viral load among people on treatment fell dramatically during the first six months. Whereas at baseline just one out of 126 participants has a viral load of less than 1,700 copies/ml, after six months of treatment 94/96 patients were below the threshold (Bunnell et al. 2008). More recent data from a well-supported research setting in Uganda show that 79 percent of index patients starting on ARVs had a plasma viral load of under 400 copies of HIV-1 RNA per ml after six months on treatment (Reynolds et al. 2009).

The lower viral loads do indeed seem to be translating into lower HIV transmission at the individual level. In a European setting, Castilla and colleagues found that 8.6 percent of steady partners of index seropositive people not treated with antiretrovirals were infected with HIV, while there were no infections in the partners of people on ARVs (Castilla et al. 2005).

Bunnell and colleagues report that only one of 49 known seronegative spouses of patients on ARVs in their Ugandan study seroconverted in a year (Bunnell et al. 2006). This is supported by more recent data from a population cohort in Uganda, in which consenting adults in the general population are tested for HIV annually, and treated with ARVs if their CD4 count falls below 250. In discordant couples in which the infected partner was not on ARVs, new infections were recorded at 8.6 per 100 person-years of observation, while none of the treated participants passed HIV on to their partners during the limited study period (Reynolds et al. 2009). In Rwanda and Zambia, Sullivan and colleagues found that the incidence of new infections in previously serodiscordant couples was 0.7 percent for those where the infected partner was on ARVs, compared with 3.4 percent where the infected partner remained untreated (Sullivan et al. 2009).

In the heterosexual transmission of HIV, which predominates in most of sub-Saharan Africa and in all of the very high-prevalence epidemics of East and Southern Africa, the amount of free virus in seminal and genital fluids is more important than blood viral load in determining whether a new infection will occur. There is emerging evidence that seminal and genital viral load show greater variability than plasma viral load and may be associated with higher infectivity of HIV in sub-Saharan Africa (Dyer et al. 1997; Vernazza et al. 1997; Chakraborty et al. 2001; Pilcher et al. 2004b; Gupta and Klasse 2006; Pilcher et al. 2007).

A number of recent studies have found that seminal viral load can persist at measurable levels even when plasma viral load is undetectable, and a handful of instances of HIV transmission from people with undetectable levels of HIV in blood have been recorded (Marcelin et al. 2009; Sheth et al. 2009). These observations are not, however, enough to call into question the core observation that when ARV treatment suppresses viral loads to very low levels as measured in plasma, HIV transmission is rare.

Other factors also affect viral load (and therefore, infectivity) for people on treatment—notably interruptions in treatment, treatment failure, and coinfection with other sexually transmitted infections. Treatment interruption can either be deliberate (in which case it is known as structured interruption), or as a result of poor adherence, intermittent access to drug supplies, etc. Sexually transmitted infections (STIs) are associated with higher viral load but are also often associated with periods of high sexual activity which ramp up transmission of new infections.

HIV virology is critical to understanding the likely effect of widespread HIV treatment on the spread of the virus in sub-Saharan Africa. The evidence suggests that ARV treatment can effectively reduce the likelihood of onward transmission

of HIV (and thus work as effective prevention) *at the individual level* in the following circumstances: the infected person has been diagnosed with HIV infection;
the infected person is taking ARVs without interruption; the ARVs are effectively
suppressing viral load; and the infected person does not have other infections
such as STIs which can cause viral load to spike upwards.

These are, essentially, the conditions that were laid out by the Swiss AIDS
Commission in a highly controversial statement on the infectiousness of people
with HIV on ARV treatment (Vernazza et al. 2008). If these conditions were met,
the authors concluded, a person could be considered not to pose any substantial
threat of onward transmission of HIV to their sex partners.

The fact that treatment is preventative at the individual level does not necessarily mean it will prevent rises in incidence at the population level—that will
depend on coverage and quality of treatment as well as on the effect that growth
in treatment might have on sexual behavior. The next section of this chapter
looks at these issues in epidemics in wealthy countries, and where data are available, in African settings.

## Diagnosis of HIV and the Role of Primary Infection

Treatment depends on diagnosis. The timing of diagnosis is extremely important
because a person's viral load (and therefore, infectiousness) varies greatly over the
course of their infection. It is now well established that recently infected people
experience a short period of very high viral load, regardless of gender or route
of transmission. Some of this time in which a person is highly infectious occurs
before the production of antibodies which are captured by common HIV tests—
in other words, before a person seroconverts and becomes "HIV positive" (Celum
et al. 2001; Chakraborty et al. 2001; Gray et al. 2004; Routy et al. 2004; Fiebig et al.
2003; Pilcher et al. 2004a,b).

In a large population of people being tested in public clinics in North Carolina, HIV was transmitted by acute HIV cases at a rate >1:13 to 1:18 unprotected
coital acts (Pilcher et al. 2006). This compares with per act infection rates during
chronic infection for heterosexuals estimated at between 1:2000 and 1:3000 (Galvin
and Cohen 2004). Recent data from a cohort of gay men in the United Kingdom
found that men with primary infection were four times more likely to pass HIV
on to an uninfected partner than those with chronic, untreated infection (Fisher
et al. 2009). However, since this period of high infection is brief compared with
chronic or latent infection (typically lasting four months or less as compared with
a median of some nine years for chronic infection among people who are not
treated), there is currently some debate about the relative contribution of the primary infection phase to the ongoing spread of HIV. Mathematical modeling and

common sense both suggest that its effect is greatest in situations where newly infected people have the highest partner turnover—for example, in commercial sex, among gay men active on the party scene, among injecting drug users, and in jail (Xiridou et al. 2004; Mastro et al. 1994; Ramalingam et al. 2000). These are the groups among whom new infections are concentrated in most of the world, with the notable exception of sub-Saharan Africa. In that region, new infections are spread more widely throughout the general population, passing through sexual networks in which a large proportion of people have a relatively small number of concurrent sexual partners, with partnerships often overlapping for long periods (Halperin and Epstein 2004). It is no surprise, then, that peak infectivity in primary infection will make a greater proportional contribution in non-African epidemics. Recent modeling work suggests that in high prevalence epidemics such as those of East and Southern Africa, lower rates of transmission over long periods of latency contribute a substantial proportion of new infections—perhaps as much as half. Another third may occur in late stage infection (Abu-Raddad and Longini 2008). These conclusions somewhat contradict empirical observations, even in well-established epidemics. Wawer and colleagues observe that 48 percent of all HIV transmission recorded in the Rakai serodiscordance study took place within five months of the infection of the index partner. They calculate that transmission probabilities per act of unprotected sex within the first five months are eight times higher than they are during established infection. They rise again to half their peak levels during late stage infection, the two years before death (Wawer et al. 2003).

Recently, phylogenetic analysis which compares viruses taken from different people has allowed for the investigation of patterns of transmission within a population, and over time. In most societies, patterns of sex and drug taking are far from constant. In their sexual lives, people have periods of high mixing, often in youth and after the break-up of a partnership, interspersed with periods of greater stability. People are more likely both to contract and to transmit HIV when they are in what Koopman and colleagues call "high contact mode" (Koopman et al. 1997).

Phylogenetic analysis of data from gay men in Britain found that where a "most likely" transmitter was identifiable, 24 percent were recent infections at the time they passed on the virus, despite the fact that just 2 percent of the person-years under study were classified as recent infections (Fisher et al. 2009). While the difference in infectivity is almost certainly largely related to viral load, it is interesting to note that people who are newly infected are significantly more likely to transmit HIV even after controlling for differences in viral load, with a rate ratio of transmission of 3.25 compared with transmission by men with untreated chronic infection. This suggests that other factors, possibly including "high contact" sexual risk behaviors, also have an influence. Of further interest, 76 percent of incident cases in this large cohort covering an entire city were unrelated to any other reported case. This suggests that many of the people from whom these men acquired infection remain undiagnosed.

A similar pattern was found in a large phylogenetic analysis in Quebec. Investigators found that though "primary infections" of less than six months in duration accounted for only 10 percent of the profiled sample, they accounted for 50 percent of onward transmission of HIV (Brenner et al. 2007). There was very little co-clustering of chronic and new infections, regardless of treatment status.

Some of these studies have been able to pinpoint time of infection relative to time of diagnosis. In many cases, at least in the UK, men were shown to have passed on HIV before any contact with the health services and any opportunity for diagnosis existed. This was true even for men who presented at health services during primary infection or soon after (Brown et al. 2009), though it is clear that only a small fraction of infections are ever identified this early, even in populations with very high awareness of HIV risk and very good access to publicly funded HIV testing and care services (Sudarshi et al. 2008). Unlinked testing data in the UK suggest that 69 percent of over 1,000 men who walked in to specialist STI clinics with an undiagnosed HIV infection from 1999–2002 left with the infection still undiagnosed. Although uptake of voluntary testing services has since risen dramatically, annual HIV incidence has not fallen (Brown et al. 2009). Among gay men in many industrial countries, including the UK and the U.S., between a fifth and a quarter of new HIV diagnoses are made at the same time as AIDS diagnoses, indicating that the infection has gone undetected for many years. People who have become sexually active since ARVs reduced both the incidence and visibility of AIDS are less likely to be tested; in the UK, three-quarters of gay men under 20 had never tested for HIV, compared with an already high 38 percent of gay men of all ages. Among men who believed they were HIV negative, only a third had tested in the last year (Sigma Research 2008). In Australia, which has one of the highest levels of testing among gay men on record, 66 percent of HIV-negative men in Sydney and 57 percent in Melbourne had their last negative test within the previous 12 months (Prestage et al. 2008).

In summary, well-educated people belonging to groups at high risk for HIV infection in well-resourced settings with near universal access to testing and ARV treatment are still seeking HIV testing only sporadically. For these men, who include most of those most likely to transmit the virus because of peak infectivity, the value of ARVs in preventing the onward spread of HIV is necessarily limited.

Among heterosexuals of African origin in the UK, there is less clustering of new infections around the time of primary infection. In the UK, phylogenetic analysis of non-B subtypes (which are mostly accounted for by heterosexual transmission, much of it among people of African origin) found that the average interval between transmissions within clusters was 27 months, twice the 14 months found with the same methods among gay men in the UK. Only 1 percent of infections happened within six months, compared with 25 percent among gay men (Hughes et al. 2009). This suggests that transmission dynamics among heterosexuals are very different from those found among gay men within the UK, with primary infection accounting for a much lower proportion of infections.

It is not clear to what extent these data can be extrapolated to heterosexuals in sub-Saharan Africa; since partner turnover tends to be lower on average in this population than in gay men in industrial countries, it seems reasonable to expect that the role of primary infection would be less pronounced. This in turn means that very early identification of new infections may be less essential to breaking the chain of transmission through testing and early treatment at the population level in Africa. Identifying prevalent infections remains, however, a *sine qua non* for using treatment to reduce new HIV infections.

Uptake of testing has historically been very low in many African settings. A switch to opt-out testing in health care settings has increased knowledge of serostatus among women in particular. A household survey conducted in Kenya in 2007, with over 15,800 participants, found that HIV testing had increased massively since 2003—26 percent of men and 45 percent of women said they knew their status. That status did not always equate with reality, however. Of true positives, only 16 percent reported being positive—56 percent of those infected had never been tested before, and 28 percent reported that their most recent test was negative.

Efforts to increase testing are underway in many countries. In Uganda, which already has higher levels of testing than many countries, door-to-door testing appears to work well for families of people who are infected, who often have a higher prevalence than the background population. However, even in this well-supported population, the proportion sharing their status with their sex partner remained at two-thirds or below (Lugada et al. 2009). This reduces the possibilities for effective prevention through ARV use, not least because there is a strong association between disclosure and being fully adherent to drug regimens (Tunthanathip et al. 2009). A study of discordant couples in South India found that partners were 5.5 times more likely to seroconvert if their partners did not disclose to them (Kumarasamy et al. 2009).

Identifying incident infections through RNA testing or other methods, challenging in very well-resourced Western settings, is likely to be more challenging still in sub-Saharan Africa. Efforts to develop an algorithm for those at highest risk have yielded some useful results; among male STI patients in Malawi, an algorithm centered on symptoms of primary infection, STI syndromes, and reported sexual behavior proved 95 percent sensitive and 60 percent specific in identifying infections before or during seroconversion, but RNA or p24 antigen testing required to confirm acute primary infections remains costly and rare in developing countries (Powers et al. 2007).

While epidemic dynamics suggest that the importance of very early testing is less pronounced in the high-prevalence epidemics of East and Southern Africa than in settings where HIV is concentrated among subpopulations with high-risk behavior, a recent paper advocating universal treatment as a prevention tool is based on the assumption that previously HIV-negative adults in sub-Saharan Africa will be tested for the virus annually. This level of testing has not been achieved anywhere in the world, even if we restrict analysis to groups at highest risk of infection such as gay men in urban areas in wealthy nations, for whom testing is freely available and heavily promoted. The likelihood that these levels of testing can be achieved in sub-Saharan Africa is frankly slim, although this would be a prerequisite for successful suppression of viral load and thus for the remainder of the "treatment as prevention" strategy.

## Effective Suppression of Viral Load

The first great success in using antiretrovirals as a tool for HIV prevention was in preventing transmission from infected women to their newborns. HIV is now very rarely transmitted to infants in wealthy countries with strong health systems. Regimens to prevent transmission from mother to child have been greatly simplified in recent years, and rolled out on a large scale in many countries with high HIV prevalence. A large trial in five sites across sub-Saharan Africa found that new regimens cut HIV transmission to infants to 5.6 percent, four-fifths lower than the 30 percent transmission rates commonly seen in pretreatment days (de Vincenzi and Kesho Bora Study Group 2009). This effect is achieved largely because treatment of the mother reduces her viral load during pregnancy, around birth, and during breastfeeding, thus lowering the likelihood that she will transmit infectious body fluids to her infant. Preventing transmission of HIV from pregnant women to their infants is popular with donors as well as African governments. Coverage of the services remains low in some countries in sub-Saharan African countries, but as regimens become easier to deliver, it is likely that services will expand rapidly.

Using antiretrovirals to prevent HIV transmission among adults is more complex. Many things about ARV treatment regimens remain unclear. First, and most hotly disputed at present, is the timing of treatment. Like most drugs, ARVs have side effects, and their long-term impact is not yet known. In addition, the threat of drug resistance grows with length of treatment. For this reason, clinicians have been trying to arrive at a model which maximizes healthy years gained, while minimizing possibly unnecessary time on treatment. Three major patterns have been advocated: (1) aggressive treatment of primary infection where identified, followed by a break in treatment until indicated; (2) structured interruption of treatment, stopping when viral load has been undetectable for some time, resuming when indicated and stopping again when recontrolled; and (3) continuous treatment from the time treatment is first indicated by virological, clinical, or (most commonly) immunological measures.

A fourth model recently proposed but not widely tested is to treat continuously from the moment of diagnosis, regardless of stage of disease. This is proposed by those advocating treatment as a means of HIV prevention (Granich et al. 2009). Some consider that this implies that the public health benefits of treatment are potentially more important than clinical benefits to individuals. The risk is that individuals will be exposed for longer than is necessary to medication that carries a risk of side effects and may limit future treatment options. In other words, the welfare of individual patients may be compromised for the public good of meeting prevention goals (Garnett and Baggaley 2009).

The "treat everyone" approach seems to be proposed in part because it avoids difficult decisions about what is the most appropriate clinical or immunological point to begin treatment. Developing countries, which have often had limited capacity to perform monitoring tests, frequently began by setting clinical criteria for treatment. Now, it is common to see national guidelines recommend treatment when CD4 cell counts fall below 200/ml. Many wealthier nations treat at CD4 <=350, and there is currently a move to increase this to CD4 <=500 (Kitahata et al. 2009).

Models that include treatment interruption usually result in a sharp rise in viral load when people stop taking medication. Patients who stop taking medication during chronic infection will experience sharper and more sustained rises in viral load than those who interrupt treatment during or shortly after primary infection. In a recent study, virtually all people interrupting treatment during chronic infection had detectable viral loads within four weeks of stopping treatment, and by 12 weeks all had plasma viral loads of over 5,000 copies/ml (Steingrover et al. 2008). In the case of treatment failure, rebounds in RNA viral load can be more sustained, and reach higher levels in genital fluids than in plasma (Cu-Uvin et al. 2009).

While viral loads do rebound if treatment given during primary infection is stopped, they do appear to stabilize at a lower set point than among people who receive no early treatment (Prazuck et al. 2008; Steingrover et al. 2008). Structured interruption appears to be of limited benefit to the patient, with high rebounds in viral load and similar disease progression. Spikes in viral load negate some of the benefit of ARVs as a prevention tool, compared with those on continuous treatment. However a phylogenetic analysis among gay men in Britain found no quantifiable evidence that people who had interrupted treatment were more likely to transmit HIV than those with untreated chronic infection (Burman et al. 2008; Fisher et al. 2009).

## Adherence

Though it is difficult to study, it is plausible to expect that unstructured interruption in the form of poor adherence would have similar effects to structured interruption. Data from wealthy countries with good access to health services show that while poor adherence is limited, it is strongly associated with virological failure and may also be associated with the emergence of drug resistance (Glass et al. 2008). Both of these would suggest that poor adherence would lead to more HIV transmission. It is also worth noting, however, that poor adherence is strongly linked with increases in mortality. To the extent that death removes those with virological failure from the sexually active population, this would reduce the risk of transmission (Lima et al. 2008).

Measures of adherence differ, but it is clear that drug taking itself varies enormously from site to site. In a large and well-supported study population in Rakai, Uganda, 45 percent of participants had less than 90 percent adherence (Reynolds et al. 2009). In a large Kenyan treatment program, 30 percent reported imperfect adherence (Wools-Kaloustian et al. 2009). Adherence to medication is strongly associated with financial position. Lack of funds for travel and the purchase of medication affect adherence, encouraging intermittent dosing only when the patient is feeling sick (Braitstein et al. 2006; Rosen, Fox, and Gill 2007b). It is interesting to note that the somewhat poor adherence in the Kenyan study was recorded even after a big ramp-up of the program which led to the opening of many clinics and a significant reduction of travel time for patients. If global economic conditions continue to deteriorate, and household budgets get squeezed yet further, it seems likely that patients on ARVs will find it harder than ever to take time off work, find the funds for travel to clinics, and finance the other expenditures associated with taking medicines regularly—even where the medication itself is provided free of charge. Global economic conditions will also inevitably affect the resources available to fund continued expansion of treatment programs, and the investment in health systems and personnel that are needed to keep those programs working effectively and to keep viral loads in check.

Many reports of adherence look only at those who are retained in the treatment program. However, it is likely that those lost to follow-up have lower rates of ongoing adherence than those who show up regularly for their medication. Many sites across sub-Saharan Africa report significant loss to follow-up, varying from a high of 85 percent at 24 months to a low of 46 percent. Loss to follow-up is highest in the first six months, which is also commonly the period when mortality among those starting ARVs late in the course of infection is highest. In a comparison of sub-Saharan African and European/North American sites, researchers found that 19 percent of clients dropped out for a year or more, four times as many as in rich countries (Braitstein et al. 2006).

In Malawi, a careful attempt to find patients recorded as "lost to follow-up" (i.e., who had not shown up for three months or more) found that 50 percent were dead. Of those still alive, two-thirds were no longer taking ARVs (Yu et al. 2007). In other words, a third of all patients lost to follow-up had interrupted treatment and were subject to the higher viremia and thus greater likelihood of passing on HIV associated with it. These breaks in treatment are not always adjusted for when considering the effect of ARVs on viral load in developing countries. One recent comparison of treatment outcomes in rich and poor countries reported similar virological outcomes: 77 percent of patients in rich countries had a viral load of under 500 copies/ml at six months, compared with 76 percent in poorer countries. However no adjustments were made for loss to follow-up; the analysis included only those whose viral load measurements were available—just 48 percent of patients in developing countries, compared with 86 percent in the industrial world. High loss to follow-up makes it likely that virological failure was in fact far higher in developing countries.

The model demonstrating the effectiveness of universal treatment as a prevention tool assumes a drop-out rate (including treatment interruption but excluding death) of 1.5 percent per year (Granich et al. 2009). In the light of the data reviewed above, this seems optimistic. Poorer adherence would lead to a reduction in infectiousness far less than the 99 percent assumed by the model. A good portion of the benefit of universal treatment as prevention at the population level is eroded if the reduction in infectiousness achieved is only 95 percent. At an 80-percent reduction in infectiousness, the added life span and the ongoing opportunities for transmission it brings could outweigh the reduced infectiousness, leading to increases in HIV incidence (Fraser 2009).

*STIs*

The association between STIs and higher HIV viral load is well described in both Western and African settings; STIs also lead to increased viral shedding. Both of these factors increase the infectivity of HIV-infected people. Genital ulcer disease (GUD) increases shedding of HIV in genital tract fluids in both men and women (Ghys et al. 1997; Schacker et al. 1998; Pilcher et al. 2004a). Non-ulcerative STIs increase shedding in men (Moss et al. 1995). Evidence for increased cervico-vaginal shedding of HIV among women infected with non-ulcerative STIs is less clear, though some studies have shown increased shedding (Ghys et al. 1997; Mostad et al. 1997).

HIV viral load in blood plasma increases in men with GUD and during acute episodes of infection with other STIs, notably Herpes Simplex Virus Type 2 (HSV-2), a common cause of GUD (Schacker et al. 1998; Gray et al. 2004). HIV viral load in seminal fluid increases in men with ulcerative and non-ulcerative STIs (Cohen et al. 1997; Dyer et al. 1998; Dyer et al. 1999).

Recent evidence from phylogenetic analysis among gay men in Europe confirms that this translates directly into HIV transmission; HIV-infected men who experienced an STI in the study interval were 12 times more likely to infect a partner with HIV than were men with no STI (Fisher et al. 2009).

Because background STI prevalence is far higher in many sub-Saharan African settings than it is among men who have sex with men in the industrial world, it is to be expected that untreated STIs will have a greater effect on the ongoing transmission of HIV. A recent study among male STI patients in Malawi found that while treatment of urethritis led to a fall in seminal viral load in chronically HIV-infected patients, treatment of GUD made no significant difference to seminal viral load (Pilcher et al. 2007). This is worrying because GUD prevalence is extremely high in many populations, and it is strongly implicated in the ongoing spread of HIV. A seroconversion study among men in an STI clinic in Malawi, where background prevalence was 37 percent, found that 1.6 percent of patients were newly infected with HIV but still antibody negative; 71 percent of these acute infections had GUD (Powers et al. 2007).

It is likely that the association between STIs and high risk of HIV transmission is not exclusively due to elevated viral load. In multivariate analysis which controlled for differences in viral load among gay men, the rate ratio for HIV transmission among those with STIs shrank from 12 to a still considerable 6 (Fisher et al. 2009). This suggests that clustering of behavioral risk, discussed below, also plays a part in rapid onward spread of HIV.

## Treatment failure and drug resistance

Imperfect adherence increases the risk of both treatment failure and the transmission of strains of HIV that are resistant to the most commonly used first-line therapies. To avoid increased risk of HIV transmission, patients must switch to second-line therapies very quickly after virological failure occurs. This may be difficult in situations, increasingly common as treatment programs expand across Africa, where virological monitoring is not available. In these cases, immunological failure is used as a proxy for virological failure. However, it is likely that a fall in CD4 counts lags rises in viral load by several months (Wools-Kaloustianet al. 2006).

Even where virological measures are available, switching to second-line therapy can be slow. In a new analysis of 17 ARV programs from 14 countries in Africa, Asia, and Latin America, only 24 per cent of the people who met either immunological or virological criteria for treatment failure were switched to second-line treatments (Keiser and ART-LINC Collaboration 2009). In a well-resourced program in South Africa, Ive and colleagues calculated the time from virological failure (defined as two consecutive detectable tests, with tests generally at intervals of close to two months) to regimen switching. The median time was 210 days—adding the time between tests, this means there was an average of nine months in which patients were at high risk of passing on HIV (Ive et al. 2009). There are undoubtedly greater challenges to come. A World Health Organization working group on treatment in 2007 estimated that the need for second-line treatment would grow by a compound 40 per cent from 2006 to 2010. This would add half a million people to those needing more expensive and complex regimens (Coutinho 2009).

There is limited evidence that there may be racial differences in response to antiretroviral treatment for HIV. In a U.S. military cohort with equal access to care and controlling for rank, sex, baseline CD4, and other factors that may affect disease progression, African Americans were twice as likely not to have viral load controlled at six months as European Americans, and the difference persisted at 12 months (Weintrob et al. 2008). If this difference were to translate to the majority population in sub-Saharan Africa, then it would be reasonable to expect that virological failure would be more common in sub-Saharan Africa than it has been among cohorts in North America, Europe, and Australasia, even if other factors such as health service access were similar.

It is worth noting that there is evidence of ongoing transmission from people with chronic infections in HIV care in wealthy countries. By tracing contacts of newly infected patients in North Carolina and performing phylogenetic analysis, McCoy and colleagues found that 72 percent of the identified transmitters were chronic cases in HIV care, and 43 percent were currently or previously on ARVs (McCoy et al. 2008). Countries with more equitable health care systems, such as Canada, report fewer transmissions from chronic infections (Brenner et al. 2007). This suggests that the strength of the health system and easy access may be important determinants of treatment outcomes. Countries with weak or inequitable health services can expect higher virological failure among those on treatment, and thus greater risk of ongoing HIV transmission. While it is fashionable these days to make declarations about the need to invest in building up health systems in developing countries, remarkably little money has been invested in this area (Ravishankar et al. 2009). It is possible that a global economic crisis will further sap the will or ability of donors in wealthy countries to plough money into health systems in other countries, with possible consequences for the delivery of HIV treatment services, and thus, for prevention.

*Mortality*

The preceding discussion points to factors which may increase viral load, and therefore, increase the possibility for onward transmission of HIV. But it is important to consider that many of these factors can work, paradoxically, to reduce the likelihood of transmission at a population level. High viral loads are associated with higher transmission probabilities, yes, but they are also associated with higher mortality. Someone with a lower viral load who survives for a longer period may infect more people over the course of their life than someone with higher viral load who dies more rapidly (Fraser 2009).

Mortality is very strongly correlated with CD4 count at initiation of treatment; it is becoming increasingly apparent that people starting ARVs when their CD4 cell counts fall below 200 are far more likely to die than those initiating earlier. Historically, the average CD4 count when a patient went on treatment in industrial countries has been 234/ml, compared to 108/ml in developing countries (Braitstein et al. 2006). Later entry into treatment, however, does not account for all the excess death in African patients. One year mortality rates were higher in developing countries than in industrial ones even after adjusting for baseline CD4 levels, perhaps because of existing comorbidities with tuberculosis (TB) and other diseases at initiation. In a South African cohort, for example, mortality was three times higher than that recorded among patients in the European Athena database, after stratifying by CD4 count. Recent research in South Africa suggests a "threshold effect" at a CD4 count of 200. Below that level, mortality ranges from 5.4–38 deaths per 100 person-years of observation (pyo). Above that level, the death rate drops sharply to 1.2–2.7 per 100 pyo (Lawn et al. 2009).

It is likely that treatment guidelines will shift to recommend earlier initiation of treatment, and that in turn will lead to lower mortality, assuming that services can be provided. A population-based survey in Kenya which measured CD4 counts was able to estimate the additional need that this change would imply. Currently, an estimated 217,000 people would be eligible for ARVs, if diagnosed. If the threshold were increased to a CD4 count of 350 cells/ml, drugs and associated support services would have to be found for another 145,000 (Mohammed et al. 2009). The "universal treatment as prevention" model proposed by Granich and colleagues suggests immediate treatment for anyone testing positive—a model not yet in place in rich countries with dramatically lower prevalence rates, and one that raises difficult questions about the welfare of individual patients versus the collective good.

If it were possible to provide services even on the currently recommended scale, it would increase the lifespan of a substantial proportion of those living with HIV in Africa—clearly, a very desirable outcome. But this result also increases the proportion of sexually active adults with HIV and time in which temporary virological failure may occur, and so potentially increases the risk of onward transmission of HIV.

## Risk Behavior in an Age of Treatment

Virology is an important and frequently overlooked factor when considering HIV prevention approaches. Changes in viremia and infectivity would, of course, be of little consequence if infected people were not having unprotected sex or sharing needles with uninfected people. Changes in risk behavior in an era of increasing access to HIV treatment are, therefore, of paramount importance in determining the future of the epidemic.

When HIV treatment first became widely available in industrial countries, the incidence of AIDS dropped very precipitously. The disfiguring and fatal syndrome ceased to be an inevitable consequence of HIV infection. Public health officials worried that once the "fear factor" associated with AIDS evaporated, people would be less concerned about avoiding HIV, and risky behavior would rise. A great deal of research focused on the effects of "treatment optimism" (the belief that partners on treatment were less likely to be infectious) and "behavioral disinhibition" (a greater willingness to take risks because HIV was no longer perceived to be life threatening). Much of the research expressed wide-eyed dismay at changes in attitudes and called for prevention messages reinforcing that all unprotected sex was risky sex (Suarez et al. 2001).

Early research among gay men and other groups in industrial countries showed that HIV-infected people did not adopt more risky behavior simply because they were taking ARVs. This research has been repeated, more recently, among men and women on HIV treatment in East Africa, with much the same results (Bunnell et al. 2008; Reynolds et al. 2009). Focusing research on those who are infected and on treatment is of little use, however, in explaining the likely dynamics of the ongoing spread of HIV. At the population level, especially where a great deal of infection is undiagnosed, the behavior of those who believe themselves to be uninfected is more important than the behavior of those who are infected and in well-monitored treatment programs.

In the early years of the HIV epidemic, gay communities in industrial countries reacted swiftly to protect themselves from infection. Condom use in anal sex rose very sharply, and new infections of both STIs and HIV fell. Shortly after effective treatment became widely available in 1995, behaviors began to change. Casual partnerships rose again, condom use fell, and the consequences of this could be seen in rising STIs (Grulich and Kaldor 2008). HIV incidence did not, however, immediately rise. This led researchers to conclude that lower infectivity in men on treatment combined with other behavioral responses were outweighing the effects of reduced condom use. These potentially protective responses included: serosorting (people only having unprotected sex with someone of the same HIV status as themselves); negotiated safety (unprotected sex only within a primary partnership; with all other sex protected); strategic positioning (negative partners always taking the insertive role in anal sex); and the avoidance of internal ejaculation (Davidovich et al. 2001; Stolte et al. 2001; Xia et al. 2006; Jin et al. 2008).

Unfortunately, the success of these strategies has proven fleeting. A decade into the age of treatment, it became clear that HIV incidence was indeed on the rise again among gay men. National surveillance and cohort data from Australia, Canada, England, Germany, Ireland, the Netherlands, New Zealand, Scotland, Spain, Switzerland, and the United States all indicate rising incidence (Grulich and Kaldor 2008). In short, increases in unprotected sex with people of opposite or unknown HIV status and the effects on viremia of rising STI prevalence (also a consequence of rising unprotected sex) are outweighing the effect of lower viral load among those on effective treatment. In many countries, including the U.S. and the UK, incidence is highest among gay men under 35. That is the generation that became sexually active after universal HIV treatment reduced AIDS to virtual invisibility. In a careful analysis of trends in infection among gay men in the Netherlands, Bezemer and colleagues attributed rising incidence to rising risk in untreated individuals, rather than in those on treatment. Had risk behavior remained at pretreatment levels rather than rising as treatment expanded, mathematical modelling suggests new infections would have been cut by close to half (Dukers et al. 2007; Bezemer et al. 2008; Fraser 2009).

It is worth noting that changes in risk behavior lagged widespread access to treatment and the consequent disappearance of AIDS by a few years in industrial countries. In Africa, treatment access is still limited in many settings—even where it is widespread, in countries such as Botswana, Malawi, and South Africa, programs are relatively new. It is therefore difficult to predict whether risk behavior across the whole population, infected and uninfected, treated and untreated, will be similarly affected. It is worth noting that rising risk behavior presupposes an earlier adoption of safer behavior. It is not possible to abandon condom use, as gay men in San Francisco have done, in a situation where condom use was never widespread.

In a study of discordant couples in Uganda, 17 percent of people on ARVs reported a non-marital partner, compared with 7 percent of those not on ARVs (p = 0.096). Interestingly, in this population of intensively counseled and supported known discordant couples, only a third used condoms consistently, suggesting that at least within marriage, there is little safe behavior that might be reversed by waning concern about HIV infection in an age of treatment (Reynolds et al. 2009).

## Summary and Conclusions

Table 10.1 attempts to summarize the potential effect of various treatment-related factors on the spread of HIV in sub-Saharan Africa, compared with the experience of industrial countries.

*Table 10.1* The effect of treatment-related factors on the likely transmission of HIV

| Influencing factor | Industrial countries | Sub-Saharan Africa |
|---|:---:|:---:|
| Infectious people are on ARVs | ↓↓ | ↓ |
| ARVs reduce viral load (VL) | ↓↓↓ | ↓↓↓ |
| ARVs increase lifespan | ↑↑↑ | ↑ |
| Treatment interruption increases VL | ↑ | ↑↑ |
| Treatment failure increases VL | ↑ | ↑↑ |
| STIs increase VL | ↑↑ | ↑↑↑ |
| AIDS disappears, risk rises | ↑↑↑ | ↑↑(?) |
| Prevention disappears, risk rises | ↑↑ | ↑(?) |

NOTE: Down arrows indicate that the factor lowers the risk of transmission, and up arrows indicate that the risk of transmission is increased. The number of arrows indicates the likely magnitude of the effect: One arrow indicates that the factor is likely to result in a modest increase or decrease in HIV transmission, two arrows indicate a more substantial increase or decrease, and three arrows a large increase or decrease. Question marks indicate that few supporting data are available.

At the moment, access to both testing and treatment, among those in need of it, is better in industrial countries than in most countries in Africa. Among those on treatment, ARVs greatly reduce the risk of onward transmission in both regions. Mortality among those treated is currently greater in Africa; this reduces the potential for onward transmission compared with industrial countries. However, unstructured treatment interruption, treatment failure, and coinfection with STIs, each leading to rises in viral load, are far more common in sub-Saharan Africa. These factors are all related to an extent to the strength of health systems. It is unclear whether they will improve or deteriorate as programs are rolled out to reach ever more people in need.

The behavioral consequences of increased access to treatment in sub-Saharan Africa are as yet unclear. Among gay men in industrial nations, the virtual disappearance of AIDS has had a clear impact. Men are less concerned about becoming infected with what they increasingly perceive as an inconvenient, chronic disease. They may also assume that any infected partner is likely to be on treatment and, therefore, not infectious. Risk behavior has risen markedly; the effect on HIV transmission is multiplied through simultaneous rises in STIs. Few communities in sub-Saharan Africa adopted safer sexual behaviors on the scale that gay men did in the pretreatment era, and denial of the direct link between unprotected sex and HIV has also been more pronounced. Some of those currently deterred from risk because of fear of AIDS may be less diligent as treatment becomes more widely available, but it seems likely that there is less scope for a "reversal" in safe behavior in Africa than there has been among gay men in other regions.

There is some evidence that HIV incidence in gay men is rising in part because prevention has been neglected as more time, attention, and money is spent on treatment. The single exception to observed rises in incidence in this group is among men in the state of New South Wales in Australia (Zablotska et al. 2008). A comparison of potential influences on transmission, between New South Wales and other Australian states where incidence is rising, suggests that the major difference is that both government and community groups in New South Wales continued to invest in substantial prevention activities, while in other states prevention budgets shrank as treatment increased (Bernard, Kippax, and Baxter 2008; Fairley et al. 2008). Concern has been expressed that an overemphasis on treatment has undermined prevention efforts in developing countries, also (Global HIV Prevention Working Group 2007; Horton and Das 2008). Since prevention campaigns have had relatively little success to date in many parts of sub-Saharan Africa, a displacement of attention paid to prevention is likely to have a relatively less detrimental effect in the high-prevalence epidemics of East and Southern Africa than elsewhere.

The effect of widespread treatment on prevention can ultimately only be measured reliably by looking at trends in incidence. These data are rare anywhere in the world and extremely rare in Africa. In rural Uganda, a large population-based cohort has reported changes in behavior and infection for many years. It appears that many years of falling incidence are now being reversed in tandem with rises in some indicators of sexual risk, although it is difficult at present to link the changes to trends in treatment (Shafer et al. 2008). A demographic surveillance site in South Africa's Hlabisa district (where one in five adults is infected with HIV) measured HIV incidence in the general population from 2003–08. In this population, HIV testing is widely available and actively promoted, and ARVs have been provided in the public sector since 2004, with very good coverage. Incidence has remained constant between 3.0 and 4.0 per 100 person-years of observation throughout the study period (Bärnighausen et al. 2009).

In countries with strong health systems, near universal access to prevention services, testing and treatment, a relatively light caseload, and relatively abundant human and financial resources, changes in behavior are outweighing the effect of reduced infectivity among those on HIV treatment. In consequence, new sexually transmitted HIV infections are on the rise. Given the evidence reviewed in this chapter, it seems implausible to expect a better outcome in countries with very high levels of HIV prevalence and generally weak health systems. This is especially the case since the data from Africa at this stage covers a population that has privileged access to treatment in well-resourced programs often in research settings. If services are expanded (even through the delivery of lower quality public sector programs), then increases in treatment will almost certainly increase the absolute number of adults living with HIV in the short term. This is desirable, since it is the result of fewer deaths. But without new investment in effective prevention programs, expanded access to HIV treatment in sub-Saharan Africa will very likely translate into more new infections.

# REFERENCES

Abebe, Y., A. Schaap, G. Mamo, A. Negussie, B. Darimo, D.Wolday, and E. J. Sanders. 2003. "HIV Prevalence in 72,000 Urban and Rural Army Recruits, Ethiopia." *AIDS* 17(12): 1835–40.

Abimiku, A., and R. C. Gallo. 1995. HIV: Basic Virology and Pathophysiology. In *HIV Infection in Women*, ed. J. A. DeHovitz and A. Duerr, 13–31. New York: Raven Press.

Abu-Raddad, L. J., and I. M. Longini, Jr. 2008. "No HIV Stage is Dominant in Driving the HIV Epidemic in Sub-Saharan Africa." *AIDS* 22(9): 1055–61.

Acemoglu, D., and S. Johnson. 2006. Disease and Development: The Effect of Life Expectancy on Economic Growth. NBER Working Paper No. 12269, National Bureau of Economic Research, Cambridge, MA.

Achmat, Z. 2004. AIDS and Human Rights: A New South African Struggle. 2004. John Foster Lecture, November 10.

Adair, T. 2007. Desire for Children and Unmet Need for Contraception among HIV-Positive Women in Lesotho. DHS Working Papers No. 32, Demographic and Health Surveys, Calverton, MD.

Adhvaryu, A. R., and K. Beegle. 2009. The Long-Run Impacts of Adult Deaths on Older Household Members in Tanzania. World Bank Policy Research Working Paper 5037, World Bank, Washington, DC.

AED (Academy for Educational Development). 2003. *Multisectoral Responses to HIV/AIDS: A Compendium of Promising Practices from Africa*. Washington, DC: AED.

Afrobarometer. 2004. Public Opinion and HIV/AIDS: Facing Up to the Future? Afrobarometer Briefing Paper No. 12, April.

Agha, S. 2002. "Quasi-experimental Study to Assess the Impact of Four Adolescent Sexual Health Interventions in Sub-Saharan Africa." *International Family Planning Perspectives* 28(2): 67–70.

Ahmed, S., T. Lutalo, M. Wawer, D. Serwadda, N. K. Sewankambo, F. Nalugoda, F. Makumbi, F. Wabwire-Mangen, N. Kiwanuka, G. Kigozi, M. Kiddugavu, and R. Gray. 2001. "HIV Incidence and Sexually Transmitted Disease Prevalence Associated with Condom Use: A Population Study in Rakai, Uganda." *AIDS* 15(16): 2171–9.

Ainsworth, M., K. Beegle, and G. Koda. 2005. "The Impact of Adult Mortality and Parental Deaths on Schooling in Northwestern Tanzania." *Journal of Development Studies* 41(3): 412–39.

Ainsworth, M., and J. Dayton. 2000. Is the AIDS Epidemic Having an Impact on the Coping Behavior and Health Status of the Elderly? Evidence from Northwestern Tanzania. World Bank, Washington, DC.

Ainsworth, M., and D. Filmer. 2006. "Inequalities in Children's Schooling: AIDS, Orphanhood, Poverty, and Gender." *World Development* 34(6): 1099–128.

Ainsworth, M., S. Ghosh, and I. Semali. 1995. The Impact of Adult Deaths on Household Composition in Kagera Region, Tanzania. Unpublished Manuscript, World Bank, Washington, DC.

Ainsworth, M., and M. Over. 1997. *Confronting AIDS: Public Priorities in a Global Epidemic.* New York: Oxford University Press.

Ainsworth, M., and I. Semali. 1998. Who is Most Likely to Die of AIDS? Socio-economic Correlates of Adult Deaths in Kagera Region, Tanzania. In *Confronting AIDS: Evidence for Developing World*, ed. M. Ainsworth, L. Fransen, and M. Over, 95–108. Brussels: European Commission.

———. 2000. The Impact of Adult Deaths on Children's Health in Northwestern Tanzania. Policy Research Working Paper 2266. World Bank, Washington, DC.

Akileswaran, C., M. A. Laurie, T. P. Flanigan, and K. H. Mayer. 2005. "Lessons Learned from Use of Highly Active Antiretroviral Therapy in Africa." *Clinical Infectious Diseases* 41(1): 376–85.

Aliber, M., and C. Walker. 2006. "The Impact of HIV/AIDS on Land Rights: Perspectives from Kenya." *World Development* 34(4): 704–27.

Allen, S., E. Karita, E. Chomba, D. L. Roth, J. Telfair, I. Zulu, L. Clark, N. Kancheya, M. Conkling, R. Stephenson, B. Bekan, K. Kimbrell, S. Dunham, F. Henderson, M. Sinkala, M. Caraël, and A. Haworth. 2007. "Promotion of Couples' Voluntary Counseling and Testing for HIV through Influential Networks in Two African Capital Cities." *BMC Public Health* 7: 349.

Allen, S., A. Serufilira, J. Bogaerts, P. Van de Perre, F. Nsengumuremyi, C. Lindan, M. Caraël, W. Wolf, T. Coates, and S. Hulley. 1992a. "Confidential HIV Testing and Condom Promotion in Africa. Impact on HIV and Gonorrhea Rates." *JAMA* 268(23): 3338–43.

Allen, S., A. Serufilira, V. Gruber, S. Kegeles, P. Van de Perre, M. Caraël, and T. J. Coates. 1993. "Pregnancy and Contraception Use among Urban Rwandan Women after HIV Testing and Counseling." *American Journal of Public Health* 83(5): 705–10.

Allen, S., J. Tice, P. Van de Perre, A. Serufilira, E. Hudes, F. Nsengumuremyi, J. Bogaerts, C. Lindan, and S. Hulley. 1992b. "Effect of Serotesting with Counselling on Condom Use and Seroconversion among HIV Discordant Couples in Africa." *BMJ* 304(6842): 1605–9.

Allen, T., and S. Heald. 2004. "HIV/AIDS Policy in Africa: What Has Worked in Uganda and What Has Failed in Botswana?" *Journal of International Development* 16(8): 1141–54.

Amuron, B., G. Namara, J. Birungi, C. Nabiryo, J. Levin, H. Grosskurth, A. Coutinho, and S. Jaffar. 2009. "Mortality and Loss-to-Follow-up during the Pre-treatment Period in an Antiretroviral Therapy Programme under Normal Health Service Conditions in Uganda." *BMC Public Health* 9: 290.

Anabwani, G., and P. Navario. 2005. "Nutrition and HIV/AIDS in Sub-Saharan Africa: An Overview." *Nutrition* 21(1): 96–9.

Anderson, R. 2003. Keynote Address. Report of the Scientific Meeting on the Empirical Evidence for the Demographic and Socio-Economic Impact of AIDS, Durban, March 26–28, 2003.

Annan, K. 2002. "In Africa, AIDS Has a Woman's Face." *International Herald Tribune*, December 29, 2002.

Aral, S. O., M. Over, L. Manhart, and K. K. Holmes. 2006. Sexually Transmitted Infections. In *Disease Control Priorities in Developing Countries.* 2nd edition, ed. D. T. Jamison, J. G. Breman, A. R. Measham, G. Alleyne, M. Claeson, D. B. Evans, P. Jha, A. Mills, and P. Musgrove, 311–30. New York: World Bank and Oxford University Press.

Arndt, C. 2006. "HIV/AIDS, Human Capital, and Economic Growth Prospects for Mozambique." *Journal of Policy Modeling* 28(5): 477–89.

Arndt, C., and J. D. Lewis. 2001. "The HIV/AIDS Pandemic in South Africa: Sectoral Impacts and Unemployment." *Journal of International Development* 13(4): 427–49.

Arpadi, S. M. 2005. Growth Failure in HIV-infected Children. *Consultation on Nutrition and HIV/AIDS in Africa: Evidence, Lessons and Recommendations for Action*. Durban, South Africa, World Health Organization, April 10–13, 2005.

Arrow, K. 1964. "The Role of Securities in the Optimal Allocation of Risk Bearing." *Review of Economic Studies* 31(86): 91–6.

ASCI (AIDS, Security and Conflict Initiative). 2009. AIDS, Conflict and Security: New Realities, New Responses. Social Science Research Council, New York, and Clingendael Institute, The Hague. Available at: http://asci.researchhub.ssrc.org/rdb/asci-hub

Au, J. T., K. Kayitenkore, E. Shutes, E. Karita, P. J. Peters, A. Tichacek, and S. A. Allen. 2006. "Access to Adequate Nutrition Is a Major Potential Obstacle to Antiretroviral Adherence among HIV-infected Individuals in Rwanda." *AIDS* 20(16): 2116–8.

Auvert, B., A. Buvé, B. Ferry, M. Caraël, L. Morison, E. Lagarde, N. J. Robinson, M. Kahindo, J. Chege, N. Rutenberg, R. Musonda, M. Laourou, and E. Akam; Study Group on Heterogeneity of HIV Epidemics in African Cities. 2001. "Ecological and Individual Level Analysis of Risk Factors for HIV Infection in Four Urban Populations in Sub-Saharan Africa with Different Levels of HIV Infection." *AIDS* 15(Suppl. 4): S15–30.

Auvert, B., D. Taljaard, E. Lagarde, J. Sobngwi-Tambekou, R. Sitta, and A. Puren. 2006. "Randomized, Controlled Intervention Trial of Male Circumcision for Reduction of HIV Infection Risk: The ANRS 1265 Trial." *PLoS Medicine* 2(11): 1112–22.

Bachmann, M. O., and F. L. Booysen. 2003. "Health and Economic Impact of HIV/AIDS on South African Households: A Cohort Study." *BMC Public Health* 3:14.

Bailey, R. C., S. Moses, C. B. Parker, K. Agot, I. Maclean, J. N. Krieger, C. F. Williams, R. T. Campbell, and J. O. Ndinya-Achola. 2007. "Male Circumcision for HIV Prevention in Young Men in Kisumu, Kenya: A Randomised Controlled Trial." *Lancet* 369(9562): 643–56.

Bailey, R. C., F. A. Plummer, and S. Moses. 2001. "Male Circumcision and HIV Prevention: Current Knowledge and Future Research Directions." *Lancet Infectious Diseases* 1(4): 223–31.

Baird, S., E. Chirwa, C. McIntosh, and B. Özler. 2009. The Short-Term Impacts of a Schooling Conditional Cash Transfer Program on the Sexual Behavior of Young Women. World Bank Policy Research Working Paper Series No. 5089, World Bank, Washington, DC.

Baird, S., C. McIntosh, and B. Özler. 2009. Sex and the Classroom. Can a Cash Transfer Program for Schooling Decrease HIV infection? Unpublished presentation made at the World Bank, November 10, 2009.

Bakaki, P., J. Kayita, J. E. Moura Machado, J. B. Coulter, D. Tindyebwa, C. M. Ndugwa, and C. A. Hart. 2001. "Epidemiologic and Clinical Features of HIV-infected and HIV-uninfected Ugandan Children Younger than 18 Months." *Journal of Acquired Immune Deficiency Syndromes* 28(1): 35–42.

Baldwin, P. 2005. *Disease and Democracy: The Industrialized World Faces AIDS*. Berkeley: University of California Press.

———. 2007. Comment on *AIDS and Power*. Available at: http://www.ssrc.org/programs/pages/african-arguments/peter-baldwin-comments-on-aids-and-power/

Banerjee, A., E. Duflo, R. Glennerster, and C. Kinnan. 2009. The Miracle of Microfinance? Evidence from a Randomized Evaluation. MIT Poverty Action Lab, Cambridge, MA.

Barnett, T. 1994. The Effects of HIV/AIDS on Farming Systems and Rural Livelihoods in Uganda, Tanzania and Zambia. Rome, FAO.

———. 2009. HIV/AIDS and State Fragility. AIDS, Security, and Conflict Initiative Synthesis Paper. Available at: http://asci.researchhub.ssrc.org/working-papers/ASCI%20Synthesis%20Paper%20State%20Fragility.pdf

Barnett, T., and P. Blaikie. 1992. *AIDS in Africa: Its Present and Future Impacts.* New York: Guilford Press.

Barnett, T., and G. Prins. 2005. *HIV/AIDS and Security: Fact, Fiction and Evidence.* Geneva: UNAIDS and London: LSEAIDS.

Barnett, T., J. Tumashabe, G. Bantebya, R. Ssebuliba, J. Ngasongwa, D. Kapunga, M. Ndelike, M. Drinkwater, G. Nitti, and M. Haslwinimer. 1995. "Field Report: The Social Impact of HIV/AIDS on Farming Systems and Livelihoods in Rural Africa: Some Experiences and Lessons from Uganda, Tanzania and Zambia." *Journal of International Development* 7(1): 163–76.

Barnett, T., and A. Whiteside. 2006. *AIDS in the Twenty-First Century: Disease and Globalization,* 2nd edition. Basingstoke, UK: Palgrave Macmillan.

Bärnighausen, T., O. Bangre, F. Tanser, G. Cooke, and M. L. Newell. 2009. HIV Incidence Time Trend and Characteristics of Recent Seroconverters in a Rural Community with High HIV Prevalence: South Africa. 16th Conference on Retroviruses and Opportunistic Infections, Montreal, February 8–11, 2009.

Bärnighausen, T., S. Biraro, J.-B. Bwanika, S. Gregson, T. Hallett, V. Hosegood, R. Isingo, T. Lutalo, M. Marston, P. Mushati, W. Mwita, A. Ndyanabo, L.-A. Shafer, J. Todd, M. Nyirenda, A. Wringe, and B. Zaba. 2008. Diverse Age Patterns of HIV Incidence Rates in Africa. Presentation at the XVII International AIDS Conference, Mexico City, August 3–8, 2008.

Bärnighausen, T., D. E. Bloom, and S. Humair. 2007. "Human Resources for Treating HIV/AIDS: Needs, Capacities, and Gaps." *AIDS Patient Care and STDs* 21(11): 799–812.

Barro, R., and X. Sala-i-Martin. 1995. *Economic Growth.* New York: McGraw-Hill.

Barry, J. 2004. *The Great Influenza: The Story of the Deadliest Pandemic in History.* Harmondsworth: Penguin.

Bashford, A., ed. 2007. *Medicine at the Border: Disease, Globalization and Security, 1850 to the Present.* London: Palgrave Macmillan.

Baum, M. K. 2000. "Role of Micronutrients in HIV-infected Intravenous Drug Users." *Journal of Acquired Immune Deficiency Syndromes* 25(Suppl. 1): S49–52.

Baum, M. K., and G. Shor-Posner. 1998. "Micronutrient Status in Relationship to Mortality in HIV-1 Disease." *Nutrition Reviews* 56(1, Pt. 2): S135–9.

Baylies, C. 2002. "The Impact of AIDS on Rural Households in Africa: A Shock Like Any Other?" *Development and Change* 33(4): 611–32.

Bechu, N. 1998. The Impact of AIDS on the Economy of Families in Côte d'Ivoire: Changes in Consumption among AIDS-affected Households. In *Confronting AIDS: Evidence from the Developing World,* ed. M. Ainsworth, L. Fransen, and M. Over, 241–53. Brussels: European Commission.

Becquet, R., L. Becquet, D. K. Ekouevi, I. Viho, C. Sakarovitch, P. Fassinou, G. Bedikou, M. Timite-Konan, F. Dabis, V. Leroy; ANRS 1201/1202 Ditrame Plus Study Group. 2007. "Two-year Morbidity and Mortality and Alternatives to Prolonged Breastfeeding among Children Born to HIV-infected Mothers in Côte d'Ivoire." *PLoS Med* 4(1): e17–31.

Beegle, K. 2005. "Labor Effects of Adult Mortality in Tanzanian Households." *Economic Development and Cultural Change* 53(3): 655–84.

Beegle, K., and D. de Walque. 2009. Demographic and Socioeconomic Patterns of HIV/AIDS Prevalence in Africa. In *The Changing HIV/AIDS Landscape,* ed. E. L. Lule, R. M. Seifman, and A. C. David, 81–104. Washington, DC: World Bank.

Beegle, K., and J. De Weerdt. 2008. "Methodological Issues in the Study of the Socio-economic Consequences of HIV/AIDS." *AIDS* 22(Suppl. 1): S89–94.

Beegle, K., J. De Weerdt, and S. Dercon. 2006a. Adult Mortality and Economic Growth in the Age of HIV/AIDS. World Bank Working Paper Series: Draft, World Bank, Washington, DC.

———. 2006b. "Orphanhood and the Long-Run Impact on Children." *American Journal of Agricultural Economics* 88(5): 1266–72.

———. 2007. "Adult Mortality and Consumption Growth in the Age of HIV/AIDS." *Economic Development and Cultural Change* 56(2): 299–326.

Beegle, K., D. Filmer, A. Stokes, and L. Tiererova. 2009. Orphanhood and the Living Arrangements of Children in Sub-Saharan Africa. Policy Research Working Paper 4889, World Bank, Washington, DC.

Behrman, J. R., and A. B. Deolalikar. 1998. Health and Nutrition. In *Handbook of Development Economics,* Vol. I, ed. J. Behrman and T. N. Srinivasan, 633–711. Amsterdam: Elsevier Science.

Beisel, W. R. 1996. "Nutrition in Pediatric HIV Infection: Setting the Research Agenda. Nutrition and Immune Function: Overview." *Journal of Nutrition* 126(10 Suppl.): 2611S–5S.

Bekker, L. G., L. Myer, C. Orrell, S. Lawn, and R. Wood. 2006. "Rapid Scale-up of a Community-based HIV Treatment Service: Programme Performance over 3 Consecutive Years in Guguletu, South Africa." *South Africa Medical Journal* 96(4): 315–22.

Bell, C., S. Devarajan, and H. Gersbach. 2003. The Long-Run Economic Costs of AIDS: Theory and an Application to South Africa. World Bank Policy Research Working Paper No. 3152, World Bank, Washington, DC.

———. 2004. Thinking about the Long-run Economic Costs of AIDS. In *The Macroeconomics of HIV/AIDS,* ed. M. Haacker, 96–133. Washington, DC: International Monetary Fund.

———. 2006. "The Long-Run Economic Costs of AIDS: A Model with an Application to South Africa." *World Bank Economic Review* 20(1): 55–89.

Benjamin, D. 1992. "Household Composition, Labor Markets, and Labor Demand: Testing for Separation in Agricultural Household Models." *Econometrica* 60(2): 287–322.

Bennett, S., and C. Chanfreau. 2005. "Approaches to Rationing Antiretroviral Treatment: Ethical and Equity Implications." *Bulletin of the World Health Organization* 83(7): 541–7.

Berhane, R., D. Bagenda, L. Marum, E. Aceng, C. Ndugwa, R. J. Bosch, and K. Olness. 1997. "Growth Failure as a Prognostic Indicator of Mortality in Pediatric HIV Infection." *Pediatrics* 100(1): E7–10.

Bernard, D., S. Kippax, and D. Baxter. 2008. "Effective Partnership and Adequate Investment Underpin a Successful Response: Key Factors in Dealing with HIV Increases." *Sexual Health* 5(2): 193–201.

Bertozzi, S. M., M. Laga, S. Bautista-Arredondo, and A. Coutinho. 2008. "Making HIV Prevention Programmes Work." *Lancet* 372(9641): 831–44.

Bezemer, D., F. de Wolf, M. C. Boerlijst, A. van Sighem, T. D. Hollingsworth, M. Prins, R. B. Geskus, L. Gras, R. A. Coutinho, and C. Fraser. 2008. "A Resurgent HIV-1 Epidemic among Men Who Have Sex with Men in the Era of Potent Antiretroviral Therapy." *AIDS* 22(9): 1071–7.

Bhargava, A., D. T. Jamison, L. J. Lau, and C. J. L. Murray. 2001. "Modeling the Effects of Health on Economic Growth." *Journal of Health Economics* 20(3): 423–40.

BIDPA (Botswana Institute for Development Policy Analysis). 2000. *Macroeconomic Impacts of the HIV/AIDS Epidemic in Botswana.* Gaborone, Botswana: BIDPA.

Biggs, T., and M. K. Shah. 1996. The Impact of the AIDS Epidemic on African Firms. Background paper for *Confronting AIDS: Public Priorities in a Global Epidemic.* 1999. Washington, DC: World Bank.

Bland, R., N. Rollins, H. Coovadia, A. Coutsoudis, and M. L. Newell. 2007. "Infant Feeding Counseling for HIV-infected and Uninfected Women: Appropriateness of Choice and Practice." *Bulletin of the World Health Organization* 85(4): 289–96.

Bloom, D. E., and D. Canning. 2000. "The Health and Wealth of Nations." *Science* 287(5456): 1207–9.

Bloom, D. E., D. Canning, and J. Sevilla. 2004. "The Effect of Health on Economic Growth: A Production Function Approach." *World Development* 32(1): 1–13.

Bloom, D. E., and A. S. Mahal. 1997. "Does the AIDS Epidemic Threaten Economic Growth?" *Journal of Econometrics* 77(1): 105–24.

Blower, S. M., H. B. Gershengorn, and R. M. Grant. 2000. "A Tale of Two Futures: HIV and Antiretroviral Therapy in San Francisco." *Science* 287(5453): 650–4.

Boerma, J. T., P. D. Ghys, and N. Walker. 2003. "Estimates of HIV-1 Prevalence from National Population-based Surveys as a New Gold Standard." *Lancet* 362(9399): 1929–31.

Boileau, C., S. Clark, M. Poulin, S. Bignami-Van-Assche, G. Reniers, S. C. Watkins, H-P. Kohler, and J. Heymann. 2009. "Sexual and Marital Trajectories and HIV Infection among Women in Rural Malawi, 2001–2004." *Sexually Transmitted Infections* 85(Suppl. 1): i27–33.

Boily, M.-C., R. F. Baggaley, L. Wang, B. Masse, R. G. White, R. J. Hayes, and M. Alary. 2009. "Heterosexual Risk of HIV-1 Infection per Sexual Act: Systematic Review and Meta-Analysis of Observational Studies." *Lancet* 9(2): 118–29.

Bolan, G., A. A. Ehrhardt, and J. N. Wasserheit. 1999. Gender Perspectives and STDs. In *Sexually Transmitted Diseases*, 3rd edition, ed. K. K. Holmes, P. F. Sparling, P.-A. Mårdh, S. M. Lemon, W. E. Stamm, P. Piot , and J. N. Wasserheit, 117–127. New York: McGraw-Hill.

Bollinger, L., J. Stover, and UNAIDS. 2007. Methodology for Care and Treatment Interventions. Available at: http://data.unaids.org/pub/Report/2007/20070925_annex_iii_treatment_care_methodology_en.pdf.

Bongaarts, J., P. Reining, P. Way, and F. Conant. 1989. "The Relationship between Male Circumcision and HIV Infection in African Populations." *AIDS* 3(6): 373–77.

Bonnel, R. 2000. "HIV/AIDS and Economic Growth: A Global Perspective." *South African Journal of Economics* 68(5): 360–79.

Bonnell, C., J. Hargreaves, V. Strange, P. Pronyk, and J. Porter. 2006. "Should Structural Interventions Be Evaluated Using RCTs? The Case of HIV Prevention." *Social Science and Medicine* 63(5): 1135–42.

Booysen, F. L. R. 2003. "HIV/AIDS and Poverty: Evidence from the Free State Province." *South African Journal of Economic and Management Sciences* 6(2): 419–38.

———. 2005. "Income and Poverty Dynamics in HIV/AIDS-affected Households in The Free State Province of South Africa." *South African Journal of Economics* 72(3): 522–45.

Booysen, F. L. R., and M. Bachmann. 2002. HIV/AIDS, Poverty and Growth: Evidence from a Household Impact Study Conducted in the Free State Province, South Africa. Paper presented at the Annual Conference of the Centre for the Study of African Economies, Oxford, March 18–19, 2002.

Bosworth, B. P., and S. M. Collins. 2003. "The Empirics of Growth: An Update." *Brookings Papers on Economic Activity* 2: 113–206.

Boutayeb, A., and S. Boutayeb. 2005. "The Burden of Non-communicable Diseases in Developing Countries." *International Journal for Equity in Health* 4: 2. Available at: http://www.pubmedcentral.nih.gov/articlerender.fcgi?artid=546417

Bracher, M., G. Santow, and S. C. Watkins. 2003. "Moving and Marrying: Estimating the Prevalence of HIV Infection among Newly-Weds in Malawi." *Demographic Research* Special Collection 1 (Article 7): 207–46. Available at: http://www.demographic-re search.org/special/1/7/

Braitstein, P., M. W. Brinkhof, F. Dabis, M. Schechter, A. Boulle, P. Miotti, R. Wood, C. Laurent, E. Sprinz, C. Seyler, D. R. Bangsberg, E. Balestre, J. A. Sterne, M. May, and M. Egger; Antiretroviral Therapy in Lower Income Countries (ART-LINC) Collaboration; ART Cohort Collaboration (ART-CC) groups. 2006. "Mortality of HIV-1-Infected Patients in the First Year of Antiretroviral Therapy: Comparison between Low-income and High-income Countries." *Lancet* 367(9513): 817–24.

Brenner, B. G., M. Roger, J. P. Routy, D. Moisi, M. Ntemgwa, C. Matte, J. G. Baril, R. Thomas, D. Rouleau, J. Bruneau, R. Leblanc, M. Legault, C. Tremblay, H. Charest, and M. A. Wainberg; Quebec Primary HIV Infection Study Group. 2007. "High Rates of Forward Transmission Events after Acute/Early HIV-1 Infection." *Journal of Infectious Diseases* 195(7): 951–9.

Brocklehurst, P. 2002. Interventions for Reducing the Risk of Mother-to-Child Transmission of HIV Infection. *Cochrane Database Systematic Reviews* (1): CD000102.

Brown, A. E., R. J. Gifford, J. P. Clewley, C. Kucherer, B. Masquelier, K. Porter, C. Balotta, N. K. Back, L. B. Jorgensen, C. de Mendoza, K. Bhaskaran, O. N. Gill, A. M. Johnson, and D. Pillay; Concerted Action on Seroconversion to AIDS and Death in Europe (CASCADE) Collaboration. 2009. "Phylogenetic Reconstruction of Transmission Events from Individuals with Acute HIV Infection: Toward More-Rigorous Epidemiological Definitions." *Journal of Infectious Diseases* 199(3): 427–31.

Brunelli, C., E. Kenefick, and F. Yamauchi. 2008. The Impacts of Adult Death on Child Growth and Nutrition: Evidence from Five Southern African Countries. RENEWAL Brief No. 12, HIV, Livelihoods, Food and Nutrition Security: Findings from RENEWAL Research (2007–2008), International Food Policy Research Institute, Washington, DC.

Buchacz, K., D. J. Hu, S. Vanichseni, P. A. Mock, T. Chaowanachan, L. O. Srisuwanvilai, R. Gvetadze, F. Van Griensven, J. W. Tappero, D. Kitayaporn, J. Kaewkungwal, K. Choopanya, and T. D. Mastro. 2004. "Early Markers of HIV-1 Disease Progression in a Prospective Cohort of Seroconverters in Bangkok, Thailand: Implications for Vaccine Trials." *Journal of Acquired Immune Deficiency Syndromes* 36(3): 853–60.

Bunnell, R., J. P. Ekwaru, P. Solberg, N. Wawai, W. Bikaako-Kajura, W. Were, A. Coutinho, C. Liechty, E. Madraa, G. Rutherford, and J. Mermin. 2006. "Changes in Sexual Behavior and Risk of HIV Transmission after Antiretroviral Therapy and Prevention Interventions in Rural Uganda." *AIDS* 20(1):85–92.

Bunnell, R., A. Opio, J. Musinguzi, W. Kirungi, P. Ekwaru, V. Mishra, W. Hladik, J. Kafuko, E. Madraa, and J. Mermin. 2008. "HIV Transmission Risk Behavior among HIV-infected Adults in Uganda: Results of a Nationally Representative Survey." *AIDS* 22(5): 617–24.

Bureau of Economic Research. 2001. The Macro-Economic Impact of HIV/AIDS in South Africa. Stellenbosch, Economic Research Note No. 10, September.

Burke, K. 2006. Orphans in Sub-Saharan Africa. Mimeo, Cortland State University of New York, Cortland, NY.

Burman, W., B. Grund, J. Neuhaus, J. Douglas, Jr., G. Friedland, E. Telzak, R. Colebunders, N. Paton, M. Fisher, and C. Rietmeijer; SMART Study Group and INSIGHT. 2008. "Episodic Antiretroviral Therapy Increases HIV Transmission Risk Compared with Continuous Therapy: Results of a Randomized Controlled Trial." *Journal of Acquired Immune Deficiency Syndromes* 49(2): 142–50.

Bussmann, H., C. W. Wester, N. Ndwapi, N. Grundmann, T. Gaolathe, J. Puvimanasinghe, A. Avalos, M. Mine, K. Seipone, M. Essex, V. Degruttola, and R. G. Marlink. 2008. "Five-year Outcomes of Initial Patients Treated in Botswana's National Antiretroviral Treatment Program." *AIDS* 22(17): 2303–11.

Byron, E., S. Gillespie, and M. Nangami. 2008. "Integrating Nutrition Security with Treatment of People Living with HIV: Lessons Being Learned in Kenya." *Food and Nutrition Bulletin* 29(2): 87–97.

Caldwell, J. C. 1997. "The Impact of the African AIDS Epidemic." *Health Transition Review* 7(Suppl. 2): 169–88.

——. 2000. "Rethinking the African AIDS Epidemic." *Population and Development Review* 26(1): 117–35.

Campbell, C. 2000. "Selling Sex in the Time of AIDS: The Psycho-Social Context of Condom Use by Sex Workers on a Southern African Mine." *Social Science and Medicine* 50(4): 4479–94.

Cantrell, R. A., M. Sinkala, K. Megazinni, S. Lawson-Marriott, S. Washington, B. H. Chi, B. Tambatamba-Chapula, J. Levy, E. M. Stringer, L. Mulenga, and J. S. Stringer. 2008. "A Pilot Study of Food Supplementation to Improve Adherence to Antiretroviral Therapy among Food-insecure Adults in Lusaka, Zambia." *Journal of Acquired Immune Deficiency Syndromes* 49(2): 190–5.

Carpenter, L. M., A. Kamali, A. Ruberantwari, S. S. Malamba, and J. A. Whitworth. 1999. "Rates of HIV-1 Transmission within Marriage in Rural Uganda in Relation to the HIV Sero-Status of the Partners." *AIDS* 13(9): 1083–9.

Carr, A., K. Samaras, S. Burton, M. Law, J. Freund, D. J. Chisholm, and D. A. Cooper. 1998. "A Syndrome of Peripheral Lipodystrophy, Hyperlipidaemia and Insulin Resistance in Patients Receiving HIV Protease Inhibitors." *AIDS* 12(7): F51–8.

Carter, M., J. May, J. Agüero, and S. Ravindranath. 2007. "The Economic Impact of Premature Adult Mortality: Panel Data Evidence from KwaZulu Natal, South Africa." *AIDS* 21(Suppl. 7): S67–73.

Case, A., and C. Ardington. 2006. "The Impact of Parental Death on School Outcomes: Longitudinal Evidence from South Africa." *Demography* 43(3): 402–20.

Case, A., and C. Paxson. 2009. The Impact of the AIDS Pandemic on Health Services in Africa: Evidence from the Demographic and Health Surveys. Princeton University, March 2009.

Case, A., C. Paxson, and J. Ableidinger. 2004. "Orphans in Africa: Parental Death, Poverty and School Enrollment." *Demography* 41(3): 483–508.

Caselli, F. 2005. Accounting for Cross-Country Income Differences. In *Handbook of Economic Growth*, Vol. 1, ed. P. Aghion, and S. N. Durlauf, 679–741. Amsterdam and Boston: Elsevier, North-Holland.

Cassell, M. M., D. T. Halperin, J. D. Shelton, and D. Stanton. 2006. "Risk Compensation: The Achilles' Heel of Innovations in HIV Prevention?" *BMJ* 332(7541): 605–7.

Castilla, J., J. Del Romero, V. Hernando, B. Marincovich, S. García, and C. Rodríguez. 2005. "Effectiveness of Highly Active Antiretroviral Therapy in Reducing Heterosexual Transmission of HIV." *Journal of Acquired Immune Deficiency Syndromes* 40(1): 96–101.

Celum, C. L., S. P. Buchbinder, D. Donnell, J. M. Douglas, Jr., K. Mayer, B. Koblin, M. Marmor, S. Bozeman, R. M. Grant, J. Flores, and H. W. Sheppard. 2001. "Early Human Immunodeficiency Virus (HIV) Infection in the HIV Network for Prevention Trials Vaccine Preparedness Cohort: Risk Behaviors, Symptoms, and Early Plasma and Genital Tract Virus Load." *Journal of Infectious Diseases* 183(1): 23–35.

Center for Global Development. 2007a. A Trickle or a Flood: Commitments and Disbursement for HIV/AIDS from the Global Fund, PEPFAR, and the World Bank's Multi-Country AIDS Program (MAP). Available at: http://www.cgdev.org/content/publications/detail/13029/

———. 2007b. HIV/AIDS Monitor: Tracking Aid Effectiveness. Available at: http://www.cgdev.org/section/initiatives/_active/hivmonitor

———. 2008a. World Bank Gives Low Marks for its HIV/AIDS Programs in Mozambique. Posted by David Wendt. Available at: http://blogs.cgdev.org/globalhealth/2008/10/world-bank-gives-low-marks-for.php

———. 2008b. Seizing the Opportunity on AIDS and Health Systems. Available at: http://www.cgdev.org/content/publications/detail/16459/

Center for Women's Global Leadership. 2007. *Action on Gender Based Violence and HIV/AIDS: Bringing Together Research, Policy, Programming and Advocacy.* Cambridge, MA: Harvard School of Public Health.

Central Bureau of Statistics, Republic of Namibia. 2006. Namibia Household Income and Expenditure Survey 2003/2004—Preliminary Report, National Planning Commission, Windhoek.

Central Statistics Office, Government of Botswana. 2006. Stats Brief – 2003 Household Income and Expenditure Survey (HIES). Central Statistics Office, Gaborone.

Chakraborty, H., P. K. Sen, R. W. Helms, P. L. Vernazza, S. A. Fiscus, J. J. Eron, B. K. Patterson, R. W. Coombs, J. N. Krieger, and M. S. Cohen. 2001. "Viral Burden in Genital Secretions Determines Male-to-Female Sexual Transmission of HIV-1: A Probabilistic Empiric Model." *AIDS* 15(5): 621–7.

Chambers, R., and G. Conway. 1992. *Sustainable Rural Livelihoods: Practical Concepts for the 21st Century.* Brighton, UK: Institute of Development Studies.

Chandisarewa, W., L. Stranix-Chibanda, E. Chirapa, A. Miller, M. Simoyi, A. Mahomva, Y. Maldonado Y, and A. K. Shetty. 2007. "Routine Offer of Antenatal HIV Testing ("Opt-out" Approach) to Prevent Mother-to-Child Transmission of HIV in Urban Zimbabwe." *Bulletin of the World Health Organization* 85(11): 843–50.

Chapoto, A., and T. S. Jayne. 2006. Socioeconomic Characteristics of Individuals Afflicted by AIDS-Related Prime-Age Mortality in Zambia. In: *AIDS, Poverty, and Hunger: Challenges and Responses*, ed. S. Gillespie, 33–55. Washington, DC: International Food Policy Research Institute.

———. 2008. "Impacts of AIDS-Related Mortality on Farm Household Welfare in Zambia." *Economic Development and Cultural Change* 56(2): 327–74.

Chapoto, A., T. S. Jayne, and N. Mason. 2010, forthcoming. "Widows' Land Security in the Era of HIV/AIDS: Panel Survey Evidence from Zambia." *Economic Development and Cultural Change.* Final version accepted: July 2009.

Cheek, R. 2001. "Playing God with HIV: Rationing HIV Treatment in Southern Africa." *African Security Review* 10(4): 19–28.

Cheluget, B., G. Baltazar, P. Orege, M. Ibrahim, L. H. Marum, and J. Stover. 2006. "Evidence for Population Level Declines in Adult HIV Prevalence in Kenya." *Sexually Transmitted Infections* 82(Suppl. 1): i21–6.

CHGA (Commission on HIV/AIDS and Governance in Africa). 2008. *Securing Our Future: Report of the Commission on HIV/AIDS and Governance in Africa.* Addis Ababa: UNECA.

Chin, J. 2007. *The AIDS Pandemic: The Collision of Epidemiology with Political Correctness.* London: Radcliffe.

———. 2008. The Myth of a General AIDS Pandemic: How Billions Are Wasted on Unnecessary AIDS Prevention Programmes. Discussion Paper No. 2, Campaign for Fighting Diseases. Available at: http://www.fightingdiseases.org/pdf/Jim_chin_AIDS.pdf

Chirambo, K., and J. Steyn. 2008. AIDS and State Fragility: The Challenge of Increased Deaths among Local Councillors in South Africa. ASCI Working Paper No. 25. Available at: http://asci.researchhub.ssrc.org/working-papers/ASCI%20Research%20Paper%2025-IDASA.pdf

Clark, S. 2004. "Early Marriage and HIV Risk in Sub-Saharan Africa." *Studies in Family Planning* 35(3): 149–60.

Clark, S., J. Bruce, and A. Dude. 2006. "Protecting Young Women from HIV/AIDS: The Case against Child and Adolescent Marriage." *International Family Planning Perspectives* 32(2): 79–88.

Clark, S., M. Poulin, and H.-P. Kohler. 2009. "Marital Aspirations, Sexual Behaviors, and HIV/AIDS in Rural Malawi." *Journal of Marriage and the Family* 71(2): 396–416.

Cleland, J., and M. M. Ali. 2006. "Sexual Abstinence, Contraception, and Condom Use by Young African Women: A Secondary Analysis of Survey Data." *Lancet* 368(9549): 1788–93.

Clemens, M., and S. Bazzi. 2008. Don't Close the Golden Door: Making Immigration Policy Work for Development. In *The White House and the World: A Global Development Agenda for the Next U.S. President*, ed. N. Birdsall, 241–72. Washington, DC: Center for Global Development.

Coates, T. J., L. Richter, and C. Caceres. 2008. "Behavioural Strategies to Reduce HIV Transmission: How to Make Them Work Better." *Lancet* 372(9639): 669–84.

Cochrane, J. H. 1991. "A Simple Test of Consumption Insurance." *Journal of Political Economy* 99(5): 957–76.

Coetzee, D., K. Hildebrand, A. Boulle, G. Maartens, F. Louis, V. Labatala, H. Reuter, N. Ntwana, and E. Goemaere. 2004. "Outcomes after Two Years of Providing Antiretroviral Treatment in Khayelitsha, South Africa." *AIDS* 18(6): 887–95.

Cohen, M. S., I. F. Hoffman, R. A. Royce, P. Kazembe, J. R. Dyer, C. C. Daly, D. Zimba, P. L. Vernazza, M. Maida, S. A. Fiscus, and J. J. Eron, Jr.; AIDSCAP Malawi Research Group.1997. "Reduction of Concentration of HIV-1 in Semen after Treatment of Urethritis: Implications for Prevention of Sexual Transmission of HIV-1." *Lancet* 349(9069): 1868–73.

Collins, D. L., and M. Leibbrandt. 2007. "Financial Impacts of HIV/AIDS on Poor Households in South Africa." *AIDS* 21(Suppl. 7): S75–81.

Connelly, P., and S. Rosen. 2005. "Will Small And Medium Enterprises Provide HIV/AIDS Services To Employees? An Analysis of Market Demand." *South African Journal of Economics* 73(S1): 613–26.

Coovadia, H., and A. Coutsoudis. 2007. "HIV, Infant Feeding, and Survival: Old Wine in New Bottles, but Brimming with Promise." *AIDS* 21(14): 1837–40.

Coovadia, H., and G. Kindra. 2008. "Breastfeeding, HIV Transmission and Infant Survival: Balancing Pros and Cons." *Current Opinion in Infectious Diseases* 21(1): 11–5.

Coovadia, H., N. C. Rollins, R. M. Bland, K. Little, A. Coutsoudis, M. L. Bennish, and M. L. Newell. 2007. "Mother-to-Child Transmission of HIV-1 Infection during Exclusive Breastfeeding in the First 6 Months of Life: An Intervention Cohort Study." *Lancet* 369(9567): 1107–16.

Corno, L., and D. de Walque. 2007. The Determinants of HIV Infection and Related Sexual Behaviors: Evidence from Lesotho. World Bank Policy Research Working Paper Series No. 4421, World Bank, Washington, DC.

Corrigan, P., G. Glomm, and F. Mendez. 2005. "AIDS Crisis and Growth." *Journal of Development Economics* 77(1): 107–24.

Coutinho, A. 2009. Limits and Realities of ART Scale-up. 16th Conference on Retroviruses and Opportunistic Infections, Montreal, February 8–11, 2009.

Coutsoudis, A., R. A. Bobat, H. M. Coovadia, L. Kuhn, W. Y. Tsai, and Z. A. Stein. 1995. "The Effects of Vitamin A Supplementation on the Morbidity of Children Born to HIV-Infected Mothers." *American Journal of Public Health* 85(8): 1076–81.

Coutsoudis, A., K. Pillay, E. Spooner, L. Kuhn, and H. M. Coovadia. 1999. "Randomized Trial Testing the Effect of Vitamin A Supplementation on Pregnancy Outcomes and Early Mother-to-Child HIV-1 Transmission in Durban, South Africa." *AIDS* 13(12): 1517–24.

Crampin, A. C., S. Floyd, J. R. Glynn, N. Madise, A. Nyondo, M. M. Khondowe, C. L. Njoka, H. Kanyongoloka, B. Ngwira, B. Zaba, B., and P. E. Fine. 2003. "The Long-term Impact of HIV and Orphanhood on the Mortality and Physical Well-being of Children in Rural Malawi." *AIDS* 17(3): 389–97.

Creek, T., W. Arvelo, A. Kim, L. Lu, A. Bowen, O. Mach, T. Finkbeiner, L. Zaks, J. Masunge, and M. Davis. 2007. A Large Outbreak of Diarrhea among Non-breastfed Children in Botswana, 2006–Implications for HIV Prevention Strategies and Child Health. The 14th Conference on Retroviruses and Opportunistic Infections, Los Angeles, CA, February 25–28, 2007.

Cross Continents Collaboration for Kids (3Cs4kids) Analysis and Writing Committee. 2008. "Markers for Predicting Mortality in Untreated HIV-infected Children in Resource-limited Settings: A Meta-analysis." *AIDS* 22(1): 97–105.

Cu-Uvin, S., A. Delong, D. Perez, J. Ingersoll, J. Kurpewski, E. Kojic, and A. Caliendo. 2009. Patterns of HIV-1 RNA Rebound in the Blood and Female Genital Tract. 16th Conference on Retroviruses and Opportunistic Infections, Montreal, February 8–11, 2009.

Cuddington, J. T. 1993a. "Modeling the Macroeconomic Effects of AIDS, with an Application to Tanzania." *World Bank Economic Review* 7(2): 173–89.

——— 1993b. "Further Results on the Macroeconomic Effects of AIDS: The Dualistic, Labor-Surplus Economy." *World Bank Economic Review* 7(3): 403–17.

Cuddington, J. T., and J. D. Hancock. 1994. "Assessing the Impact of AIDS on the Growth Path of the Malawian Economy." *Journal of Development Economics* 43(2): 363–68.

———. 1995. "The Macroeconomic Impact of AIDS in Malawi: A Dualistic, Labor Surplus Economy." *Journal of African Economics* 4(1): 1–28.

Davenport, C., and C. E. Loyle. 2009. The Conflict and HIV/AIDS Nexus: An Empirical Assessment. ASCI Working Paper no. 21. Available at: http://asci.researchhub.ssrc.org/working-papers/ASCI%20Research%20Paper%2021-Davenport%20and%20Loyle.pdf

Davey, G., D. Fekade, and E. Parry. 2006. "Must Aid Hinder Attempts to Reach the Millennium Development Goals?" *Lancet* 367(9511): 629–31.

Davidovich, U., J. de Wit, N. Albrecht, R. Geskus, W. Stroebe, and R. Coutinho. 2001. "Increase in the Share of Steady Partners as a Source of HIV Infection: A 17-Year Study of Seroconversion among Gay Men." *AIDS* 15(10): 1303–8.

Davis, C., and M. Feshbach. 1980. "Rising Soviet Infant Mortality." INTERCOM 8(17): 12–4.

Davis, M. 2001. *Late Victorian Holocausts: El Niño Famines and the Making of the Third World*. London: Verso.

De Cock, K. 2007. WHO/UNAIDS Guidance on Provider-Initiated HIV Testing and Counseling in Health Care Settings. Presentation at 4th IAS Conference, Sydney, July 24, 2007. Available at: http://www.ias2007.org/PAG/ppt/TUSY201.ppt

De Cock, K., and A. Johnson. 1998. "From Exceptionalism to Normalisation: A Reappraisal of Attitudes and Practice around HIV Testing." *BMJ* 316(7127): 290–3.

De Cock, K., D. Mbori-Ngacha, and E. Marum. 2002. "Shadow on the Continent: Public Health and HIV/AIDS in Africa in the 21st Century." *Lancet* 360(9326): 67–72.

de Vincenzi, I. 1994. "A Longitudinal Study of Human Immunodeficiency Virus Transmission by Heterosexual Partners." European Study Group on Heterosexual Transmission of HIV [see comments]. *New England Journal of Medicine* 331(6): 341–6.

de Vincenzi, I., and Kesho Bora Study Group. 2009. Triple-antiretroviral (ARV) Prophylaxis during Pregnancy and Breastfeeding Compared to Short-ARV Prophylaxis to Prevent Mother-to-Child Transmission of HIV-1 (MTCT): The Kesho Bora Randomized Controlled Clinical Trial in Five Sites in Burkina Faso, Kenya and South Africa. 5th IAS Conference on HIV Pathogenesis Treatment and Prevention, July 19–22, 2009.

de Waal, A. 2003. "How Will HIV/AIDS Transform African Governance?" *African Affairs* 102(406): 1–23.

———. 2006. *AIDS and Power: Why There Is No Political Crisis—Yet.* London: Zed Books.

de Waal, A., and A. Whiteside. 2003. "'New Variant Famine': AIDS and Food Crisis in Southern Africa." *Lancet* 362(9391): 1234–7.

de Walque, D. 2006. Who Gets AIDS and How? The Determinants of HIV Infection and Sexual Behaviors in Burkina Faso, Cameroon, Ghana, Kenya, and Tanzania. World Bank Policy Research Working Paper 3844, World Bank, Washington, DC.

———. 2007. "How Does the Impact of an HIV/AIDS Information Campaign Vary with Educational Attainment? Evidence from Rural Uganda." *Journal of Development Economics* 84(2): 686–714.

———. 2009. "Does Education Affect HIV Status? Evidence from Five African Countries." *World Bank Economic Review* 23(2): 209–33.

Deaton, A. 2006. Global Patterns of Income and Health: Facts, Interpretations, and Policies. NBER Working Paper No. 12269, National Bureau of Economic Research, Cambridge, MA.

Deininger, K., M. Garcia, and K. Subbarao. 2003. "AIDS-induced Orphanhood as a Systemic Shock: Magnitude, Impact and Program Interventions in Africa." *World Development* 31(7): 1201–20.

Devarajan, S., M. J. Miller, and E. V. Swanson. 2002. *Goals for Development: History, Prospects, and Costs.* Washington, DC: World Bank, Human Development Network, Office of the Vice President, and, Development Data Group.

DFID (United Kingdom Department for International Development). 2004. DFID Knowledge Programme on HIV/AIDS and STIs. *MEMA kwa Vijana: Community Randomized Trial of an Adolescent Sexual Health Programme in Rural Mwanza, Tanzania.* Department for International Development, London, UK.

Dieffenbach, C. W., and A. S. Fauci. 2009. "Universal Voluntary Testing and Treatment for Prevention of HIV Transmission." *JAMA* 301(22): 2380–2.

Dinkelman, T., D. Lam, and M. Leibbrandt. 2007. "Household and Community Income, Economic Shocks, and Risky Sexual Behavior of Young Adults: Evidence from the Cape Area Panel Study 2002 and 2005." *AIDS* 21(Suppl. 7): S49–56.

Dionne, K. Y., P. Gerland, and S. C. Watkins. 2009. "AIDS Exceptionalism: The View From Below." Unpublished manuscript, under review.

Dixon, S., S. McDonald, and J. Roberts. 2001. "AIDS and Economic Growth in Africa: A Panel Data Analysis." *Journal of International Development* 13(4): 411–26.

———. 2002. "The Impact of HIV and AIDS on Africa's Economic Development." *BMJ* 324(7331): 232–4.

Docking, T. 2001. AIDS and Violent Conflict in Africa. Special Report No. 75, U.S. Institute of Peace, Washington, DC.

Doctor, H. V., and A. A. Weinreb. 2003. "Estimation of AIDS Adult Mortality by Verbal Autopsy in Rural Malawi." *AIDS* 17(17): 2509–13.

Doherty, T. 2006. "HIV and Infant Feeding: Operational Challenges of Achieving Safe Infant Feeding Practices". Digital Comprehensive Summaries of Uppsala Dissertations from the Faculty of Medicine. University dissertation, Acta Universitatis Upsaliensis, Uppsala, Sweden.

Donoval, B. A., A. L. Landay, S. Moses, K. Agot, J. O. Ndinya-Achola, E. A. Nyagaya, I. MacLean, and R. C. Bailey. 2006. "HIV-1 Target Cells in Foreskins of African Men With Varying Histories of Sexually Transmitted Infections." *American Journal of Clinical Pathology* 125(3): 386–91.

Donovan, C., and L. A. Bailey. 2006. Understanding Rwandan Agriculture Households' Strategies to Deal with Prime-Age Illness and Death: A Propensity Score Matching Approach. In *AIDS, Poverty, and Hunger: Challenges and Responses. Highlights of the International Conference on HIV/AIDS and Food and Nutrition Security, Durban, South Africa, April 14–16, 2005,* ed. S. Gillespie, 109–28. Washington, DC: International Food Policy Research Institute.

Dorward, A. R., I. Mwale, and R. Tueso. 2006. "Labor Market and Wage Impacts of HIV/AIDS in Rural Malawi." *Review of Agricultural Economics* 28(3): 429–39.

Downs, A. M., and I. de Vincenzi. 1996. "Probability of Heterosexual Transmission of HIV: Relationship to the Number of Unprotected Sexual Contacts." European Study Group in Heterosexual Transmission of HIV [see comments]. *Journal of Acquired Immune Deficiency Syndromes and Human Retrovirology* 11(4): 388–95.

Drain, P. K., D. T. Halperin, J. P. Hughes, J. D. Klausner, and R. C. Bailey. 2006. "Male Circumcision, Religion, and Infectious Diseases: An Ecologic Analysis of 118 Developing Countries." *BMC Infectious Diseases* 6: 172.

Dreyfuss, M. L., G. I. Msamanga, D. Spiegelman, E. Duflo, P. Dupas, M. Kremer, and S. Sinei. 2006. Education and HIV/AIDS Prevention: Evidence from a Randomized Evaluation in Western Kenya. Policy Research Working Paper No. 4024, World Bank, Washington, DC.

Drinkwater, M. 1993. The Effects of HIV/AIDS on Agricultural Production Systems in Zambia. An Analysis and Field Reports of Case Studies out in Mpongwe, Ndola Rural District and Teta, Serenje District. FAO, Rome.

Druce, N., and A. Nolan. 2007. "Seizing the Big Missed Opportunity: Linking HIV and Maternity Care Services in Sub-Saharan Africa." *Reproductive Health Matters* 15(30): 190–201. Available at: http://options.co.uk/images/stories/resources/options/rhm_hiv.pdf

du Guerny, J. 1999. AIDS and Agriculture in Africa: Can Agriculture Policy Make a Difference? FAO, Rome.

Duflo, E., P. Dupas, M. Kremer, and S. Sinei. 2006. Education and HIV/AIDS Prevention: Evidence from a Randomized Evaluation in Western Kenya. World Bank Research Policy Working Paper No. 4024. World Bank, Washington, DC.

Dukers, N. H., H. S. Fennema, E. M. van der Snoek, A. Krol, R. B. Geskus, M. Pospiech, S. Jurriaans, W. I. van der Meijden, R. A. Coutinho, and M. Prins. 2007. "HIV Incidence and HIV Testing Behavior in Men Who Have Sex with Men: Using Three Incidence Sources, The Netherlands, 1984–2005." *AIDS* 21(4): 491–9.

Dunbar, M. S., C. Maternowska, M. J. Kang, S. M. Laver, I. Mudekunye, and N. S. Padian. Forthcoming. "Findings from SHAZ!: A Feasibility Study of a Microcredit and Lifeskills HIV Prevention Intervention to Reduce Risk among Adolescent Female Orphans in Zimbabwe." *Journal of Prevention and Intervention in the Community.*

Dunkle, K. L., R. K. Jewkes, H. C. Brown, M. Yoshihama, G. E. Gray, J. A. McIntyre, and S. D. Harlow. 2004. "Gender-based Violence, Relationship Power, and Risk of HIV Infection among Women Attending Antenatal Clinics in South Africa." *Lancet* 363(9419): 1415–21. Quoted in UNAIDS 2004, 22.

Dunkle, K. L., R. K. Jewkes, M. Nduna, J. Levin, N. Jama, N. Khuzwayo, M. P. Koss, and N. Duwury. 2006. "Perpetration of Partner Violence and HIV Risk Behaviour among Young Men in the Rural Eastern Cape, South Africa." *AIDS* 20(16): 2107–14.

Dupas, P. 2009. Do Teenagers Respond to HIV Risk Information? Evidence from a Field Experiment in Kenya. NBER Working Paper No. 14707, National Bureau of Economic Research, Cambridge, MA.

Durlauf, S. N., P. A. Johnson, and J. R. W. Temple. 2005. Growth Econometrics. In *Handbook of Economic Growth*, Vol. 1, ed. P. Aghion, and S. N. Durlauf, 555–677. Amsterdam and Boston: Elsevier, North-Holland.

Dyer, J. R., J. J. Eron, I. F. Hoffman, P. Kazembe, P. L. Vernazza, E. Nkata, C. Costello Daly, S. A. Fiscus, and M. S. Cohen. 1998. "Association of CD4 Cell Depletion and Elevated Blood and Seminal Plasma Human Immunodeficiency Virus Type 1 (HIV-1) RNA Concentrations with Genital Ulcer Disease in HIV-1-infected Men in Malawi." *Journal of Infectious Diseases* 177(1): 224–7.

Dyer, J. R., B. L. Gilliam, J. J. Eron, Jr., M. S. Cohen, S. A. Fiscus, and P. L. Vernazza. 1997. "Shedding of HIV-1 in Semen during Primary Infection." *AIDS* 11(4): 543–5.

Dyer, J. R., I. F. Hoffman, J. J. Eron, Jr., S. A. Fiscus, and M. S. Cohen. 1999. "Immune Activation and Plasma Viral Load in HIV-infected African Individuals." *AIDS* 13(10): 1283–5.

Eberstadt, N. 1988. *The Poverty of Communism.* New York: Transaction Publishers.

———. 2002. "The Future of AIDS." *Foreign Affairs* 81(6): 22–42.

*Economist.* 2007. "Replenishing the Fund: Finding the Money to Fight AIDS." *Economist*, September 26, 2007.

Egger, M. 2007. Outcomes of ART in Resource Limited and Industrialized Countries. Presented at the 14th Conference on Retroviruses and Opportunistic Infections, Los Angeles, CA, February 25–28, 2007.

Egger, M., M. May, G. Chene, A. N. Phillips, B. Ledergerber, F. Dabis, D. Costagliola, A. D'Arminio Monforte, F. de Wolf, P. Reiss, J. D. Lundgren, A. C. Justice, S. Staszewski, C. Leport, R. S. Hogg, C. A. Sabin, M. J. Gill, B. Salzberger, and J. A. Sterne; ART Cohort Collaboration. 2002. "Prognosis of HIV-1 Infected Patients Starting Highly Active Antiretroviral Therapy: A Collaborative Analysis of Prospective Studies." *Lancet* 360(9327): 119–29.

Eholie, S.-P., M. Nolan, A. P. Gaumon, J. Mambo, Y. Kouamé-Yebouet, R. Aka-Kakou, E. Bissagnene, and A. Kadio. 2003. Antiretroviral Treatment Can Be Cost Saving for Industry and Life-saving for Workers: A Case Study from Côte d'Ivoire's Private Sector. In *Economics of AIDS and Access to HIV/AIDS Care in Developing Countries, Issues and Challenges.* ed. J.-P. Moatti, B. Coriat, Y. Souteyrand, T. Barnett, J. Dumoulin, and Y.-A. Flori, 311–28. Paris: Agence Nationale de Recherches sur le Sida.

Elbe, S. 2009. *Virus Alert: Security, Governmentality and the AIDS Pandemic.* New York: Columbia University Press.

Ellis, L., P. Laubscher, and B. Smit. 2006. The Macroeconomic Impact of HIV/AIDS Under Alternative Intervention Scenarios (With Specific Reference to ART) on the South African Economy. Bureau for Economic Research, University of Stellenbosch, Stellenbosch, South Africa.

Ellis, L., and J. Terwin. 2005. The Impact of HIV/AIDS on Selected Business Sectors in South Africa. Bureau for Economic Research, Stellenbosch, South Africa.

England, R. 2006. "World Spends Too Much in the Fight against AIDS." *Financial Times*, August 14, 2006.

———. 2007. "Are We Spending Too Much on HIV?" *BMJ* 334(7589): 344. Available at: http://www.bmj.com/cgi/content/full/334/7589/344

————. 2008a. Provider Purchasing and Contracting Mechanisms. Based on a review commissioned by Rockefeller Foundation. HLSP Institute.

————. 2008b. "The Writing Is on the Wall for UNAIDS." *BMJ* 336(7652): 1072.

Englund, H. 2006. *Prisoners of Freedom: Human Rights and the African Poor*. Berkeley CA: University of California Press.

Epstein, H. 2007. *The Invisible Cure: Africa, the West and the Fight against AIDS*. New York: Farrar, Straus and Giroux.

Epstein, H., and J. Kim. 2007. "AIDS and the Power of Women." *New York Review of Books* 54(2): 39–41.

Erulkar, A. S., and E. Chong. 2005. *Evaluation of a Savings & Micro-Credit Program for Vulnerable Young Women in Nairobi*. New York: Population Council. Available at: http://www.popcouncil.org/pdfs/TRY_evaluation.pdf

Esacove, A. 2010. "Good Sex / Bad Sex. A Historical Analysis of U.S. Global AIDS Prevention Policy from 1995–2005." Unpublished manuscript, under review.

Esty, D., J. Goldstone, T. R. Gurr, P. Surko, and A. Unger. 1995. State Failure Task Force Report. Washington, DC.

Etard, J. F., I. Ndiaye, M. Thierry-Mieg, N. F. Guèye, P. N. Guèye, I. Lanièce, A. B. Dieng, A. Diouf, C. Laurent, S. Mboup, P. S. Sow, and E. Delaporte. 2006. "Mortality and Causes of Death in Adults Receiving Highly Active Antiretroviral Therapy in Senegal: A 7-year Cohort Study." *AIDS* 20(8): 1181–9.

Ethiopia and ORC Macro. Central Statistical Agency. 2006. *Ethiopia Demographic and Health Survey 2005*. Addis Ababa, Ethiopia and Calverton, Maryland.

European Collaborative Study. 2003. "Height, Weight, and Growth in Children Born to Mothers with HIV-1 Infection in Europe." *Pediatrics* 111(1): e52–60.

European Union. 2005. World AIDS Day—EU Statement on HIV Prevention for an AIDS Free Generation. Available at: http://data.unaids.org/Topics/UniversalAccess/EU Statement_24nov2005_en.pdf

Evans, D., and E. Miguel. 2007. "Orphans and Schooling in Africa: A Longitudinal Analysis." *Demography* 44(1): 35–57.

Exner, T. M., J. E. Mantell, L. A. Adeokun, I. A. Udoh, O. A. Ladipo, G. E. Delano, J. Faleye, and K. Akinpelu. 2009. "Mobilizing Men as Partners: The Results of an Intervention to Increase Dual Protection among Nigerian Men." *Health Education Research* 24(5): 846–54.

Fairley, C., A. E. Grulich, J. C. Imrie, and M. Pits. 2008. "Investment in HIV Prevention Works: A Natural Experiment." *Sexual Health* 5(2): 207–10.

FAO (United Nations Food and Agriculture Organization). 1993. The Effects of HIV/AIDS on Agriculture Production System in Zambia: Analysis and Field Report of Case Studies Carried out in Mpongue, Ndola Rural District and Serenje District: Adaptive Research Planning Team Report, Ministry of Agriculture, FAO, Rome.

————. 1995. The Effects of HIV/AIDS on Farming Systems in Eastern Africa. FAO, Rome.

————. 2003. AIDS—A Threat to Rural Africa. Available at: http://www.fao.org/focus/e/aids/aids1-e.htm

————. 2004. HIV/AIDS, Gender Inequality and Rural Livelihoods. The Impact of HIV/AIDS on Rural Livelihoods in Northern Province, Zambia. FAO, Rome.

Farquhar, C., J. N. Kiarie, B. A. Richardson, M. N. Kabura, F. N. John, R. W. Nduati, D. A. Mbori-Ngacha, and G. C. John-Stewart. 2004. "Antenatal Couple Counseling Increases Uptake of Interventions to Prevent HIV-1 Transmission." *Journal of Acquired Immune Deficiency Syndromes* 37(5): 1620–6.

FASAZ (Farming System Association of Zambia). 2003. *Inter-linkages between HIV/AIDS, Agricultural Production, and Food Security*. Rome: Integrated Support to Sustainable

Development and Food Security Programme, Food and Agriculture Organization of the United Nations (FAO).

Fawzi, W., G. Msamanga, D. Hunter, B. Renjifo, G. Antelman, H. Bang, K. Manji, S. Kapiga, D. Mwakagile, M. Essex, and D. Spiegelman. 2002. "Randomized Trial of Vitamin Supplements in Relation to Transmission of HIV-1 through Breastfeeding and Early Child Mortality." *AIDS* 16(14): 1935–44.

Fawzi, W., G. Msamanga, D. Spiegelman, R. Wei, S. Kapiga, E. Villamor, D. Mwakagile, F. Mugusi, E. Hertzmark, M. Essex, and D. Hunter. 2004. "A Randomized Trial of Multivitamin Supplements and HIV Disease Progression and Mortality." *New England Journal of Medicine* 351(1): 23–32.

Ferradini, L., A. Jeannin, L. Pinoges, J. Izopet, D. Odhiambo, L. Mankhambo, G. Karungi, E. Szumilin, S. Balandine, G. Fedida, M. P. Carrieri, B. Spire, N. Ford, J. M. Tassie, P. J. Guerin, and C. Brasher. 2006. "Scaling Up of Highly Active Antiretroviral Therapy in a Rural District of Malawi: An Effectiveness Assessment." *Lancet* 367(9519): 1335–42.

Ferreira, P. C., and S. Pessoa. 2003. The Long-Run Economic Impact of AIDS. Graduate School of Economics, Fundação Getulio Vargas, Rio de Janeiro.

Feshbach, M. 2008. Russian Demography, Health and the Military: Current and Future Issues. ASCI Research Report No. 8. Available at: http://asci.researchhub.ssrc.org/russian-demography-health-and-the-military-current-and-future-issues/attachment

Fiebig, E. W., D. J. Wright, B. D. Rawal, P. E. Garrett, R. T. Schumacher, L. Peddada, C. Heldebrant, R. Smith, A. Conrad, S. H. Kleinman, and M. P. Busch. 2003. "Dynamics of HIV Viremia and Antibody Seroconversion in Plasma Donors: Implications for Diagnosis and Staging of Primary HIV Infection." *AIDS* 17(13): 1871–9.

Fink, C., and K. Elliot. 2007. Tripping over Health: U.S. Policy toward Patents and Drug Access in Developing Countries. Center for Global Development, Washington, DC.

Fisher, M., D. Sudarshi, A. Brown, D. Pao, J. Parry, A. Johnson, P. Cane, N. Gill, C. Sabin, and D. Pillay. 2009. HIV Transmission among Men Who Have Sex with Men: Association with ART, Infection Stage, Viremia, and Sexually Transmitted Diseases, a Longitudinal Phylogenetic Study. 16th Conference on Retroviruses and Opportunistic Infections, Montreal, February 8–11, 2009.

Fleming, D. T., and J. N. Wasserheit. 1999. "From Epidemiological Synergy to Public Health Policy and Practice: the Contribution of Other Sexually Transmitted Diseases to Sexual Transmission of HIV Infection." *Sexually Transmitted Infections* 75(1): 3–17.

Foreit, J. 2001. Improving Reproductive Health by Involving Men in Community-based Distribution. Programme Briefs, 2001, No. 2, Population Council/FRONTIERS, Washington, DC.

Fortson, J. 2008a. "The Gradient in Sub-Saharan Africa: Socioeconomic Status and HIV/AIDS." *Demography* 45(2): 303–22.

——. 2008b. Mortality Risk and Human Capital Investment: The Impact of HIV/AIDS in Sub-Saharan Africa. Mimeo.

——. 2009. "HIV/AIDS and Fertility." *American Economic Journal: Applied Economics* 1(3): 170–94.

——. 2010 (forthcoming). "Mortality Risk and Human Capital Investment: The Impact of HIV/AIDS in Sub-Saharan Africa." *Review of Economics and Statistics*.

Fox, M. P., S. Rosen, W. B. MacLeod, M. Wasunna, M. Bii, G. Foglia, and J. L. Simon. 2004. "The Impact of HIV/AIDS on Labour Productivity in Kenya." *Tropical Medicine and International Health* 9(3): 318–24.

Frankenberger, T. 1996. "Measuring Household Livelihood Security: An Approach for Reducing Absolute Poverty." *Food Forum* No. 34, Food Aid Management, Washington, DC.

Fraser, C. 2009. The Effect of HIV Treatment on Transmission. 16th Conference on Retroviruses and Opportunistic Infections, Montreal, February 8–11, 2009.

Friis, H. 2005. Micronutrients and HIV Infection: A Review of Current Evidence. Consultation on Nutrition and HIV/AIDS in Africa: Evidence, lessons and recommendations for action Durban, South Africa, World Health Organization, April 10–13, 2005.

Friis, H., E. Gomo, N. Nyazema, P. Ndhlovu, H. Krarup, P. Kæstel, and K. F. Michaelsen. 2004. "Effect of Multimicronutrient Supplementation on Gestational Length and Birth Size: A Randomized, Placebo-controlled, Double-blind Effectiveness Trial in Zimbabwe." *American Journal of Clinical Nutrition* 80(1): 178–84.

Fylkesnes, K., R. Musonda, M. Sichone, Z. Ndhlovu, F. Tembo, and M. Monze. 2001. "Declining HIV Prevalence and Risk Behaviours in Zambia: Evidence from Surveillance and Population-based Surveys." *AIDS* 15(7): 907–16.

Fylkesnes, K., and S. Siziya. 2004. "A Randomised Trial on Acceptability of Voluntary HIV Counselling and Testing." *Tropical Medicine and International Health* 9(5): 566–72.

Gallant, M., and E. Maticka-Tyndale. 2004. "School-based HIV Prevention Programmes for African Youth." *Social Science and Medicine* 58(7): 1337–51.

Galvin, S. R., and M. S. Cohen. 2004. "The Role of Sexually Transmitted Diseases in HIV Transmission." *Nature Reviews Microbiology* 2(1): 33–42.

Garenne, M., K. Kahn, S. Tollman, and J. Gear. 2000. "Causes of Death in a Rural Area of South Africa: An International Perspective." *Journal of Tropical Pediatrics* 46(3): 183–90.

Garnett, G. P., and R. F. Baggaley. 2009. "Treating Our Way Out of the HIV Pandemic: Could We, Would We, Should We?" *Lancet* 373(9657): 9–11.

Garrett, L. 1994. *The Coming Plague: Newly-Emerging Diseases in a World out of Balance.* New York: Farrar, Straus and Giroux.

Gavin, L., C. Galavotti, H. Dube, A. D. McNaghten, M. Murwirwa, R. Khan, and M. St. Louis. 2006. "Factors Associated with HIV Infection in Adolescent Females in Zimbabwe." *Journal of Adolescent Health* 39(4): 596.e11–8.

Gerland, P. 2008. Age Pattern of HIV Incidence by Sex and Country, Derived from DHS HIV Prevalence (Computations by P. Gerland, UNPD, September 1, 2008). New York: United Nations Population Division.

Gersovitz, M. 2005. "The HIV Epidemic in Four African Countries Seen through the Demographic and Health Surveys." *Journal of African Economies* 14(2): 191–246.

Gertler, P., and J. Gruber. 2002. "Insuring Consumption against Illness." *American Economic Review* 92(1): 51–70.

Gertler, P. J., S. Martinez, D. Levine, and S. Bertozzi. 2003. Losing the Presence and Presents of Parents: How Parental Death Affects Children. Haas School of Business, Berkeley, CA.

GFATM (The Global Fund to Fight AIDS, Tuberculosis and Malaria). 2008. Guidelines and Application Form for Round 8. Available at: http://www.theglobalfund.org/en/rounds/8/single/?lang=en

Ghys, P. D., K. Fransen, M. O. Diallo, V. Ettiègne-Traoré, I. M. Coulibaly, K. M. Yeboué, M. L. Kalish, C. Maurice, J. P. Whitaker, A. E. Greenberg, and M. Laga. 1997. "The Associations between Cervicovaginal HIV Shedding, Sexually Transmitted Diseases and Immunosuppression in Female Sex Workers in Abidjan, Côte d'Ivoire." *AIDS* 11(12): F85–93.

Gillespie, S., and S. Drimie. 2009. Hyperendemic AIDS, Food Insecurity and Vulnerability in Southern Africa: A Conceptual Evolution. Working paper prepared for the Global Environmental Change and Human Security Conference, Oslo, Norway, June 23, 2009. Washington, DC: International Food Policy Research Institute. Available at: http://programs.ifpri.org/renewal/pdf/gechoslo200906.pdf

Gillespie, S., R. Greener, A. Whiteside, and J. Whitworth. 2007. "Investigating the Empirical Evidence for Understanding Vulnerability and Associations between Poverty, HIV infection and AIDS Impact." *AIDS* 21(Suppl. 7): S1–4.

Gillespie, S., and S. Kadiyala. 2005a. HIV/AIDs and Food and Nutrition Security: From Evidence to Action. Food Policy Review 7, International Food Policy Research Institute (IFPRI), Washington, DC.

———. 2005b. "HIV/AIDS and Food and Nutrition Security: Interactions and Response." *American Agricultural Economics Association* 87(5): 1282–8.

Gillespie, S., S. Kadiyala, and R. Greener. 2007. "Is Poverty or Wealth Driving HIV Transmission?" *AIDS* 21(Suppl. 7): S5–S16.

Glass, T. R., S. De Geest, B. Hirschel, M. Battegay, H. Furrer, M. Covassini, P. L. Vernazza, E. Bernasconi, M. Rickenboch, R. Weber, and H. C. Bucher; Swiss HIV Cohort Study. 2008. "Self-reported Non-adherence to Antiretroviral Therapy Repeatedly Assessed by Two Questions Predicts Treatment Failure in Virologically Suppressed Patients." *Antiviral Therapy* 13(1): 77–85.

Glewwe, P., H. Jacoby, and E. King. 2001. "Early Childhood Nutrition and Academic Achievement: A Longitudinal Analysis." *Journal of Public Economics* 81(3): 345–68.

Glick, P. 2005. "Scaling Up HIV Voluntary Counseling and Testing in Africa. What Can Evaluation Studies Tell Us about Potential Prevention Impacts?" *Evaluation Review* 29(4): 331–57.

Glick, P., and D. E. Sahn. 2007. "Changes in HIV/AIDS Knowledge and Testing Behavior in Africa: How Much and for Whom?" *Journal of Population Economics* 20(2): 382–422.

———. 2008. "Are Africans Practicing Safer Sex? Evidence from Demographic and Health Surveys for Eight Countries." *Economic Development and Cultural Change* 56(2): 397–439.

Global HIV/AIDS Initiatives Network. 2008. Briefing Sheet 3: The Challenge of Coordination. Available at: http://www.ghinet.org/briefing%203_coordination.pdf

Global HIV Prevention Working Group. 2007. Bringing HIV Prevention to Scale: An Urgent Global Priority. Bill and Melinda Gates Foundation.

———. 2008. Behavior Change and HIV Prevention: (Re)Considerations for the 21st Century. Available at: http://www.globalhivprevention.org/pdfs/PWG_behavior%20report_FINAL.pdf

Glynn, J. R., M. Caraël, M. B. Auvert, M. Kahindo, J. Chege, R. M. Musonda, F. Kaona, and A. Buvé; Study Group on the Heterogeneity of HIV Epidemics in African Cities. 2001. "Why Do Young Women Have a Much Higher Prevalence of HIV than Young Men? A Study in Kisumu, Kenya and Ndola, Zambia." *AIDS* 15(Suppl. 4): S51–60.

Glynn, J. R., M. Caraël, A. Buvé, S. Anagonou, L. Zekeng, M. Kahindo, and R. Musonda. 2004. "Does Increased General Schooling Protect against HIV Infection? A Study in Four African Cities." *Tropical Medicine and International Health* 9(1): 4–14.

Goetz, A. M., and R. S. Gupta. 1995. "Who Takes the Credit: Gender, Power, and Control over Loan Use in Rural Credit Programs in Bangladesh." *World Development* 24(1): 45–63.

Graff Zivin, J., H. Thirumurthy, and M. Goldstein. 2006. AIDS Treatment and Intrahousehold Resource Allocations: Children's Nutrition and Schooling in Kenya. NBER Working Paper 12689, National Bureau of Economic Research, Cambridge, MA.

————. 2009. AIDS Treatment and Intrahousehold Resource Allocation: Children's Nutrition and Schooling in Kenya. *Journal of Public Economics* 97(7–8): 1008–15.

Granich, R. M. 2009. HAART as Prevention. Presented at the 5th IAS Conference on HIV Pathogenesis, Treatment and Prevention, Cape Town, South Africa, July 21, 2009.

Granich, R. M., C. F. Gilks, C. Dye, K. M. De Cock, and B. G. Williams. 2009. "Universal Voluntary HIV Testing with Immediate Antiretroviral Therapy as a Strategy for Elimination of HIV Transmission: A Mathematical Model." *Lancet* 373(9657): 48–57.

Grant, M. 2008. "Children's School Participation and HIV/AIDS in Rural Malawi: The Role of Parental Knowledge and Perceptions." *Demographic Research* 19(Article 45): 1603–34. Available at: http://www.demographic-research.org/volumes/vol19/45/

Gray, R. H., G. Kigozi, D. Serwadda, F. Makumbi, S. Watya, F. Nalugoda, N. Kiwanuka, L. H. Moulton, M. A. Chaudhary, M. Z. Chen, N. K. Sewankambo, F. Wabwire-Mangen, M. C. Bacon, C. F. Williams, P. Opendi, S. J. Reynolds, O. Laeyendecker, T. C. Quinn, and M. J. Wawer. 2007. "Male Circumcision for HIV Prevention in Men in Rakai, Uganda: A Randomised Trial." *Lancet* 369(9562): 657–66.

Gray, R. H., X. Li, M. J. Wawer, D. Serwadda, N. K. Sewankambo, F. Wabwire-Mangen, T. Lutalo, N. Kiwanuka, G. Kigozi, F. Nalugoda, M. P. Meehan, M. Robb, and T. C. Quinn. 2004. "Determinants of HIV-1 Load in Subjects with Early and Later HIV Infections, in a General-population Cohort of Rakai," Uganda. *Journal of Infectious Diseases* 189(7): 1209–15.

Gray, R. H., D. Serwadda, G. Kigozi, F. Nalugoda, and M. J. Wawer. 2006. "Uganda's HIV Prevention Success: The Role of Sexual Behavior Change and the National Response. Commentary on Green et al." *AIDS and Behavior* 10(4): 347–50.

Gray, R. H., M. J. Wawer, R. Brookmeyer, N. K. Sewankambo, D. Serwadda, F. Wabwire-Mangen, T. Lutalo, X. Li, T. vanCott, and T. C. Quinn; Rakai Project Team. 2001. "Probability of HIV-1 Transmission per Coital Act in Monogamous, Heterosexual, HIV-1 Discordant Couples in Rakai, Uganda." *The Lancet* 357(9263): 1149–53.

Green, E. C., D. T. Halperin, V. Nantulya, and J. Hogle. 2006. "Uganda's HIV Prevention Success: The Role of Sexual Behavior Change and the National Response." *AIDS and Behaviour* 10(4): 335–46.

Greener, R. 2004. Impact of HIV/AIDS on Poverty and Inequality. In *The Macroeconomics of HIV/AIDS*, ed. M. Haacker, 167–81. Washington, DC: International Monetary Fund.

Greener, R., K. Jefferis, and H. Siphambe. 2000. "The Impact of HIV/AIDS on Poverty and Inequality in Botswana." *South African Journal of Economics* 68(5): 888–915.

Greenhalgh, S. 1988. "Fertility as Mobility: Sinic Transitions." *Population and Development Review* 14(4): 629–74.

Gregson, S., and G. P. Garnett. 2000. "Contrasting Gender Differentials in HIV-1 Prevalence and Associated Mortality Increase in Eastern and Southern Africa: Artefact of Data or Natural Course of Epidemics?" *AIDS* 14(Suppl. 3): S85–99.

Gregson, S., G. P. Garnett, C. A. Nyamukapa, T. B. Hallett, J. J. C. Lewis, P. R. Mason, S. K. Chandiwana, and R. M. Anderson. 2006. "HIV Decline Associated with Behavior Change in Eastern Zimbabwe." *Science* 311(5761): 664–6.

Gregson, S., C. A. Nyamukapa, G. P. Garnett, P. R. Mason, T. Zhuwau, M. Caraël, S. K. Chandiwana, and R. M. Anderson. 2002. "Sexual Mixing Patterns and Sex-Differentials in Teenage Exposure to HIV Infection in Rural Zimbabwe." *Lancet* 359(9321): 1896–903.

Greig, A., D. Peacock, R. Jewkes, and S. Msimang. 2008. "Gender and AIDS: Time to Act." *AIDS* 22(Suppl. 2): S35–43.

Grepin, K. 2009. Too Much of a Good Thing: Is HIV/AIDS Funding Strengthening African Health Systems? Ph.D. thesis, Harvard University, April 2009.

Grosskurth, H., J. Todd, E. Mwijarubi, P. Mayaud, A. Nicoll, G. ka-Gina, J. Newell, D. Mabey, R. Hayes, F. Mosha, K. Senkoro, J. Changalucha, A. Klokke, E. Mwijarubi, and K. Mugeye. 1995. "Impact of Improved Treatment of Sexually Transmitted Diseases on HIV Infection in Rural Tanzania: Randomised Controlled Trial." *Lancet* 346(8974): 530–6.

Grulich, A. E., and J. M. Kaldor. 2008. "Trends in HIV Incidence in Homosexual Men in Developed Countries." *Sexual Health* 5(2): 113–8.

Guinea and ORC Macro. Direction Nationale de la Statistique Ministère du Plan Conakry, Guinée. 2006. *Guinea Demographic and Health Survey 2005.* Calverton, Maryland.

Gupta, G. R., J. O. Parkhurst, J. A. Ogden, P. Aggleton, and A. Mahal. 2008. "Structural Approaches to HIV Prevention." *Lancet* 372(9640): 764–75.

Gupta, K., and P. J. Klasse. 2006. "How Do Viral and Host Factors Modulate the Sexual Transmission of HIV? Can Transmission Be Blocked?" *PLoS Medicine* 3(2): e79.

Habyarimana, J., B. Mbakile, and C. Pop-Eleches. 2007. HIV/AIDS, ARV Treatment and Worker Absenteeism: Evidence from a Large African Firm. 10th Bureau for Research and Economic Analysis of Development (BREAD) Conference on Development Economics, Princeton, NJ, April 27–28, 2007.

————. 2009. The Impact of HIV/AIDS and ARV Treatment on Worker Absenteeism: Implications for African Firms. Mimeo.

Haddad, L., and S. Gillespie. 2001. "Effective Food and Nutrition Policy Responses to HIV/AIDS: What We Know and What We Need to Know." *Journal of International Development* 13(4): 487–511.

Hall, N., D. Webb, Southern Africa AIDS Information Dissemination Service, and G. Mutangadura. 1998. *Socio-Economic Impact of Adult Mortality and Morbidity on Households in Kafue District, Zambia.* Harare, Zimbabwe: SAfAIDS.

Hallett, T. B., J. Aberle-Grasse, G. Bello, L-M. Boulos, M. P. A. Cayemittes, B. Cheluget, J. Chipeta, R. Dorrington, S. Dube, A. K. Ekra, J. M. Garcia-Calleja, G. P. Garnett, S. Greby, S. Gregson, J. T. Grove, S. Hader, J. Hanson, W. Hladik, S. Ismail, S. Kassim, W. Kirungi, L. Kouassi, A. Mahomva, L. Marum, C. Maurice, M. Nolan, T. Rehle, J. Stover, and N. Walker. 2006. "Declines in HIV Prevalence Can Be Associated with Changing Sexual Behaviour in Uganda, Urban Kenya, Zimbabwe, and Urban Haiti." *Sexually Transmitted Infections* 82(Suppl. 1): i1–8.

Hallett, T. B., S. Gregson, J. J. C. Lewis, B. A. Lopman, and G. P. Garnett. 2007. "Behavior Change in Generalized HIV Epidemics: Impact of Reducing Cross-Generational Sex and Delaying Sexual Debut." *Sexually Transmitted Infections* 83: 150–4.

Hallman, K. 2004. Socioeconomic Disadvantage and Unsafe Sexual Behaviors among Young Women and Men in South Africa. Working Paper No. 190, Population Council, Policy Research Division, New York.

Halperin, D. T. 2008. "Putting a Plague in Perspective." *New York Times,* January 1, 2008. Available at: http://www.nytimes.com/2008/01/01/opinion/01halperin.html?_r=1

Halperin, D. T., N. Andersson, M. Mavuso, and B. George. 2006. Assessing a National HIV Behavior Change Campaign Focusing on Multiple Concurrent Partnerships in Swaziland. Oral presentation abstract, XVI International AIDS Conference, Toronto, August 13–18, 2006. Available at: http://www.aids2006.org/abstract.aspx?elementId=2199617

Halperin, D. T., and H. Epstein. 2004. "Concurrent Sexual Partnerships Help to Explain Africa's High HIV Prevalence: Implications for Prevention." *Lancet* 364(9428): 4–6.

Hammer, S., K. E. Squires, M. D. Hughes, J. M. Grimes, L. M. Demeter, J. S. Currier, J. J. Eron, J. E. Feinberg, H. H. Balfour, L. R. Deyton, J. A. Chodakewitz, M. A. Fischl, J. P. Phair, L. Pedneault, B.-Y. Nguyen, and J. C. Cook. 1997. "A Controlled Trial of

Two Nucleoside Analogues Plus Indinavir in Persons with Human Immuno-deficiency Virus Infection and CD4 Cell Counts of 200 Per Cubic Millimeter or Less." *New England Journal of Medicine* 337(11): 725–33.

Hamoudi, A., and N. Birdsall. 2004. "AIDS and the Accumulation and Utilisation of Human Capital in Africa." *Journal of African Economies* 13(Suppl. 1): i96–136.

Hardon, A, P., D. Akurut, C. Comoro, C. Ekezie, H. F. Irunde, T. Gerrits, J. Kglatwane, J. Kinsman, R. Kwasa, J. Maridadi, T. M. Moroka, S. Moyo, A. Nakiyemba, S. Nsimba, R. Ogenyi, T. Oyabba, F. Temu, and R. Laing. 2007. "Hunger, Waiting Time and Transport Costs: Time to Confront Challenges to ART Adherence in Africa." *AIDS Care* 19(5): 658–65.

Hargreaves, J. R., C. P. Bonell, T. Boler, D. Boccia, I. Birdthistle, A. Fletcher, P. M. Pronyk, and J. R. Glynn. 2008a. "Systematic Review Exploring Time Trends in the Associa-tion between Educational Attainment and Risk of HIV Infection in Sub-Saharan Africa." *AIDS* 22: 403–14.

Hargreaves, J. R., and J. R. Glynn. 2002."Educational Attainment and HIV-1 Infection in Developing Countries: A Systematic Review." *Tropical Medicine and International Health* 7(6): 489–98.

Hargreaves, J. R., L. A. Morison, J. C. Kim, C. P. Bonell, J. D. H. Porter, C. Watts, J. Busza, G. Phetla, and P. M. Pronyk. 2008b. "The Association between School Attendance, HIV Infection and Sexual Behaviour among Young People in Rural South Africa." *Journal of Epidemiology and Community Health* 62: 113–9.

Harries, A. D., E. J. Schouten, and E. Libamba. 2006. "Scaling Up Antiretroviral Treatment in Resource-poor Settings." *Lancet* 367(9525): 1870–2.

Harvey, P. 2004. HIV/AIDS and Humanitarian Action. Humanitarian Policy Group Report 16. London: Overseas Development Institute. Available at: http://www.odi.org.uk/hpg/papers/hpgreport16.pdf

Haslwimmer, M. 1994. The Social and Economic Impact of HIV/AIDS on Nakambala Sugar Estate. FAO, Rome.

Health System Strengthening Workshop, 2009. The World Bank (Health Nutrition, and Population (HNP), World Bank Institute (WBI), Health Systems Global Expert Team (HSGET)), GAVI Alliance, and The Global Fund to Fight AIDS, Tuberculosis, and Malaria (Global Fund). June 25–27, 2009. Available at: http://web.worldbank.org/WBSITE/EXTERNAL/TOPICS/EXTENERGY2/EXTRENENERGYTK/0,,contentMDK:22231443~menuPK:5138518~pagePK:64020865~piPK:51164185~theSitePK:5138247,00.html

Hearst, N., and S. Chen. 2004. "Condom Promotion for AIDS Prevention in the Develop-ing World: Is it Working?" *Studies in Family Planning* 35(1): 39–47.

Heinecken, L. 2001. "HIV/AIDS, the Military and the Impact on National and International Security." *Society in Transition* 32(1): 120–47.

Hertog, S. 2009. Sex Ratios of HIV Prevalence: Uniting Demographic, Epidemiological and Sociological Perspectives to Understand Gender Imbalances in Generalized HIV/AIDS Epidemics. Ph.D. Dissertation, University of Wisconsin-Madison, Madison, Wisconsin.

Hickey, C. 1999. *Factors Explaining Observed Patterns of Sexual Behavior. Phase 2—Longi-tudinal Study, Final Report.* Zomba: Centre for Social Research, University of Malawi.

Higgins, D. L., C. Galavotti, K. R. O'Reilly, D. J. Schnell, M. Moore, D. L. Rugg, and R. John-son. 1991. "Evidence for the Effects of HIV Antibody Counseling and Testing on Risk Behaviors." *JAMA* 266(17): 2419–29.

Hirsch, J., S. Meneses, B. Thompson, M. Negroni, B. Pelcastre, and C. del Rio. 2007. "The Inevitability of Infidelity: Sexual Reputation, Social Geographies, and Marital Risk in Rural Mexico." *American Journal of Public Health* 97(6): 986–96.

Hisada, M., T. R. O'Brien, P. S. Rosenberg, and J. J. Goedert. 2000. "Virus Load and Risk of Heterosexual Transmission of Human Immunodeficiency Virus and Hepatitis C Virus by Men with Hemophilia." The Multicenter Hemophilia Cohort Study. *Journal of Infectious Diseases* 181(4): 1475–8.

HIV Prevention Trials Network. 2009. HPTN052 Study Information. Available at: http://www.hptn.org/research_studies/HPTN052.asp

Hoddinott, J., and B. Kinsey. 2001. "Child Growth in the Time of Drought." *Oxford Bulletin of Economics and Statistics* 63(4): 409–36.

Hoddinott, J., J. A. Maluccio, J. R. Behrman, R. Flores, and R. Martorell. 2008. "Effect of a Nutrition Intervention during Early Childhood on Economic Productivity in Guatemalan Adults." *Lancet.* 371(9610): 411–6.

Hogg, R. S., B. Yip, C. Kully, K. J. Craib, M. V. O'Shaughnessy, M. T. Schechter, and J. S. Montaner. 1998. "Improved Survival Among HIV-infected Individuals Following Initiation of Antiretroviral Therapy." *Journal of the American Medical Association* 279(6):450–54.

Hogle, J. A., ed., E. Green, V. Nantulya, R. Stoneburner, and J. Stover. 2002. *What Happened in Uganda? Declining HIV Prevalence, Behavior Change, and the National Response.* Washington, DC: USAID. Available at: http://www.usaid.gov/our_work/global_health/aids/Countries/africa/uganda_report.pdf

Holbrooke, R., and R. Furman. 2004. "A Global Battle's Missing Weapon." *New York Times*, February 10, 2004.

Holmes, K. K., P. F. Sparling, P.-A. Mårdh, S. M. Lemon, W. E. Stamm, P. Piot, and J. N. Wasserheit. 1999. *Sexually Transmitted Disease,* 3rd edition. New York: McGraw-Hill.

Holtgrave, D. R. 2007. "Costs and Consequences of the U.S. Centers for Disease Control and Prevention's Recommendations for Opt-out HIV Testing." *PLoS Medicine* (6): e194.

Hooper, E. 2000. *The River: A Journey to the Source of HIV and AIDS.* Harmondsworth: Penguin.

Hope, R. 2007. *Addressing Cross-Generational Sex.* Washington, DC: Population Reference Bureau.

Horton, R., and P. Das. 2008. "Putting Prevention at the Forefront of HIV/AIDS." *Lancet* 372(9637): 421–2.

Hosegood, V., N. McGrath, K. Herbst, and I. M. Timaeus. 2004. "The Impact of AIDS Mortality on Household Dissolution and Migration in Rural South Africa." *AIDS* 18(11): 1585–90.

Hughes, G., A. Leigh Brown, J. Bollback, A. Rambaut, E. Fearnhill, and D. Dunn; UK Collaborative Group on HIV Drug Resistance. 2009. Phylodynamic Analysis of Non-B HIV in the United Kingdom Reveals Substantial Post-immigration Transmission but Longer Intervals between Transmissions than for Subtype B. 16th Conference on Retroviruses and Opportunistic Infections, Montreal, February 8–11, 2009.

ICRW (International Center for Research on Women). 2004. To Have and to Hold: Women's Property and Inheritance Rights in the Context of HIV/AIDS in Sub-Saharan Africa. Information Brief, ICRW, Washington, DC. Available at: http://www.icrw.org/docs/2004_info_haveandhold.pdf

IHP+ (International Health Partnership). 2008a. Expanding Predictable Financing for Health Systems Strengthening and Delivering Results. Terms of reference. Available at: http://www.internationalhealthpartnership.net/pdf/Expanding_HSS_investments_TORs_August_2008_EN_FINAL.pdf

———. 2008b. Update on the International Health Partnership and Related Initiatives (IHP+). Prepared for the Health 8 Meeting, January 28, 2008. Available at: http://www.who.int/healthsystems/IHP+progress_report_H8.pdf

Iliff, P. J., E. G. Piwoz, N. V. Tavengwa, C. D. Zunguza, E. T. Marinda, K. J. Nathoo, L. H. Moulton, B. J. Ward, and J. H. Humphrey; ZVITAMBO Study Group. 2005. "Early Exclusive Breastfeeding Reduces the Risk of Postnatal HIV-1 Transmission and Increases HIV-free Survival." *AIDS* 19(7): 699–708.

Iliffe, J. 2006. *The African AIDS Epidemic: A History.* Oxford: James Currey.

IMF (International Monetary Fund). 2007. Botswana: Botswana: Selected Issues and Statistical Appendix. International Monetary Fund, Washington, DC.

———. 2008a. Botswana: 2007 Article IV Consultation – Staff Report. International Monetary Fund, Washington, DC.

———. 2008b. Zambia: Statistical Appendix. International Monetary Fund, Washington, DC.

———. 2008c. Namibia: Selected Issues and Statistical Appendix. International Monetary Fund, Washington, DC.

———. 2008d. Namibia: 2007 Article IV Consultation—Staff Report. International Monetary Fund, Washington, DC.

———. 2009. World Economic Outlook Database, October 2009 Edition. International Monetary Fund, Washington, DC.

ING Barings South African Research. 2000. Economic Impact of AIDS in South Africa: A Dark Cloud on the Horizon. ING Barings South Africa, Johannesburg, South Africa.

Institute of Medicine (IOM). 2007. *PEPFAR Implementation: Progress and Promise.* Washington, DC: The National Academy Press.

International Crisis Group. 2001. HIV/AIDS as a Security Issue. Issues Report No. 1, June 19, Washington, DC.

Iqbal, Z., and C. Zorn. 2010."Violent Conflict and the Spread of HIV/AIDS in Africa." *Journal of Politics* 72(1): 149–162.

Ive, P., B. Malope-Kgokong, M. Fox, M. Maskew, P. MacPhail, and I. Sanne. 2009. Time from Virologic Failure to Switching to Second-line Therapy in Patients Receiving ART in Johannesburg, South Africa. 16th Conference on Retroviruses and Opportunistic Infections, Montreal, February 8–11, 2009.

Ivory Coast Government, Enquête Démographique et de Santé and ORC Macro. 1998/99. *Ivory Coast Demographic and Health Survey 1998/99.* Calverton, Maryland, USA.

Izumi, K. 2009. Reclaiming Rights – Reclaiming Livelihoods. A Brief on Secure Land and Property Rights for Women in Sub-Saharan Africa in the Era of AIDS. Available at: http://www.kubatana.net/html/archive/landr/090626fao.asp?sector=LANDR&year=0&range_start=1

Jackson, D. J., A. E. Goga, T. Doherty, and M. Chopra. 2009. "An Update on HIV and Infant Feeding Issues in Developed and Developing Countries." *Journal of Obstetric, Gynecologic, and Neonatal Nursing* 38(2): 219–29.

Jacob, H. 2008. Impact of HIV/AIDS on Governance in Manipur and Nagaland. ASCI Research Report No. 6. Available at: http://asci.researchhub.ssrc.org/impact-of-hiv-aids-on-governance-in-manipur-and-nagaland/attachment

Jacobson, L. 2000. "The Family as Producer of Health—An Extended Grossman Model." *Journal of Health Economics* 19(5): 611–37.

Jamison, D. T., J. G. Breman, A. R. Measham, G. Alleyne, M. Claeson, D. B. Evans, P. Jha, A. Mills, and P. Musgrove. 2006. *Disease Control Priorities in Developing Countries,* 2nd edition. New York: Oxford University Press.

Jayne, T. S., A. Chapoto, E. Byron, M. Ndiyoi, P. Hamazakaza, S. Kadiyala, and S. Gillespie. 2006. "Community-level Impacts of AIDS-related Mortality: Panel Survey Evidence from Zambia." *Review of Agricultural Economics* 28(3): 440–57.

Jayne, T. S., M. Villarreal, P. Pingali, and G. Hemrich. 2005. HIV/AIDS and the Agricultural Sector in Eastern and Southern Africa: Anticipating the Consequences. FAO, Rome.

Jefferis, K., A. Kinghorn, H. Siphambe, and J. Thurlow. 2008. "Macroeconomic and Household-level Impacts of HIV/AIDS in Botswana." *AIDS* 22 (Suppl. 1): S113–9.

Jejeebhoy, S. J., I. Shah, and S. Thapa. 2006. *Sex Without Consent: Young People in Developing Countries.* New York: Zed Books.

Jewkes, R., K. Dunkle, M. Nduna, J. Levin, N. Jama, N. Khuzwayo, K. Moss, A. Puren, and N. Duvvury, N. 2006a. "Factors Associated with HIV Sero-status in Young Rural South African Women: Connections between Intimate Partner Violence and HIV." *International Journal of Epidemiology* 35(6): 1461–8.

Jewkes, R., M. Nduna, J. Levin, N. Jama, K. Dunkle, N. Khuzwayo, M. Koss, A. Puren, K. Wood, and N. Duwury. 2006b. "A Cluster Randomised Controlled Trial to Determine the Effectiveness of Stepping Stones in Preventing HIV Infections and Promoting Safer Sexual Behaviour amongst Youth in the Rural Eastern Cape, South Africa: Trial Design, Methods and Baseline Findings." *Tropical Medicine and International Health* 11(1): 3–16.

Jewkes, R., M. Nduna, J. Levin, N. Jama, K. Dunkle, A. Puren, and N. Duwury. 2008. "Impact of Stepping Stones on Incidence of HIV and HSV-2 and Sexual Behaviour in Rural South Africa: Cluster Randomised Controlled Trial." *BMJ* 337: a506.

Jewkes, R., M. Nduna, J. Levin, N. Jama, K. Dunkle, K. Wood, M. Koss, A. Puren, and N. Duwury. 2007. Evaluation of Stepping Stones: A Gender Transformative HIV Prevention Intervention. MRC Policy Brief, Gender and Health Research Unit, Medical Research Council, South Africa.

Jha, P., and Mills, A., chairs of Working Group 5. 2002. Improving Outcomes of the Poor. Report of Working Group 5 of the Commission on Macroeconomics and Health. Geneva: World Health Organization. (cited in Over et al. 2004).

Jin, F., G. P. Prestage, A. McDonald, T. Ramacciotti, J. C. Imrie, S. C. Kippax, J. M. Kaldor, and A. E. Grulich. 2008. "Trend in HIV Incidence in a Cohort of Homosexual Men in Sydney: Data from the Health in Men Study." *Sexual Health* 5(2): 109–12.

Johannessen, A., E. Naman, B. J. Ngowi, L. Sandvik, M. I. Matee, H. E. Aglen, S. G. Gundersen, and J. N. Bruun. 2008. "Predictors of Mortality in HIV-infected Patients Starting Antiretroviral Therapy in a Rural Hospital in Tanzania." *BMC Infectious Diseases* 8: 52.

Johnson, J., and B. Rogaly. 1997. *Microfinance and Poverty Reduction.* Oxford: Oxfam and London: Action Aid.

Johnson, W., C. Alons, L. Fidalgo, E. Piwoz, S. Kahn, A. Macombe, R. Catarina, A. Briend, R. Lovich, E. Warming, F. Floriano, and V. Chavane. 2006. The Challenge of Providing Adequate Infant Nutrition Following Early Breastfeeding Cessation by HIV-positive, Food Insecure Mozambican Mothers. 16th International AIDS Conference, Toronto, August 13–18, 2006.

Juhn, C., S. Kalemli-Ozcan, and B. Turan. 2008a. HIV and Fertility in Africa: First Evidence from Population Based Surveys. NBER Working Paper No. 14248, National Bureau of Economic Research, Cambridge, MA.

———. 2008b. HIV and Fertility in Africa: What Do the New Data Say? Available at: http://www.voxeu.org/index.php?q=node/1734

Jukes, M., S. Simmons, and D. Bundy. 2008. "Education and Vulnerability: The Role of Schools in Protecting Young Women and Girls from HIV in Southern Africa." *AIDS* 22(Suppl. 4): S1–16.

Kabeer, N. 2001. "Conflicts over Credit: Re-evaluating the Empowerment Potential of Loans to Women in Rural Bangladesh." *World Development* 29(1): 63–84.

Kadiyala, S. 2006. Prime Age Adult Mortality in Rural Ethiopia: Determinants and Impacts on Households and Children. Friedman School of Nutrition Science and Policy, Tufts University, Boston.

Kadiyala, S., A. Quisumbing, B. L. Rogers, and P. Webb. 2009. "The Impact of Prime Age Adult Mortality on Child Survival and Growth in Rural Ethiopia." *World Development* 37(6): 1116–28.

Kagimu, M., E. Marum, F. Wabwire-Mangen, N. Nakyanjo, Y. Walakira, and J. Hogle. 1998. "Evaluation of the Effectiveness of AIDS Health Education Interventions in the Muslim Community in Uganda." *AIDS Education and Prevention* 10(3): 215–28.

Kajoba, G. M. 2006. "Women and Land in Zambia: A Case Study of Small-Scale Farmers in Chinema Village, Chibombo District, Central Zambia." *Eastern Africa Social Science Research Review* 28(1): 35–61.

Kajubi, P., M. R. Kamya, S. Kamya, S. Chen, W. McFarland, and N. Hearst. 2005. "Increasing Condom Use without Reducing HIV Risk: Results of a Controlled Community Trial in Uganda." *Journal of Acquired Immune Deficiency Syndromes* 40(1): 77–82.

Kalemli-Ozcan, S. 2002. "Does the Mortality Decline Promote Economic Growth?" *Journal of Economic Growth* 7(4): 411–39.

———. 2008. AIDS, "Reversal" of the Demographic Transition and Economic Development: Evidence from Africa. NBER Working Paper 12181, National Bureau of Economic Research, Cambridge, MA.

Kalemli-Ozcan, S., H. E. Ryder, and D. N. Weil. 2000. "Mortality Decline, Human Capital Investment, and Economic Growth." *Journal of Development Economics* 62(1): 1–23.

Kalichman, S. C., L. Eaton, and S. Pinkerton. 2007. "Circumcision for HIV Prevention: Failure to Fully Account for Behavioral Risk Compensation." *PLoS Medicine* 4(3): e138.

Kamali, A., M. Quigley, J. Nakiyingi, J. Kinsman, J. Kengeya-Kayondo, R. Gopal, A. Ojwiya, P. Hughes, L. M. Carpenter, and J. Whitworth. 2003. "A Community Randomized Trial of Sexual Behaviour and Syndromic STI Management Interventions on HIV-1 Transmission in Rural Uganda." *Lancet* 361(9358): 645–52.

Kambou, G., S. Devarajan, and M. Over. 1992. "The Economic Impact of AIDS in an African Country: Simulations with a Computable General Equilibrium Model of Cameroon." *Journal of African Economies* 1(1): 109–30.

Kang-Dufour, M., M .S. Dunbar, I. Mudekunye, D. Nhamo, and N. S. Padian. 2009. Evaluation of SHAZ! Phase II: Potential Efficacy to Mitigate Structural Risk Factors and Prevent HIV/STI and Pregnancy. Presentations at the Conference of the International Society for Sexually Transmitted Diseases Research, London, June 28–July1, 2009.

Kapiga, S., and I. Aitken. 2003. *Role of Sexually Transmitted Diseases in HIV-1 Transmission.* New York: Kluwer Academic Publisher.

Kaplan, R. 1994. "The Coming Anarchy." *Atlantic Monthly* 273(2): 44–77.

Kardam, N. 1991. *Bringing Women In: Women's Issues in International Development Programs.* Boulder and London: Lynne Rienner Publishers.

Karlan, D., and J. Zinman. 2009. Expanding Microenterprise Credit Access: Using Randomized Supply Decisions to Estimate the Impacts in Manila. New Haven, CT: Innovations for Poverty Action, July.

Kates, J., J.-A. Izazola, and E. Lief. 2007. Financing the Response to AIDS in Low- and Middle Income Countries: International Assistance from the G8, European Commission and Other Donor Governments, 2006. The Kaiser Family Foundation and UNAIDS. Available at: http://www.kff.org/hivaids/upload/7347_03.pdf

Katzenstein, D., M. Laga, and J. P. Moatti. 2003. "The Evaluation of the HIV/AIDS Drug Access Initiatives in Cote d'Ivoire, Senegal and Uganda: How Access to Antiretroviral Treatment Can Become Feasible in Africa." *AIDS* 17(Suppl. 3): S1–4.

Keiser, O., and ART-LINC Collaboration of the International Epidemiological Databases to Evaluate AIDS (IeDEA). 2009. Switching to Second-line ART, and Mortality in Resource-limited Settings: Collaborative Analysis of Treatment Programs in Africa, Asia, and Latin America. 16th Conference on Retroviruses and Opportunistic Infections, Montreal, February 8–11, 2009.

Keller, B. 2000. *Women's Access to land in Zambia.* International Federation of Surveyors (FIG) Commission of (Cadastre and Land Management) Task Force on Women Access to Land, Köln, Germany.

Kelly, R. J., R. H. Gray, N. K. Sewankambo, D. Serwadda, F. Wabwire-Mangen, T. Lutalo, and M. J. Wawer. 2003. "Age Differences in Sexual Partners and Risk of HIV Infection in Rural Uganda." *Journal of Acquired Immune Deficiency Syndromes* 32(4): 446–51.

Kharas, H. 2008. *A Reality Check on African Aid.* Washington, DC: The Brookings Institution.

Kim, J. C., P. Pronyk, T. Barnett, and C. Watts. 2008. "Exploring the Role of Economic Empowerment in HIV Prevention." *AIDS* 22(Suppl. 4): S57–71.

Kim, J. C., C. H. Watts, J. R. Hargreaves, L. X. Ndhlovu, G. Phetla, L. A. Morison, J. Busza, J. D. Porter, and P. Pronyk. 2008. "Understanding the Impact of a Microfinance Based Intervention on Women's Empowerment and the Reduction of Intimate Partner Violence in South Africa." *American Journal of Public Health* 97(10): 1794–802.

Kinsman, J., J. Nakiyingi, A. Kamali, L. Carpenter, M. Quigley, R. Pool, and J. Whitworth. 2001. "Evaluation of a Comprehensive School-based AIDS Education Programme in Rural Masaka, Uganda." *Health Education Research* 16(1): 85–100.

Kirby, D. 2001. *Emerging Answers: Research Findings on Programs to Reduce Teen Pregnancy.* Washington, DC: National Campaign to Prevent Teen Pregnancy.

Kirby, D., B. Laris, and L. Rolleri. 2005. Impact of Sex and HIV Education Programs on Sexual Behaviors of Youth in Developing and Developed Countries. Youth Research Working Paper No. 2, Family Health International (FHI), Research Triangle Park, NC.

Kirimi, L. W. 2008. Essays on Disease-related Working-Age Adult Mortality: Evidence from Rural Kenya. Unpublished Ph.D. Dissertation. Michigan State University, Department of Agricultural, Food, and Resource Economics. East Lansing. Michigan.

Kitahata, M., S. Gange, and R. Moore; North American AIDS Cohort Collaboration on Research and Design. 2009. Initiating Rather than Deferring HAART at a CD4+ Count >500 Cells/mm3 Is Associated with Improved Survival. 16th Conference on Retroviruses and Opportunistic Infections, Montreal, February 8–11, 2009.

Klag, M. J. 2007. "Shift Tactics in AIDS Battle." *Baltimore Sun*, November 29, 2007.

Koenig, S. P., F. Léandre, and P. E. Farmer. 2004. "Scaling-up HIV Treatment Programmes in Resource-limited Settings: The Rural Haiti Experience." *AIDS* 18(Suppl. 3): S21–5.

Kohler, H.-P., J. R. Behrman, and S. C. Watkins. 2007. "Social Networks and HIV/AIDS Risk Perceptions." *Demography* 44(1): 1–33.

Koopman, J. S., J. A. Jacquez, G. W. Welch, C. P. Simon, B. Foxman, S. M. Pollock, D. Barth-Jones, A. L. Adams, and K. Lange. 1997. "The Role of Early HIV Infection in the Spread of HIV through Populations." *Journal of Acquired Immune Deficiency Syndromes and Human Retrovirology* 14(3): 249–58.

Korenromp, E. L., R. G. White, K. K. Orroth, R. Bakker Maggwa, A. Kamali, D. Serwadda, R. H. Gray, H. Grosskurth, J. D. Habbema, and R. J. Hayes. 2005. "Determinants of the Impact of Sexually Transmitted Infection Treatment on Prevention of HIV

Infection: A Synthesis of Evidence from the Mwanza, Rakai, and Masaka Intervention Trials." *Journal of Infectious Diseases* 191(Suppl. 1): S168–78.

Kotler, D. P., A. R. Tierney, J. Wang, and R. N. Pierson, Jr. 1989. "Magnitude of Body-cell-mass Depletion and the Timing of Death from Wasting in AIDS." *American Journal of Clinical Nutrition* 50(3): 444–7.

Ksoll, C. 2007. Family Networks and Orphan Caretaking in Tanzania. Economics Series Working Paper 361, University of Oxford, Department of Economics.

Kuhn, L., M. Sinkala, C. Kankasa, K. Semrau, P. Kasonde, N. Scott, M. Mwiya, C. Vwalika, J. Walter, W. Y. Tsai, G. M. Aldrovandi, and D. M. Thea. 2007. "High Uptake of Exclusive Breastfeeding and Reduced Early Post-natal HIV Transmission." *PLoS* 2(12): e1363.

Kumarasamy, N., K. Venkatesh, A. Srikrishnan, L. Prasad, P. Balakrishnan, E. Thanburaj, J. Sharma, S. Solomon, and K. Maye. 2009. Risk Factors for HIV Transmission among Heterosexual Discordant Couples in South India. 16th Conference on Retroviruses and Opportunistic Infections, Montreal, February 8–11, 2009.

Kumwenda, N., P. G. Miotti, T. E. Taha, R. Broadhead, R. J. Biggar, J. B. Jackson, G. Melikian, and R. D. Semba. 2002. "Antenatal Vitamin A Supplementation Increases Birth Weight and Decreases Anemia among Infants Born to Human Immunodeficiency Virus–infected Women in Malawi." *Clinical Infectious Diseases* 35(5): 618–24.

Kwaramba, P. 1997. The Socio-Economic Impact of HIV/AIDS on Communal Agricultural Systems in Zimbabwe. ZFU, Friedrich Ebert Stifting Economic Advisory Project, Working Paper 19, Harare, Zimbabwe.

Lagakos, S. W., and A. R. Gable. 2008. "Challenges to HIV Prevention—Seeking Effective Measures in the Absence of a Vaccine." *New England Journal of Medicine* 358(15): 1543–5.

Larson, B. A., G. Barnes, G. Rogers, and J. G. Larson. 1995. "Forests, Agriculture, and Child Health in Zaire: A Household Modeling Approach." *Forest Science* 42(1): 3–9.

Larson, B. A., M. P. Fox, S. Rosen, M. Bii, C. Sigei, D. Shaffer, F. Sawe, M. Wasunna, J. L. Simon. 2008. "Early Effects of Antiretroviral Therapy on Work Performance: Preliminary Results from a Cohort Study of Kenyan Agricultural Workers." *AIDS* 22(3): 421–5.

Laubscher, P., L. Visagie, and B. Smit. 2001. The Macro-Economic Impact of HIV/AIDS in South Africa. Economic Research Note No. 10, Bureau for Economic Research, University of Stellenbosch, Stellenbosch, South Africa.

Laurent, C., N. Diakhaté, F. N. Gueye, M. A. Touré, P. S. Sow, M. A. Faye, M. Gueye, I. Lanièce, C. Touré Kane, F. Liégeois, L. Vergne, S. Mboup, S. Badiane, I. Ndoye, and E. Delaporte. 2002. "The Senegalese Government's Highly Active Antiretroviral Therapy Initiative: An 18-month Follow-up Study." *AIDS* 16(10): 1363–70.

Lawn, S., F. Little, L.-G. Bekker, R. Kaplan, E. Campbel, C. Orrell, and R. Wood. 2009. Changing Mortality Risk Associated with CD4 Cell Response to Long-term ART: Sub-Saharan Africa. 16th Conference on Retroviruses and Opportunistic Infections, Montreal, February 8–11, 2009.

Laxminarayan, R., A. J. Mills, J. G. Bremen, A. R. Measham, G. Alleyne, M. Claeson, P. Jha, P. Musgrove, J. Chow, S. Shahid-Salles, and D. T. Jamison. 2006. "Advancement of Global Health: Key Messages from the Disease Control Priorities Project." *Lancet* 367(9517): 1193–208.

Lesotho Bureau of Statistics. n.d. HBS Summary Table. Obtained from website of Lesotho Bureau of Statistics: http://www.bos.gov.ls/

Levine, R. 2004. *Millions Saved: Proven Successes in Global Health*. Washington, DC: Center for Global Development.

———. 2008. Healthy Foreign Policy: Bringing Coherence to the Global Health Agenda. In *The White House and the World: A Global Development Agenda for the Next U.S. President*, ed. N. Birdsall, 43–61. Washington, DC: Center for Global Development.

Lewis, S. 2004. Keynote Lecture by Stephen Lewis, UN Special Envoy for HIV/AIDS in Africa, 11th Conference on Retroviruses and Opportunistic Infections, San Francisco, CA, February 8, 2004. Available at: http://www.who.int/3by5/partners/slewis/en/print.html

Leynaert, B., A. M. Downs, and I. de Vincenzi. 1998. "Heterosexual Transmission of Human Immunodeficiency Virus: Variability of Infectivity throughout the Course of Infection." European Study Group on Heterosexual Transmission of HIV. *American Journal of Epidemiology* 148(1): 88–96.

Lima, V. D., R. Harrigan, M. Murray, D. M. Moore, E. Wood, R. S. Hogg, and J. S. Montaner. 2008. "Differential Impact of Adherence on Long-term Treatment Response among Naive HIV-infected Individuals." *AIDS* 22(17): 2371–80.

Lorentzen, P., J. McMillan, and R. Wacziarg. 2005. Death and Development. NBER Working Paper No. 11620, National Bureau of Economic Research, Cambridge, MA.

Lovász, E., and B. Schipp. 2009. "The Impact of HIV/AIDS on Economic Growth in Sub-Saharan Africa." *South African Journal of Economics* 77(2): 245–56.

Lowicki-Zucca, M., S. Karmin, and K. L. Dehne. 2009. "HIV among Peacekeepers and Its Likely Impact on Prevalence on Host Countries' HIV Epidemics." *International Peacekeeping* 16(3): 352–63.

Lugada, E., S. Jaffar, J. Levin, B. Abang, J. Mermin, G. Namara, H. Grosskurth, E. Mugalanzi, S. Gupta, and R. Bunnell. 2009. Comparison of Home- and Clinic-based HIV Counseling and Testing among Household Members of Persons Taking ART: Uganda. 16th Conference on Retroviruses and Opportunistic Infections, Montreal, February 8–11, 2009.

Luke, N. 2005. "Confronting the 'Sugar Daddy' Stereotype: Age and Economic Asymmetries and Risky Sexual Behavior in Urban Kenya." *International Family Planning Perspectives* 31(1): 6–14.

Luke, N, and K. M. Kurz. 2002. *Cross-Generational and Transactional Sexual Relations in Sub-Saharan Africa: Prevalence of Behavior and Implications for Negotiating Safer Sexual Practice*. Washington, DC: ICRW.

Lunney, K. M., A. L. Jenkins, N. V. Tavengwa, F. Majo, D. Chidhanguro, P. Iliff, G. T. Strickland, E. Piwoz, E. L. Iannotti, and J. H. Humphrey. 2008. "HIV-Positive Poor Women May Stop Breast-feeding Early to Protect Their Infants from HIV Infection Although Available Replacement Diets Are Grossly Inadequate." *Journal of Nutrition* 138(2): 351–7.

MacFarlan, M., and S. Sgherri. 2001. The Macroeconomic Impact of HIV/AIDS in Botswana. IMF Working Paper No. 01/80, International Monetary Fund, Washington, DC.

Machina, H. 2002. Women's Land Rights in Zambia: Policy Provisions, Legal Framework and Constraints. Paper presented at the Regional Conference on Women's Land Rights, Harare, Zimbabwe, May 26–30, 2002. Available at: http://www.oxfam.org.uk/what_we_do/issues/livelihoods/landrights/downloads/womenzam.rtf

Mahal, A. 2004. "Economic Implications of Inertia on HIV/AIDS and Benefits of Action." *Economic and Political Weekly* 39(10): 1049–63.

Mahal, A., D. Canning, K. Odumosou, and P. Okonkwo. 2008. "Assessing the Economic Impact of HIV/ AIDS on Nigerian Households: A Propensity Score Matching Approach." *AIDS* 22(Suppl. 1): S95–101.

Mahlungulu, S., L. A. Grobler, M. E. Visser, and J. Volmink. 2007. Nutritional Interventions for Reducing Morbidity and Mortality in People with HIV. *Cochrane Database of*

*Systematic Reviews 2007,* Issue 3. Art. No.: CD004536. DOI: 10.1002/14651858.CD-004536.pub2.

Malawi and ORC Macro. National Statistical Office. 2005. *Malawi Demographic and Health Survey 2004.* Calverton, Maryland: NSO and ORC Macro.

Maman, S., J. K. Mbwambo, N. M. Hogan, G. P. Kilonzo, J. C. Campbell, E. Weiss, and M. D. Sweat. 2002. "HIV-positive Women Report More Lifetime Partner Violence: Findings from a Voluntary Counselling and Testing Clinic in Dares Salaam, Tanzania." *American Journal of Public Health* 92(8): 1331–7.

Mamlin, J., S. Kimaiyo, S. Lewis, H. Tadayo, F. K. Jerop, C. Gichunge, T. Petersen, Y. Yih, P. Braitstein, and R. Einterz. 2009. "Integrating Nutrition Support for Food-insecure Patients and Their Dependents into an HIV Care and Treatment Program in Western Kenya." *American Journal of Public Health* 99(2): 215–21.

Mankiw, N. G., D. Romer, and D. N. Weil. 1992. "A Contribution to the Empirics of Economic Growth." *Quarterly Journal of Economics* 107(2): 407–37.

Manning, R. 2003. The Impact of HIV/AIDS on Local-level Democracy: A Case Study of the eThekweni Municipality, KwaZulu-Natal, South Africa. Democracy in Africa Research Unit, CSSR Working Paper No. 35.

Manzi, M., R. Zachariah, R. Teck, L. Buhendwa, J. Kazima, E. Bakali, P. Firmenich, and P. Humblet. 2005. "High Acceptability of Voluntary Counselling and HIV-Testing But Unacceptable Loss to Follow Up in a Prevention of Mother-to-Child HIV Transmission Programme in Rural Malawi: Scaling-up Requires a Different Way of Acting." *Tropical Medicine and International Health* 10(12): 1242–50.

Marcelin, A.-G., R. Tubiana, S. Lambert-Niclot, G. Lefebvre, S. Dominguez, M. Bonmarchand, D. Vauthier-Brouzes, F. Marguet, G. Peytavin, and C. Poirot; Pitie-Salpetriere AMP a Risque Viral Study Group. 2009. Detection of HIV-1 RNA in Seminal Plasma Samples from Treated Patients with Undetectable HIV-1 RNA in Blood Plasma. 16th Conference on Retroviruses and Opportunistic Infections, Montreal, February 8–11, 2009.

Marins, J. R., L. F. Jamal, S. Y. Chen, M. B. Barros, E. S. Hudes, A. A. Barbosa, P. Chequer, R. Teixeira, and N. Hearst. 2003. "Dramatic Improvement in Survival among Adult Brazilian AIDS Patients." *AIDS* 17(11): 1675–82.

Marum, E., M. Taegtmeyer, and K. Chebet. 2006. "Scale-up of Voluntary HIV Counseling and Testing in Kenya." *JAMA* 296(7): 859–62.

Mason, J. B., A. Bailes, K. E. Mason, O. Yambi, U. Jonsson, C. Hudspeth, P. Hailey, A. Kendle, D. Brunet, and P. Martel. 2005. "AIDS, Drought and Child Malnutrition in Southern Africa." *Public Health Nutrition* 8(6): 551–63.

Mason, N. M., A. Chapoto, T. S. Jayne, and R. J. Myers. 2010. "A Test of the New Variant Famine Hypothesis: Panel Survey Evidence from Zambia." *World Development* 38(3): 356–68.

Mastro, T. D., and I. de Vincenzi. 1996. "Probabilities of Sexual HIV-1 Transmission." *AIDS* 10(Suppl. A): S75–82.

Mastro, T. D., G. A. Satten, T. Nopkesorn, S. Sangkharomya, and I. M. Longini, Jr. 1994. "Probability of Female-to-Male Transmission of HIV-1 in Thailand." *Lancet* 343(8891): 204–7.

Masuku, T. 2007. AIDS in the South African Police Service: A Threat to the State? Justice Africa, London. Available at: http://www.justiceafrica.org/wp-content/uploads/2007/10/policing-south-africa.pdf

Mather, D., and C. Donovan. 2008. The Impacts of Prime-Age Adult Mortality on Rural Household Income, Assets, and Poverty in Mozambique. Research Report, Ministry of Agriculture and Rural Development, Republic of Mozambique.

Mather D., C. Donovan, and T. Jayne. 2005. "Using Empirical Information in the Era of HIV/AIDS to Inform Mitigation and Rural Development Strategies: Selected Results from African Country Studies." *American Journal of Agricultural Economics* 87(5): 1289–97.

Mather, D., C. Donovan, T. S. Jayne, M. Weber, A. Chapoto, E. Mazhangara, L. Bailey, K. Yoo, T. Yamano, and E. Mghenyi. 2004. A Cross-Country Analysis of Household Responses to Adult Mortality in Rural Sub-Saharan Africa: Implications for HIV/AIDS Mitigation and Rural Development Policies. International Development Working Papers 82, Department of Agricultural Economics, Michigan State University.

Matovu, J. K., R. H. Gray, N. Kiwanuka, G. Kigozi, F. Wabwire-Mangen, F. Nalugoda, D. Serwadda, N. K. Sewankambo, and M. J. Wawer. 2007. "Repeat Voluntary HIV Counseling and Testing (VCT), Sexual Risk Behavior and HIV Incidence in Rakai, Uganda." *AIDS and Behavior* 11(1): 71–8.

Matovu, J. K., R. H. Gray, F. Makumbi, M. J. Wawer, D. Serwadda, G. Kigozi, N. K. Sewankambo, and F. Nalugoda. 2005. "Voluntary HIV Counseling and Testing Acceptance, Sexual Risk Behavior and HIV Incidence in Rakai, Uganda." *AIDS* 19(5): 503–11.

Matovu, J. K., G. Kigozi, F. Nalugoda, F. Wabwire-Mangen, and R. H. Gray. 2002. "The Rakai Project Counselling Programme Experience." *Tropical Medicine and International Health* 7(12): 1064–7.

Maxwell, D., K. Sadler, A. Sim, M. Mutonyi, and R. Egan, and M. Webster. 2008. Emergency Food Security Interventions. Humanitarian Practice Network Paper Number 10, Overseas Development Institute, London.

McCarthy, O., and A. M. Over. 2009. Projecting the Future Budgetary Cost of AIDS Treatment (Manual, Software Package, and Dataset). 6-5-2009.

McCoy, S. I., F. F. Fikree, and N. S. Padian. 2009. What Will it Take to Prevent HIV? Constructing an Effective Prevention Program Disease Control Priorities Project. Available at: http://www.dcp2.org/file/240/dcpp-twphiv_web.pdf

McCoy, S. I., J. Kuruc, C. Gay, C. Hurt, J. Anderson, C. Pilcher, J. Barnhart, J. Eron, and P. Leone; the North Carolina STAT Team. 2008. Partner Counseling and Referral Outcomes after Acute HIV Identification in North Carolina. 15th Conference on Retroviruses and Opportunistic Infections, Boston, February 3–6, 2008.

McDermott, A. Y., A. Shevitz, T. Knox, R. Roubenoff, J. Kehayias, and S. Gorbach. 2001. "Effect of Highly Active Antiretroviral Therapy on Fat, Lean, and Bone Mass in HIV-Seropositive Men and Women." *American Journal of Clinical Nutrition* 74(5): 679–86.

McDonald, S., and J. Roberts. 2006. "AIDS and Economic Growth: A Human Capital Approach." *Journal of Development Economics* 80(1): 228–50.

McGough, L., S. Reynolds, C. Quinn, and M. Zenilman. 2005. "Which Patient First? Setting Priorities for Antiretroviral Therapy Where Resources Are Limited." *American Journal of Public Health* 95(7): 1173–80.

Medlin, C., and D. de Walque. 2008. Potential Applications of Conditional Cash Transfers for Prevention of Sexually Transmitted Infections and HIV in Sub-Saharan Africa. Policy Research Working Paper 4673, World Bank, Washington, DC.

Mehta, S., and W. Fawzi. 2007. "Effects of Vitamins, Including Vitamin A, on HIV/AIDS Patients." *Vitamins and Hormones* 75: 355–83.

Mekonnen, Y., E. Sanders, M. Aklilu, A. Tsegaye, T. F. Rinke de Wit, A. Schaap, D. Wolday, R. Geskus, R. A. Coutinho, and A. L. Fontanet. 2003. "Evidence of Changes in Sexual Behaviours among Male Factory Workers in Ethiopia." *AIDS* 17(2): 223–31.

Mensch, B. S., P. C. Hewett, R. Gregory, and S. Helleringer. 2008. "Sexual Behavior and STI/HIV Status among Adolescents in Rural Malawi: An Evaluation of the Effect of Interview Mode on Reporting." *Studies in Family Planning* 39(4): 321–34.

Merson, M., J. M. Dayton, and K. O'Reilly. 2000. "Effectiveness of HIV Prevention Interventions in Developing Countries." *AIDS* 14(Suppl. 2): S68–84.

Merson, M., N. Padian, T. J. Coates, G. R. Gupta, S. M. Bertozzi, P. Piot, P. Mane, and M. Bartos; Lancet HIV Prevention Series Authors. 2008. "Combination HIV Prevention." *Lancet* 372(9652): 1805–6.

Michelo, C., I. F. Sandøy, and K. Fylkesnes. 2006. "Marked HIV Prevalence Declines in Higher Educated Young People: Evidence from Population-based Surveys (1995–2003) in Zambia." *AIDS* 20(7): 1031–8.

Minnis, A. M., M. J. Steiner, M. F. Gallo, L. Warner, M. H. Hobbs, A. van der Straten, T. Chipato, M. Macaluso, and N. S. Padian. 2009. "Biomarker Validation of Reports of Recent Sexual Activity: Results of a Randomized Controlled Study in Zimbabwe." *American Journal of Epidemiology* 170(70): 918–24.

Mishra, V., S. B-V. Assche, R. Greener, M. Vaessen, R. Hong, P. D. Ghys, J. T. Boerma, A. Van Assche, S. Khan, and S. Rutstein. 2007a. "HIV Infection Does Not Disproportionately Affect the Poorer in Sub-Saharan Africa." *AIDS* 21(Suppl. 7): S17–28. Available at: http://www.aidsonline.com/pt/re/aids/abstract.00002030-200711007-00003.htm; jsessionid=LvZQn7v517bKnh1ZGjBp7Vf4LrqXTNc35BFL3R4GJ5XtW5dgYym1!542 054210!181195628!8091!-1

Mishra, V., S. Bignami, R. Greener, M. Vaessen, R. Hong, P. Ghys, T. Boerma, A. Van Assche, S. Khan, and S. Rutstein. 2007b. A Study of the Association of HIV Infection with Wealth in Sub-Saharan Africa. DHS Working Paper 31, Macro International, Calverton, MD.

Mkolokosa, M. 2004. "Women, Girls and HIV/Aids: Making Interventions to Stop the Scourge." *The Nation* (Malawi), World Aids Day, Supplement, December 1, 2004, 1.

Moatti, J. P., I. N'Doye, S. M. Hammer, P. Hale, and M. D. Kazatchkine. 2002. Antiretroviral Treatment for HIV-infected Adults and Children in Developing Countries: Some Evidence in Favor of Expanded Diffusion. In *State of the Art: AIDS and Economics*, ed. S. Forsythe, 96–117. International AIDS-Economics Network (IAEN). Available at: http://www.policyproject.com/pubs/other/SOTAecon.pdf

Mogae, F. 2008. Interview at XVII International AIDS Conference, Mexico City. Available at: http://www.kaisernetwork.org/health_cast/uploaded_files/080508_ias_interview _mogae_transcript.pdf

Mohammed, I., S. Dadabhai, C. Omolo, T. Galgalo, T. Oluoch, G. Kichamu, R. Bunnell, P. Muriithi, J. Mermin, and R. Kaiser. 2009. HIV Prevalence and Unmet Need for HIV Testing, Care and Treatment in Kenya: Results of a Nationally Representative Survey. 16th Conference on Retroviruses and Opportunistic Infections, Montreal, February 8–11, 2009.

Montana, L. S., V. Mishra, and R. Hong. 2008. "Comparison of HIV Prevalence Estimates from Antenatal Care Surveillance and Population-based Surveys in Sub-Saharan Africa." *Sexually Transmitted Infections* 84: 178–84.

Moore, D., C. Yiannoutsos, B. Musick, R. Downing, W. Were, R. Degerman, L. Alexander, and J. Mermin. 2007. "Determinants of Mortality among HIV-infected Individuals Receiving Home-based ART in Rural Uganda [abstract 34]. In *Program and Abstracts of the 14th Conference on Retroviruses and Opportunistic Infections*, Los Angeles, CA, February 25–28, 2007.

Moore, H. L., and T. Sanders. 2006. *Anthropology in Theory: Issues in Epistemology.* Oxford: Blackwell Publishing.

Moore, S. F. 1994. *Anthropology and Africa: Changing Perspectives on a Changing Scene*. Charlottesville, Virginia: University of Virginia Press.

Morgan, D., C. Mahe, B. Mayanja, J. M. Okongo, R. Lubega, and J. A. Whitworth. 2002. "HIV-1 Infection in Rural Africa: Is There a Difference in Median Time to AIDS and Survival Compared with that in Industrialized Countries?" *AIDS* 16(4): 597–603.

Morris, C. N., D. R. Burdge, and E. J. Cheevers. 2001. "Economic Impact of HIV Infection in a Cohort of Male Sugar Mill Workers in South Africa." *South African Journal of Economics* 68(5): 933–46.

Morris, M., and M. Kretzschmar. 1997. "Concurrent Partnerships and the Spread of HIV." *AIDS* 11(5): 641–8.

Moss, G. B., D. Clemetson, L. D'Costa, F. A. Plummer, J. O. Ndinya-Achola, M. Reilly, K. K. Holmes, P. Piot, G. M. Maitha, S. L. Hillier, N. C. Kiviat, C. W. Cameron, I. A. Wamola, and J. K. Kreiss. 1991. "Association of Cervical Ectopy with Heterosexual Transmission of Human Immunodeficiency Virus: Results of a Study of Couples in Nairobi, Kenya." *Journal of Infectious Diseases* 164(3): 588–91.

Moss, G. B., J. Overbaugh, M. Welch, M. Reilly, J. Bwayo, F. A. Plummer, J. O. Ndinya-Achola, M. A. Malisa, and J. K. Kreiss 1995. "Human Immunodeficiency Virus DNA in Urethral Secretions in Men: Association with Gonococcal Urethritis and CD4 Cell Depletion." *Journal of Infectious Diseases* 172(6): 1469–74.

Mostad, S. B., J. Overbaugh, D. M. DeVange, M. J. Welch, B. Chohan, K. Mandaliya, P. Nyange, H. L. Martin, Jr., J. Ndinya-Achola, J. J. Bwayo, and J. K. Kreiss. 1997. "Hormonal Contraception, Vitamin A Deficiency, and Other Risk Factors for Shedding of HIV-1 Infected Cells from the Cervix and Vagina." *Lancet* 350(9082): 922–7.

Muirhead, D., L. Kumaranayake, C. Hongoro, S. Charalambous, A. Grant, K. Fielding, and G. Churchyard. 2006. Health Care Costs, Savings and Productivity Benefits Resulting from a Large Employer Sponsored ART Program in South Africa. In 16th International AIDS Conference, Toronto, August 13–18, 2006.

Murphy, E. M., M. E. Greene, A. Mihailovic, and P. Olupot-Olupot. 2006. "Was the "ABC" Approach (Abstinence, Being Faithful, Using Condoms) Responsible for Uganda's Decline in HIV?" *PLoS Medicine* 3(9): e379.

Murphy, L. L., P. Harvey, and E. Silvestre. 2005. "How Do We Know What We Know about the Impact of AIDS on Food and Livelihood Insecurity? A Review of Empirical Research from Rural Sub Saharan Africa." *Human Organization* 64(3): 265–75.

Mushati, P., G. M. Mlilo, J. Lewis, and C. Zvidzai. 2003. Adult Mortality and Economic Sustainability of Households in Towns, Estates, and Villages in AIDS-affected Eastern Zimbabwe. Paper presented at the Scientific Meeting on Empirical Evidence for the Demographic and Socio-Economic Impact of AIDS, Durban, South Africa, University of Durban, March 26–28, 2003.

Mutangadura, G. B. 2004. Women and Land Tenure Rights in Southern Africa: A Human Rights-based Approach. A paper presented to the Land in Africa: Market Asset, or Secure Livelihood? Westminster, London, November 8–9, 2004. Available at: http://www.iied.org/pubs/pdfs/G00173.pdf

Mutangadura, G. B., and D. Webb. 1999. "Socio-Economic Impact of Adult Mortality and Morbidity on Urban Households in Zambia." *AIDS Analysis Africa* 9(4): Dec. 98/Jan. 99.

Myer, L., C. Mathews, F. Little, and S. S. Abdool Karim. 2001. "The Fate of Free Male Condoms Distributed to the Public in South Africa." *AIDS* 15(6): 789–93.

Naidu, V., and G. Harris. 2005. "The Impact of HIV/AIDS Morbidity and Mortality on Households – a Review of Household Studies." *South African Journal of Economics* 73(s1): 533–44.

Ndekha, M. J., J. J. G. van Oosterhout, E. E. Zijlstra, M. Manary, H. Saloojee, and M. J. Manary. 2009. "Supplementary Feeding with Either Ready-to-Use Fortified Spread or Corn-Soy Blend in Wasted Adults Starting Antiretroviral Therapy in Malawi: Randomised, Investigator Blinded, Controlled Trial." *BMJ* 338: b1867.

Newell, M.-L., H. Coovadia, M. Cortina-Borja, N. Rollins, P. Gaillard, and F. Dabis; Ghent International AIDS Society (IAS) Working Group on HIV Infection in Women and Children. 2004. "Mortality of Infected and Uninfected Infants Born to HIV-infected Mothers in Africa: A Pooled Analysis." *Lancet* 364(9441): 1236–43.

Ngom, P., and S. Clark. 2003. Adult Mortality in the Era of HIV/AIDS: Sub Saharan Africa. Workshop on HIV/AIDS and Adult Mortality in Developing Countries, Population Division, Dept. of Economic and Social Affairs, United Nations Secretariat, New York, September 8–13, 2003.

NIAID (National Institute of Allergy and Infectious Diseases). 2009. Anti-HIV Gel Shows Promise in Large-scale Study in Women. February 9, 2009. Available at: http://www3.niaid.nih.gov/news/newsreleases/2009/HPTN_035_gel.htm

NIC (National Intelligence Council). 2000. The Global Infectious Disease Threat and Its Implications for the United States. NIE 99-17D, January, Washington, DC.

———. 2002. The Next Wave of HIV/AIDS: Nigeria, Ethiopia, Russia, India and China. ICA 2002-04D, September, Washington, DC.

———. 2008. Strategic Implications of Global Health. ICA 2008-10 D, December, Washington, DC.

Ntonya, G. 2005. "Aids Fight Calling for Innovations." *The Nation* (Malawi), April 20, 2005, 19.

Ntozi, J. P. M. 1997. "Widowhood, Remarriage and Migration during the HIV/AIDS Epidemic in Uganda." *Health Transition Review* 7(Suppl.): 125–144.

Nyamukapa, C., and S. Gregson. 2005. "Extended Family's and Women's Roles in Safeguarding Orphans' Education in AIDS-afflicted Rural Zimbabwe." *Social Science and Medicine* 60(10): 2155–67.

Nyblade, L., R. Gray, F. Makumbi, T. Lutalo, J. Menken, M. Wawer, N. Sewankambo, and D. Serwadda. 2000. HIV Risk Characteristics and Participation in Voluntary Counseling and Testing in Rural Rakai District, Uganda. Paper presented at the 13th International Conference on HIV/AIDS, Durban, South Africa, July 9–14, 2000.

Obare, F., P. Fleming, P. Anglewicz, R. Thornton, F. Martinson, A. Kapatuka, M. Poulin, S. Watkins, and H.-P. Kohler. 2009. "Acceptance of Repeat Population-based Voluntary Counseling and Testing for HIV and the Socio-Demographic Variations in HIV Incidence in Rural Malawi." *Sexually Transmitted Infections* 85(2): 139–44.

Obimbo, E. M., D. A. Mbori-Ngacha, J. O. Ochieng, B. A. Richardson, P. A. Otieno, R. Bosire, C. Farquhar, J. Overbaugh, and G. C. John-Stewart. 2004. "Predictors of Early Mortality in a Cohort of Human Immunodeficiency Virus Type 1-infected African Children." *Pediatric Infectious Disease Journal* 23(6): 536–43.

OECD (Organisation for Economic Co-operation and Development) (1). International Development Statistics (IDS) online, DAC online, CRS online. Available at: http:/www.oecd.org/dataoecd/50/17/5037721.htm

——— (2). Focus on Aid in Support of HIV/AIDS Control. Available at: http://www.oecd.org/document/34/0,3343,en_2649_34447_32124066_1_1_1,00.html

——— (3). HIV/AIDS Aid Activities online database. Available at: http://www.oecd.org/dataoecd/3/56/36252360.pdf

——— (4). Creditor Reporting System 2007: Aid Activities in Support of HIV/AIDS Control, 2000–2007. Available at: http://www.oecd.org/document/36/0,3343,en_2649_34447_39967140_1_1_1,00.html

OECD (Organisation for Economic Co-operation and Development). 2007. Table 1: Net Official Development Assistance in 2006, Preliminary Data for 2006. 4-3-2007. Available at: http://www.oecd.org/dataoecd/14/5/38354517.pdf

———. 2008. Survey on Monitoring the Paris Declaration: Making Aid More Effective By 2010. Available at: http://www.oecd.org/dataoecd/58/41/41202121.pdf

O'Farrell, N. 2001. "Enhanced Efficiency of Female to Male Transmission in Core Groups in Developing Countries: The Need to Target Men." *Sexually Transmitted Diseases* 28(2): 84–91.

Office of Mission Support, Department of Peacekeeping Operations (DPKO). 2004. HIV Testing Policy for Uniformed Peacekeepers [Online]. Available at: http://www.un.org/Depts/dpko/medical/pdfs/441dpkohiv.pdf

OGAC (Office of the U. S. Global AIDS Coordinator). 2004. *The President's Emergency Plan for AIDS Relief: U.S. Five Year Global HIV/AIDS Strategy.* Washington, DC: Office of the United States Global AIDS Coordinator.

———. 2007. *PEPFAR Third Annual Report to Congress.* Washington, DC: Office of the United States Global AIDS Coordinator.

———. 2008. *The Power of Partnerships: The U.S. President's Emergency Plan for AIDS Relief. Fourth Annual Report to Congress on PEPFAR.* Washington, DC: Office of the United States Global AIDS Coordinator.

O'Keeffe, M. 2008. State Fragility and AIDS in the South Pacific. ASCI Research Report No. 9. Available at: http://asci.researchhub.ssrc.org/state-fragility-and-aids-in-the-south-pacific/attachment

Olupot-Olupot, P., A. Katawera, C. Cooper, W. Small, A. Anema, and E. Mills. 2008. Adherence to Antiretroviral Therapy among a Conflict-affected Population in Northeastern Uganda: A Qualitative Study. *AIDS* 22(14): 1882–4.

Oomman, N., M. Bernstein, and S. Rosenzweig. 2007a. Following the Funding for HIV/AIDS. Center for Global Development, Washington, DC.

———. 2007b. What is the Effect of Funding Restrictions (i.e. "Earmarks") on PEPFAR Funding for Prevention, Treatment and Care? Center for Global Development, Washington, DC.

Oster, E. 2005. "Sexually Transmitted Infections, Sexual Behavior, and the HIV/AIDS Epidemic." *The Quarterly Journal of Economics* 120(2): 467–515.

———. 2009. HIV and Sexual Behavior Change: Why Not Africa? Mimeo.

Over, M. 1992. The Macroeconomic Impact of HIV/AIDS in Sub-Saharan Africa. AFTPN Technical Working Paper 3, Population, Health, and Nutrition Division, Africa Technical Department, World Bank, Washington, DC.

———.1998. The Effects of Societal Variables on Urban Rates of HIV Infection in Developing Countries. In Confronting AIDS Evidence from the Developing World: Selected Background Papers for the World Bank Policy Research Report, *Confronting AIDS: Public Priorities in a Global Epidemic,* ed. M. Ainsworth, L. Fransen, and M. Over, 39–52. Brussels, Belgium: European Commission.

———. 1999. The Public Interest in a Private Disease: Why Should the Government Play a Role in STD Control? In *Sexually Transmitted Diseases,* ed. K. K. Holmes, P. F. Sparling, P.-A. Mårdh, S. M. Lemon, W. E. Stamm, P. Piot, and J. N. Wasserheit, 3–14. New York: McGraw-Hill.

———. 2004. Impact of the HIV/AIDS Epidemic on the Health Sectors of Developing Countries. In *The Macroeconomics of HIV/AIDS,* ed. M. Haacker, 311–44. Washington, DC: International Monetary Fund.

———. 2010. Prevention Failure: The Ballooning Entitlement Burden of U.S. Global AIDS Treatment Spending and What to Do About It. In *The Socioeconomic Dimensions of*

*HIV/AIDS in Africa: Challenges, Opportunities and Misconceptions*, ed. D. E. Sahn, Chapter 8. Ithaca, NY: Cornell University Press.

Over, M., P. Heywood, E. Marseille, I. Gupta, S. Hira, N. Nagelkerke, and A. S. Rao. 2004. *HIV/AIDS Treatment and Prevention in India: Modeling the Costs and Consequences.* Washington, DC: World Bank.

Over, M., E. Marseille, K. Sudhakar, J. Gold, I. Gupta, A. Indrayan, S. Hira, N. Nagelkerke, A. S. Rao , and P. Heywood. 2006. "Antiretroviral Therapy and HIV Prevention in India: Modeling Costs and Consequences of Policy Options." *Sexually Transmitted Diseases* 33(Suppl. 10): S145–52.

Over, M., and P. Piot. 1993. HIV Infection and Sexually Transmitted Diseases. In *Disease Control Priorities in Developing Countries*, ed. D. T. Jamison, W. H. Mosley, A. R. Measham, and J. L. Bobadilla, 455–527. New York: Oxford University Press.

Over, M., A. Revenga, E. Masaki, W. Peerapatanapokin, J. Gold, V. Tangcharoensathien, and S. Thanprasertsuk. 2007. "The Economics of Effective AIDS Treatment in Thailand." *AIDS* 21 (Suppl. 4): S105–16.

Pacht, E. R., P. Diaz, T. Clanton, J. Hart, and J. E. Gadek. 1997. "Serum Vitamin E Decreases in HIV-Seropositive Subjects over Time." *Journal of Laboratory and Clinical Medicine* 130(3): 293–6.

Padian, N. S., T. R. O'Brien, Y. Chang, S. Glass, and D. P. Franci. 1993. "Prevention of Heterosexual Transmission of Human Immunodeficiency Virus through Couple Counseling." *Journal of Acquired Immune Deficiency Syndromes* 6(9): 1043–8.

Palella, F. J., K. M. Delaney, A. C. Moorman, M. O. Loveless, J. Fuhrer, G. A. Satten, D. J. Aschman, and S. D. Holmberg. 1998. "Declining Morbidity and Mortality among Patients with Advanced Human Immunodeficiency Virus Infection." *New England Journal of Medicine* 338(13): 853–60.

Palombi, L., M. Marazzi, A. Voetberg, and N. A. Magid. 2007. "Treatment Acceleration Program and the Experience of the DREAM Program in Prevention of Mother-to-Child Transmission of HIV." *AIDS* 21(Suppl. 4): S65–71.

Papageorgiou, C., and P. Stoytcheva. 2009. What Is the Impact of AIDS on Cross-Country Income So Far? A Macro Perspective. Unpublished draft, July 2009.

Parikh, A., M. B. DeSilva, M. Cakwe, T. Quinlan, J. L. Simon, A. Skalicky, and T. Ahuwau. 2007. "Exploring the Cinderella Myth: Intrahousehold Differences in Child Well-being between Orphans and Non-Orphans in Amajuba District, South Africa." *AIDS* 21(Suppl. 7): S95–103.

Paxton, N. 2009. Rapid Politico-Economic Transitions and HIV/AIDS: An Exploratory Analysis. aids2031, New York.

Pearson, M. 2008. Assessing the Implications of Vertical Financing for Health. Unpublished. DFID Health Resource Centre, London.

———. 2009. Achieving the MDGs: At What Cost? HLSP Institute, London. http://www.hlspinstitute.org/projects/?mode=type&id=247091

Pearson, M., K. Buse, and S. Pun. 2008. Global Health Partnerships and Health Systems Strengthening in Cambodia. Summary Briefing Paper, DFID Health Resource Centre, London.

Pearson, M., K. Buse, S. Pun, and C. Dickinson. 2009. Global Health Partnerships and Country Health Systems: The Case of Cambodia. HLSP Institute, London, July 2009. Available at: http://www.hlspinstitute.org/files/project/269109/CambodiaGHPs_July09.pdf

Pedraza, M. A., J. del Romero, F. Roldán, S. García, M. C. Ayerbe, A. R. Noriega, and J. Alcamí. 1999. "Heterosexual Transmission of HIV-1 Is Associated with High Plasma Viral Load Levels and a Positive Viral Isolation in the Infected Partner." *Journal of Acquired Immune Deficiency Syndromes* 21(2): 120–5.

Perez, F., T. Mukotekwa, A. Miller, J. Orne-Gliemann, M. Glenshaw, I. Chitsike, and F. Dabis. 2004. "Implementing a Rural Programme of Prevention of Mother-to-Child transmission of HIV in Zimbabwe: First 18 Months of Experience." *Tropical Medicine and International Health* 9(7): 774–83.

Perez, F., C. Zvandaziva, B. Engelsmann, and F. Dabis. 2006. "Acceptability of Routine HIV Testing ("Opt-out") in Antenatal Services in Two Rural Districts of Zimbabwe." *Journal of Acquired Immune Deficiency Syndromes* 41(4): 514–20.

Peters, P. E., P. Walker, and D. Kambewa. 2008. "Striving for Normality in a Time of AIDS in Malawi." *Journal of Modern African Studies* 46(4): 659–87.

Pettifor, A. E., H. V. Rees, I. Kleinschmidt, A. E. Steffenson, C. MacPhail, L. Hlongwa-Madikizela, K. Vermaak, and N. S. Padian. 2005. "Young People's Sexual Health in South Africa: HIV Prevalence and Sexual Behaviors from a Nationally Representative Household Survey." *AIDS* 19(14): 1525–34.

Philipson, T. J., and R. A. Posner. 1993. *Private Choices and Public Health: The AIDS Epidemic in an Economic Perspective.* Cambridge, MA: Harvard University Press.

Pilcher, C. D., J. J. Eron, Jr., S. Galvin, C. Gay, and M. S. Cohen. 2004a. "Acute HIV Revisited: New Opportunities for Treatment and Prevention." *Journal of Clinical Investigation* 113(7): 937–45.

Pilcher, C. D., E. Foust, R. Ashby, J. Kuruc, T. Nguyen, L. Hightow, N. Harrison, S. McCoy, D. Williams, and P. Leone. 2006. Sexual Transmission Risk and Rapid Public Health Intervention in Acute HIV Infection. 13th Conference on Retroviruses and Opportunistic Infections, Denver, February 5–8, 2006.

Pilcher, C. D., G. Joaki, I. F. Hoffman, F. E. Martinson, C. Mapanje, P. W. Stewart, K. A. Powers, S. Galvin, D. Chilongozi, S. Gama, M. A. Price, S. A. Fiscus, and M. S. Cohen. 2007. "Amplified Transmission of HIV-1: Comparison of HIV-1 Concentrations in Semen and Blood during Acute and Chronic Infection." *AIDS* 21(13): 1723–30.

Pilcher, C. D., H. C. Tien, J. J. Eron, Jr., P. L. Vernazza, S. Y. Leu, P. W. Stewart, L. E. Goh, and M. S. Cohen; Quest Study; Duke-UNC-Emory Acute HIV Consortium. 2004b. "Brief but Efficient: Acute HIV Infection and the Sexual Transmission of HIV." *Journal of Infectious Diseases* 189(10): 1785–92.

Piller, C., and D. Smith. 2007. "Unintended Victims of Gates Foundation Generosity." *Los Angeles Times*, December 16, 2007.

Piot, P. 2008. AIDS Exceptionalism Revisited. Lecture at the London School of Economics, May 15.

Piot, P., M. Bartos, H. Larson, D. Zewdie, and P. Mane. 2008. "Coming to Terms with Complexity: A Call to Action for HIV Prevention." *Lancet* 372(9641): 845–59.

Piot, P., R. Greener, and S. Russell. 2007. "Squaring the Circle: AIDS, Poverty, and Human Development." *PLoS Medicine* 4(10): 1571–5.

Pisani, E. 2008. *The Wisdom of Whores: Brothels, Bureaucrats and the Business of AIDS.* Cambridge: Granta.

Poku, N., and B. Sandkjaer. 2007. HIV/AIDS and the African State. In *AIDS and Governance*, eds. N. Poku, A. Whiteside, and B. Sandkjaer, 9–28. Aldershot: Ashgate.

Population Action International. 2008. U.S. HIV/AIDS and Family Planning/Reproductive Health Assistance: A Growing Disparity within PEPFAR Focus Countries. Available at: http://www.populationaction.org/Issues/U.S._Policies_and_Funding/FPRH/Summary.shtml

Potts, M., D. T. Halperin, D. Kirby, A. Swidler, E. Marseille, J. D. Klausner, N. Hearst, R. G. Wamai, J. G. Kahn, and J. Walsh. 2008. "Reassessing HIV Prevention." *Science* 320(5877): 749–50.

Poulin, M. 2006. "The Sexual and Social Relations of Youth in Rural Malawi: Strategies for AIDS Prevention." Ph.D. Dissertation, Boston College, Department of Sociology.

———. 2007. "Sex, Money and Premarital Relationships in Southern Malawi." *Social Science and Medicine* 65(11): 2383–93.

———. 2009. Social Networks and Sexual Activity among Unmarried Young Women: The Role of School Environment. Paper Presented at the Population Association of America Annual Meeting, Detroit, Michigan, May, 2009.

Powers, K. A., W. C. Miller, C. D. Pilcher, C. Mapanje, F. E. Martinson, S. A. Fiscus, D. A. Chilongozi, D. Namakhwa, M. A. Price, S. R. Galvin, I. F. Hoffman, and M. S. Cohen; Malawi UNC Project Acute HIV Study Team. 2007. "Improved Detection of Acute HIV-1 Infection in Sub-Saharan Africa: Development of a Risk Score Algorithm." *AIDS* 21(16): 2237–42.

Prazuck, T., A. Lafeuillade, L. Hocqueloux, J.-P. Viard, V. Avettand-Fènoël, and C. Rouzioux. 2008. Can HAART Initiation at Early Acute HIV Infection Benefit the Immune-virology Outcome Despite Subsequent Treatment Cessation? The ANRS Reservoirs' Study Group. 15th Conference on Retroviruses and Opportunistic Infection, Boston, February 3–6, 2008.

Prestage, G., F. Jin, I. B. Zablotska, J. Imrie, A. E. Grulich, and M. Pitts. 2008. "Trends in HIV Testing among Homosexual and Bisexual Men in Eastern Australian States." *Sexual Health* 5(2): 119–23.

Price, J., E. Micomyiza, V. Nyeimana, and P. Tchupo. 2007. Integrating HIV Clinical Services in Primary Health Centers in Rwanda. Available at: http://www.iom.edu/.

Price-Smith, A. 2002. *The Health of Nations: Infectious Disease, Environmental Change, and Their Effects on National Security and Development.* Cambridge, MA: MIT Press.

Project Concern International. 2009. Africa Forum: Sharing Integrated Solutions for HIV/AIDS & Food Insecurity. Available at: http://www.projectconcern.org/africa forum2009

Pronyk, P., J. R. Hargreaves, J. C. Kim, L. A. Morison, G. Phetla, C. Watts, J. Busza, and J. D. Porter. 2006. "Effect of a Structural Intervention for the Prevention of Intimate Partner Violence and HIV in Rural South Africa: Results of a Cluster Randomized Trial." *Lancet* 368(9551): 1973–83.

Pronyk, P., J. Kim, T. Abramsky, G. Phetla, J. R. Hargreaves, L. A. Morison, C. Watts, J. Busza, and J. D. Porter. 2008. "A Combined Microfinance and Training Intervention Can Reduce HIV Risk Behavior in Young Female Participants." *AIDS* 22(13): 1659–65.

Quinn, T. C., M. J. Wawer, N. Sewankambo, D. Serwadda, C. Li, F. Wabwire-Mangen, M. O. Meehan, T. Lutalo, and R. H. Gray. 2000. "Viral Load and Heterosexual Transmission of Human Immunodeficiency Virus Type 1." Rakai Project Study Group. *New England Journal of Medicine* 342(13): 921–9.

Radelet, S. 2003. *Challenging Foreign Aid: A Policymaker's Guide to the Millennium Challenge Account.* Washington, DC: Center for Global Development.

Rahman, A. 1999. *Women and Microcredit and Rural Bangladesh: An Anthropological Study of Grameen Bank Lending.* Boulder: Westview Press.

Ram, R., and T. Schultz. 1979. "Life-Span, Health, Savings, and Productivity." *Economic Development and Cultural Change* 27(3): 399–421.

Ramalingam, S., R. Kannangai, K. J. Prakash, M. V. Jesudason, and G. Sridharan. 2000. "Per-exposure Rate of Transmission of HIV-1, HIV-1/2, and HIV-2 from Women to Men May Be Higher in India." *Journal of Acquired Immune Deficiency Syndromes* 25(1): 97–8.

Rapid Responses to England, R. 2008. "The Writing is on the Wall for UNAIDS." *BMJ* 336: 1072. Available at: http://www.bmj.com/cgi/eletters/336/7652/1072#196337

Ravishankar, N., P. Gubbins, R. J. Cooley, K. Leach-Kemon, C. M. Michaud, D. T. Jamison, and C. J. Murray. 2009. "Financing of Global Health: Tracking Development Assistance for Health from 1990 to 2007." *Lancet* 373(9681): 2113–24.

Rawat, R., S. Kadiyala, and P. McNamara. 2010. "The Impact of Food Assistance on Weight Gain and Disease Progression among HIV-infected Individuals Accessing AIDS Care and Treatment Services in Uganda." *BMC Public Health* 10:316.

RCQHC (Regional Centre for Quality of Health Care) and FANTA/AED. 2008. Nutrition, Food Security and HIV: A Compendium of Promising Practices. Washington, DC.

Reardon, T., E. Crawford, and V. Kelly. 1995. Promoting Farm Investment for Sustainable Intensification of Agriculture. International Development Paper 18, Department of Agricultural Economics, Michigan State University, East Lansing, MI.

Reich, M. R., and K. Takemi. 2009. "G8 and Strengthening of Health Systems: Follow-up to the Toyako Summit." *Lancet* 373(9662): 508–15.

Reniers, G. 2003. "Divorce and Remarriage in Rural Malawi." *Demographic Research* Special Collection 1(Article 6): 175–206. Available at: http://www.demographic-research.org/special/1/6/

———. 2008. "Marital Strategies for Regulating Exposure to HIV." *Demography* 45(2): 417–38.

Reniers, G., and J. Eaton. 2009. "Refusal Bias in HIV Prevalence Estimates from Nationally Representative Seroprevalence Surveys." *AIDS* 23(5): 621–9.

Republic of Malawi and the World Bank. 2007. *Malawi Poverty and Vulnerability Assessment – Investing in Our Future.* Washington, DC: The World Bank.

Republic of Rwanda. Ministry of Finance and Economic Planning and Ministry of Health. 2006. Scaling up to Achieve the Health MDGs in Rwanda. Background Study for the High-Level Forum Meeting in Tunis, June 12–13, 2006. Available at: http://www.dev partners.gov.rw/docs/index.php?dir=Coordination+Structures%2FClusters%2F Health+Sector%2FPolicies+%26+Reports%2F&download=Scaling_Up_to_Achiev e_Health_MDGs.pdf

Revenga, A., M. Over, E. Masaki, W. Peerapatanapokin, J. Gold, V. Tangcharoensathien, and S. Thanprasertsuk. 2006. *The Economics of Effective AIDS Treatment: Evaluating Policy Options for Thailand.* Washington, DC: World Bank.

Reynolds, H. W., B. Janowitz, R. Homan, and L. Johnson. 2006. "The Value of Contraception to Prevent Perinatal HIV Transmission." *Sexually Transmitted Diseases* 33(6): 350–6.

Reynolds, H. W., M. J. Steiner, and W. Cates. 2005. "Contraception's Proved Potential to Fight HIV." *Sexually Transmitted Infections* 81(2): 184–5.

Reynolds, S., F. Makumbi, J. Kagaayi, G. Nakigozi, R. Galiwongo, T. Quinn, M. Wawer, R. Gray, and D. Serwadda. 2009. ART Reduced the Rate of Sexual Transmission of HIV among HIV-Discordant Couples in Rural Rakai, Uganda. 16th Conference on Retroviruses and Opportunistic Infections, Montreal, February 8–11, 2009.

Robalino, D. A., A. Voetberg, and O. Picazo. 2002. "The Macroeconomic Impacts of AIDS in Kenya Estimating Optimal Reduction Targets for the HIV/AIDS Incidence Rate." *Journal of Policy Modeling* 24(2): 195–218.

Robinson, J., and E. Yeh. 2009. Transactional Sex as a Response to Risk in Western Kenya. MPRA Paper 7350, University Library of Munich, Germany.

Rohde, J., S. Cousens, M. Chopra, V. Tangcharoensathien, R. Black, Z. A. Bhutta, and J. E. Lawn. 2008. "30 years after Alma-Ata: Has Primary Health Care Worked in Countries?" *Lancet* 372(9642): 50–61.

Rohter, L. 2005. "Prostitution Puts U.S. and Brazil at Odds on AIDS Policy." *New York Times,* July 24, 2005.

Rosen, S., F. Feeley, P. Connelly, and J. Simon. 2006. The Private Sector and HIV/AIDS in Africa: Taking Stock of Six Years of Applied Research. Health and Development Discussion Paper No. 7, Center for International Health and Development, Boston University School of Public Health.

———. 2007a. "The Private Sector and HIV/AIDS in Africa: Taking Stock of 6 years of Applied Research." *AIDS* 21(Suppl. 3): S41–51.

Rosen, S., M. P. Fox, and C. J. Gill. 2007b. "Patient Retention in Antiretroviral Therapy Programs in Sub-Saharan Africa: A Systematic Review." *PLoS Medicine* 4(10): e298.

Rosen, S., P. Hamazakaza, F. Feeley, and M. Fox. 2007c. "The Impact of AIDS on Government Service Delivery: The Case of the Zambia Wildlife Authority." *AIDS* 21(Suppl. 3): S53–9.

Rosen, S., M. Ketlhapile, I. Sanne, and M. B. DeSilva. 2007d. "Cost to Patients of Obtaining Treatment for HIV/AIDS in South Africa." *South African Medical Journal* 97(7): 524–9.

———. 2008a. "Characteristics of Patients Accessing Care and Treatment for HIV/AIDS at Public and Nongovernmental Sites in South Africa." *Journal of the International Association of Physicians in AIDS Care* 7 (4): 200–7.

———. 2008b. "Differences in Normal Activities, Job Performance and Symptom Prevalence between Patients Not Yet on Antiretroviral Therapy and Patients Initiating Therapy in South Africa." *AIDS* 22(Suppl. 1): S131–9.

Rosen, S., I. Sanne, A. Collier, and J. L. Simon. 2005. "Rationing Antiretroviral Therapy for HIV/AIDS in Africa: Choices and Consequences." *PLoS Medicine* 2(11): 1098–104.

Rosen, S., J. R. Vincent, W. MacLeod, M. Fox, D. M. Thea, and J. L. Simon. 2004. "The Cost of HIV/AIDS to Businesses in Southern Africa." *AIDS* 18(2): 317–24.

Rosenzweig, M. R. 1988. "Risk, Implicit Contracts and the Family in Rural Areas of Low-income Countries." *Economic Journal* 98(393): 1148–70.

Ross, D. A., J. Changalucha, A. I. N. Obasi, J. Todd, M. L. Plummer, B. Cleophas-Mazige, A. Anemona, D. Everett, H. A. Weiss, D. C. Maybey, H. Grosskurth, and R. J. Hayes. 2007. "Biological and Behavioural Impact of an Adolescent Sexual Health Intervention in Tanzania: A Community Randomized Trial." *AIDS* 21(14): 1943–55.

Roth, D. L., K. E. Stewart, O. J. Clay, A. van der Straten, E. Karita, and S. Allen. 2001. "Sexual Practices of HIV Discordant and Concordant Couples in Rwanda: Effects of a Testing and Counselling Programme for Men." *International Journal of STD and AIDS* 12(3): 181–8.

Rottingen, J.-A., D. Cameron, and G. P. Garnett. 2001. "A Systematic Review of the Epidemiologic Interactions between Classic Sexually Transmitted Diseases and HIV: How Much Is Really Known?" *Sexually Transmitted Diseases* 28(10): 579–97.

Rousseau, M. C., C. Molines, J. Moreau, and J. Delmont. 2000. "Influence of Highly Active Antiretroviral Therapy on Micronutrient Profiles in HIV-Infected Patients." *Annals of Nutrition and Metabolism* 44(5–6): 212–6.

Routy, J. P., N. Machouf, M. D. Edwardes, B. G. Brenner, R. Thomas, B. Trottier, D. Rouleau, C. L. Tremblay, P. Côté, J. G. Baril, R. S. Remis, R. P. Sékaly, and M. A. Wainberg. 2004. "Factors Associated with a Decrease in the Prevalence of Drug Resistance in Newly HIV-1 Infected Individuals in Montreal." *AIDS* 18(17): 2305–12.

Ruark, A., J. D. Shelton, D. T. Halperin, M. J. Wawer, and R. H. Gray. 2009. Correspondence on Granich, R. M. et al., "Universal Voluntary HIV Testing with Immediate Antiretroviral Therapy as a Strategy for Elimination of HIV Transmission: A Mathematical Model." *Lancet* 373(9669): 1078.

Rugalema, G. 1998. It Is Not Only the Loss of Labor: HIV/AIDS, Loss of Household Assets and Household Livelihood in Bukoba District, Tanzania. Paper Presented at the East and Southern Africa Regional Conference on Responding to HIV/AIDS: Development Needs of Africa Smallholder Agriculture, Harare, Zimbabwe, June 8–12, 1998.

Rupiya, M., ed. 2006. *The Enemy Within—Southern African Militaries' Quarter-Century Battle with HIV/AIDS*. Pretoria: Institute of Security Studies.

Rwanda (Institut National de la Statistique du Rwanda) and ORC Macro. 2006. *Rwanda Demographic and Health Survey 2005*. Calverton, Maryland.

SADC PF (Southern Africa Development Community Parliamentary Forum). 2006. Report of Expert Think Tank Meeting on HIV Prevention in High HIV Prevalence Countries in Southern Africa. Maseru, Lesotho, May 10–12, 2006. Gaborone, Botswana: SADC. Available at: http://data.unaids.org/pub/Report/2006/20060601_sadc_meeting_report_en.pdf

SADC PF (Southern Africa Development Community Parliamentary Forum). 2008. Report on the Forum for Members of Parliament with, Traditional Leaders and Civil Society; Towards a More Inclusive Political Culture and Effective HIV and AIDS Responses. May 19–21, 2008, Matsapha, Swaziland. Available at: http://www.sadccitizen.net/aids/new/downloads/Swaziland%20Workshop%20Evaluation%20Report.pdf

Sala-i-Martin, X. 2005. On the Health-Poverty Trap. In *Health and Economic Growth – Findings and Policy Implications*, ed. G. López-Casasnovas, B. Rivera, and L. Currais, 95–114. Cambridge MA and London: MIT Press.

Salinas, G., and M. Haacker. 2006. HIV/AIDS: The Impact on Poverty and Inequality. IMF Working Paper No. 06/126, International Monetary Fund, Washington, DC.

Santow, G., M. Bracher, and S. Watkins. 2008. Implications for Behavioural Change in Rural Malawi of Popular Understandings of the Epidemiology of AIDS. Paper presented at the International Union for the Scientific Study of Population (IUSSP) Seminar on Potential and Actual Contributions of Behavioural Change to Curbing the Spread of HIV, Entebbe, Uganda, February 18–20, 2008.

Schacker, T., J. Zeh, H. L. Hu, E. Hill, and L. Corey. 1998. "Frequency of Symptomatic and Asymptomatic Herpes Simplex Virus Type 2 Reactivations among Human Immunodeficiency Virus-infected Men." *Journal of Infectious Diseases* 178(6): 1616–22.

Schatz, E. 2005. "Take Your Mat and Go!: Rural Malawian Women's Strategies in the HIV/AIDS Era." *Culture, Health and Sexuality* 7(5): 479–92.

Schönteich, M. 2000. Age and AIDS: South Africa's Crime Time Bomb. Institute for Security Studies, Pretoria.

Schwenk, A., A. Beisenherz, G. Kremer, V. Diehl, B. Salzberger, and G. Fätkenheuer. 1999. "Bioelectrical Impedance Analysis in HIV-infected Patients Treated with Triple Antiretroviral Treatment." *Journal of Clinical Nutrition* 70(5): 867–73.

Scott, V. E., M. Chopra, L. Conrad, and A. Ntuli. 2005. "How Equitable is the Scaling Up of HIV Service Provision in South Africa?" *South African Medical Journal* 95(2): 109–13.

Scrimshaw, N. S., and J. P. SanGiovanni. 1997. "Synergism of Nutrition, Infection, and Immunity: An Overview." *American Journal of Clinical Nutrition* 66(2): 464S–77S.

Seckinelgin, H., J. Bigirumwami, and J. Morris. 2008. HIV/AIDS, Conflict and the Gendered Implications of Transition in Burundi. ASCI Research Report No. 13. Available at: http://asci.researchhub.ssrc.org/working-papers/No.%2013%20Seckinelgin%20Gender%20Burundi.pdf

Semba, R. D., N. Shah, R. S. Klein, K. H. Mayer, P. Schuman, L. I. Gardner, and D. Vlahov; HER (Human Immunodeficiency Virus Epidemiology Research) Study Group. 2001. "Highly Active Antiretroviral Therapy Associated with Improved Anemia among HIV-infected Women." *AIDS Patient Care and STDs* 15(9): 473–80.

Semba, R. D., N. Shah, R. S. Klein, K. H. Mayer, P. Schuman, and D. Vlahov; Human Immunodeficiency Virus Epidemiology Research Study Group. 2002. "Prevalence and Cumulative Incidence of and Risk Factors for Anemia in a Multicenter Cohort Study of Human Immunodeficiency Virus-Infected and -Uninfected Women." *Clinical Infectious Diseases* 34(2): 260–6.

Semba, R. D., and A. M. Tang. 1999. "Micronutrients and the Pathogenesis of Human Immunodeficiency Virus Infection." *British Journal of Nutrition* 81(3): 181–9.

Senefeld, S., and K. Polsky. 2006. Chronically Ill Households, Food Security, and Coping Strategies in Rural Zimbabwe. In *AIDS, Poverty, and Hunger: Challenges and Responses. Highlights of the International Conference on HIV/AIDS and Food and Nutrition Security, Durban, South Africa, April 14–16, 2005,* ed. S. Gillespie, 129–40. Washington, DC: International Food Policy Research Institute.

Shafer, L. A., S. Biraro, J. Nakiyingi-Miiro, A. Kamali, D. Ssematimba, J. Ouma, A. Ojwiya, P. Hughes, L. Van der Paal, J. Whitworth, A. Opio, and H. Grosskurth. 2008. "HIV Prevalence and Incidence Are No Longer Falling in Southwest Uganda: Evidence from a Rural Population Cohort 1989–2005." *AIDS* 22(13): 1641–9.

Shell, R. 2000. The Silent Revolution: HIV/AIDS and Military Bases in Sub-Saharan Africa. In *Consolidating Democracy,* 29–41. Seminar Report Series. East London: Konrad Adenauer Foundation.

Shelton, J. D., M. M. Cassell, and J. Adetunji. 2005. "Is Poverty or Wealth at the Root of HIV?" *Lancet* 366(9491): 1057–8.

Shelton, J. D., D. T. Halperin, V. Nantulya, M. Potts, H. D. Gayle, and K. K. Holmes, 2004. "Partner Reduction is Crucial for Balanced 'ABC' Approach to HIV Prevention." *BMJ* 328(7444): 891–3.

Shelton, J. D., D. T. Halperin, and D. Wilson. 2006. "Has Global HIV Incidence Peaked?" *Lancet* 367(9517): 1120–2.

Sheth, P., C. Kovacs, K. Kemal, B. Jones, C. Laporte, M. Loutfy, H. Burger, B. Weiser, R. Pilon, and R. Kaul; Toronto Mucosal HIV Research Group. 2009. Persistent HIV RNA Shedding in Semen despite Effective ART. 16th Conference on Retroviruses and Opportunistic Infections, Montreal, February 8–11, 2009.

Shezongo-Macmillan, J. 2005. Women's Property Rights in Zambia. Paper presented at the Strategic Litigation Workshop, Johannesburg, South Africa, August 14–18, 2005.

Shiffman, J. 2006. HIV/AIDS and the Rest of the Global Health Agenda. *Bulletin of the World Health Organization* 84(12): 923. Available at: http://www.who.int/bulletin/volumes/84/12/06-036681.pdf

Sigma Research. 2008. Multiple Chances: Findings from the United Kingdom Gay Men's Sex Survey 2006. London, Sigma Research.

Silva, M., P. R. Skolnik, S. L. Gorbach, D. Spiegelman, I. B. Wilson, M. G. Fernández-DiFranco, and T. A. Knox. 1998. "The Effect of Protease Inhibitors on Weight and Body Composition in HIV-infected Patients." *AIDS* 12(13): 1645–51.

Simelane, H., S. Kunene, and T. Magongo. 2006. HIV/AIDS in the Umbufto Swaziland Defence Force. In *The Enemy Within—Southern African Militaries' Quarter-Century Battle with HIV/AIDS,* ed. M. Rupiya, 65–90. Pretoria: Institute of Security Studies.

Singh, S., J. E. Darroch, and A. Bankole. 2003. ABC in Uganda: The role of Abstinence, Monogamy and Condom Use in HIV Decline. Occasional Report No. 9, The Allan Guttmacher Institute.

Singh, I., L. Squire, and J. Strauss, eds. 1986. *Agricultural Household Models: Extensions, Application and Policy.* Baltimore, MD: Johns Hopkins University Press.

Slutkin, G., S. Okware, W. Naamara, D. Sutherland, D. Flanagan, M. Caraël, E. Blas, P. Delay, and D. Tarantola. 2006. "How Uganda Reversed Its HIV Epidemic." *AIDS and Behavior* 10(4): 351–60.

Smith, C. 2008. Indigenous Welfare and HIV/AIDS Risks: The Impacts of Government Reform in the Papua Region, Indonesia. ASCI Research Report No. 12.

Smith, J., F. Nalagoda, M. J. Wawer, D. Serwadda, N. Sewankambo, J. Konde-Lule, T. Lutalo, C. Li, and R. H. Gray. 1999. "Education Attainment as a Predictor of HIV Risk in Rural Uganda: Results from a Population-based Study." *International Journal of STD and AIDS* 10(7): 452–9.

Smith, K. P., and S. C. Watkins. 2005. "Perceptions of Risk and Strategies for Prevention: Responses to HIV/AIDS in Rural Malawi." *Social Science and Medicine* 60(3): 649–60.

Soares, R. R. 2005. "Mortality Reductions, Educational Attainment, and Fertility Choice." *American Economic Review* 95(3): 580–601.

Spiegel, P. 2004. "HIV/AIDS among Conflict-affected and Displaced Populations: Dispelling Myths and Taking Action." *Disasters* 28(4): 322–39.

Spiegel, P., A. R. Bennedsen, J. Claass, L. Bruns, N. Patterson, D. Yiweza, and M. Schilperoord. 2007. "Prevalence of HIV Infection in Conflict-affected and Displaced People in Seven Sub-Saharan African Countries: A Systematic Review." *Lancet* 369(9580): 2187–95.

Stangl, A. L., N. Wamai, J. Mermin, A. C. Awor, and R. E. Bunnell. 2007. "Trends and Predictors of Quality of Life among HIV-infected Adults Taking Highly Active Antiretroviral Therapy in Rural Uganda." *AIDS Care* 19(5): 626–36.

Steinberg, M., S. Johnson, G. Schierhout, and D. Ndegwa. 2002. Hitting Home: How Households Cope with the Impact of the HIV/AIDS Epidemic. Publication No. 6059, Kaiser Family Foundation, Washington, DC. As cited in UNICEF (2004).

Steingrover, R., K. Pogány, E. Fernandez Garcia, S. Jurriaans, K. Brinkman, H. Schuitemaker, F. Miedema, J. M. Lange, and J. M. Prins. 2008. "HIV-1 Viral Rebound Dynamics after a Single Treatment Interruption Depends on Time of Initiation of Highly Active Antiretroviral Therapy." *AIDS* 22(13): 1583–8.

Stokes, C. S. 2003. Measuring Impacts of HIV/AIDS on Rural Livelihoods and Food Security. Sustainable Development Department (SD), FAO. Rome.

Stolte, I. G., N. H. Dukers, J. B. de Wit, J. S. Fennema, and R. A. Coutinho. 2001. "Increase in Sexually Transmitted Infections among Homosexual Men in Amsterdam in Relation to HAART." *Sexually Transmitted Infections* 77(3): 184–6.

Stoneburner, R., and D. Low-Beer. 2004. "Population-level HIV Declines and Behavioral Risk Avoidance in Uganda." *Science* 304(5671): 714–8.

Stover, J. 2004. "Projecting the Demographic Consequences of HIV Prevalence Trends: The Spectrum Projection." *Sexually Transmitted Infections* 80 (Suppl. 1): i14–8.

Stover, J., N. Fuchs, D. Halperin, A. Gibbons, and D. Gillespie. 2003. Adding Family Planning to PMTCT Sites Increases the Benefits of PMTCT. Available at: http://www.fhi.org/NR/rdonlyres/earf7d7i4up5roh7hrpbxekmx55tprl5t5bcqq3tf4kfpprm3oprt3j4i6ztqznwv5g3qthqjk7zfc/FPPMTCTissuebriefrev102203enrh.pdf.

Strauss, J. 1982. "Determinants of Food Consumption in Rural Sierra Leone: Application of the Quadratic Expenditure System to the Consumption-leisure Component of a Household-firm Model." *Journal of Development Economics* 11(3): 327–53.

Strauss, J., and D. Thomas. 1995. Human Resources: Empirical Modeling of Household and Family Decisions. In *Handbook of Development Economics* Vol. 3, Part 1, ed. J. Behrman and T.N. Srinivasan, 1883–2023. Amsterdam: Elsevier/North-Holland.

———. 1998. "Health, Nutrition, and Economic Development." *Journal of Economic Literature* 36(2): 766–817.

Stringer, J. S., L. Zulu, J. Levy, E. M. Stringer, A. Mwango, B. H. Chi, M. Mtonga, S. Reid, R. A. Cantrell, M. Bulterys, M. S. Saag, R. G. Marlink, A. Mwinga, T. V. Ellerbrock, and M. Sinkala. 2006. "Rapid Scale-up of Antiretroviral Therapy at Primary Care Sites in Zambia: Feasibility and Early Outcomes." *JAMA* 296(7): 782–93.

Suarez, T. P., J. A. Kelly, S. D. Pinkerton, Y. L. Stevenson, M. Hayat, M. D. Smith, and T. Ertl. 2001. "Influence of a Partner's HIV Serostatus, Use of Highly Active Antiretroviral Therapy, and Viral Load on Perceptions of Sexual Risk Behavior in a Community Sample of Men Who Have Sex with Men." *Journal of Acquired Immune Deficiency Syndromes* 28(5): 471–7.

Sudarshi, D., D. Pao, G. Murphy, J. Parry, G. Dean, and M. Fisher. 2008. "Missed Opportunities for Diagnosing Primary HIV Infection." *Sexually Transmitted Infections* 84(1): 14–6.

Sullivan, P., K. Kayitenkore, E. Chomba, E. Karita, L. Mwananyanda, C. Vwalika, M. Conkling, N. Luisi, A. Tichacek, and S. Allen. 2009. Reduction of HIV Transmission Risk and High Risk Sex While Prescribed ART: Results from Discordant Couples in Rwanda and Zambia. 16th Conference on Retroviruses and Opportunistic Infections, Montreal, February 8–11, 2009.

Suskind, R. 2006. *The One Percent Doctrine: Deep Inside America's Pursuit of Its Enemies Since 9/11*. New York: Simon and Schuster.

Susser, I., and Z. Stein. 2000. "Culture, Sexuality, and Women's Agency in the Prevention of HIV/AIDS in Southern Africa." *American Journal of Public Health* 90(7): 1042–8.

Suttmann, U., J. Ockenga, O. Selberg, L. Hoogestraat, H. Deicher, and M. J. Muller. 1995. "Incidence and Prognostic Value of Malnutrition and Wasting in Human Immunodeficiency Virus-infected Outpatients." *Journal of Acquired Immune Deficiency Syndromes and Human Retrovirology* 8(3): 239–46.

Sweat, M. D., K. R. O'Reilly, G. P. Schmid, J. Denisona, and I. de Zoysa. 2004. "Cost-effectiveness of Nevirapine to Prevent Mother-to-Child HIV Transmission in Eight African Countries." *AIDS* 18(12): 1661–71.

Swidler, A. 1986. "Culture in Action: Symbols and Strategies." *American Sociological Review* 51(2): 273–86.

Swidler, A., and S. C. Watkins. 2007. "Ties of Dependence: AIDS and Transactional Sex in Rural Malawi." *Studies in Family Planning* 38(3): 147–62.

Tang, A. M. 2003. "Weight Loss, Wasting, and Survival in HIV-Positive Patients: Current Strategies." *AIDS Reader* 13(Suppl. 12): S23–7.

Tang, A. M., N. M. Graham, A. J. Kirby, L. D. McCall, W. C. Willett, and A. J. Saah. 1993. "Dietary Micronutrient Intake and Risk of Progression to Acquired Immunodeficiency Syndrome (AIDS) in Human Immunodeficiency Virus Type 1 (HIV-1)–infected Homosexual Men." *American Journal of Epidemiology* 138(11): 937–51.

Tang, A. M., N. M. Graham, and A. J. Saah. 1996. "Effects of Micronutrient Intake on Survival in Human Immunodeficiency Virus Type 1 Infection." *American Journal of Epidemiology* 143(12): 1244–56.

Tang, A. M., N. M. Graham, R. D. Semba, and A. J. Saah. 1997. "Association between Serum Vitamin A and E Levels and HIV-1 Disease Progression." *AIDS* 11(5): 613–20.

Taskforce for Innovative International Financing for Health Systems. 2009. Working Group 1: Constraints and Costs. First Report to Taskforce, March 13, 2009. Available at: http://www.internationalhealthpartnership.net//CMS_files/documents/working _group_1_-_report_EN.pdf

Tavory, I., and A. Swidler. 2009. "Condom Semiotics: Meaning and Condom Use in Rural Malawi." *American Sociological Review* 74(2): 171–89.

Tawfik, L. 2003. Soap, Sweetness, and Revenge: Patterns of Sexual Onset and Partnerships Amidst AIDS in Rural Southern Malawi. Ph.D. Dissertation, Bloomberg School of Public Health, Johns Hopkins University, Baltimore, MD.

Tawfik, L., and S. C. Watkins. 2007. "Sex in Geneva, Sex in Lilongwe, Sex in Balaka." *Social Science and Medicine* 64(5): 1090–101.

Temmerman, M., A. Quaghebeur, F. Mwanyumba, and K. Mandaliya. 2003. "Mother-to-Child HIV Transmission in Resource Poor Settings: How to Improve Coverage?" *AIDS* 17(8): 1239–42.

Thior, I., S. Lockman, L. M. Smeaton, R. L. Shapiro, C. Wester, S. J. Heymann, P. B. Gilbert, L. Stevens, T. Peter, S. Kim, E. van Widenfelt, C. Moffat, P. Ndase, P. Arimi, P. Kebaabetswe, P. Mazonde, J. Makhema, K. McIntosh, V. Novitsky, T. H. Lee, R. Marlink, S. Lagakos, and M. Essex; Mashi Study Team. 2006. "Breastfeeding Plus Infant Zidovudine Prophylaxis for 6 Months vs. Formula Feeding Plus Infant Zidovudine for 1 Month to Reduce Mother-to-Child HIV Transmission in Botswana: A Randomized Trial: The MASHI Study." *JAMA* 296(7): 794–805.

Thirumurthy, H., J. Graff Zivin, and M. Goldstein. 2008. "The Economic Impact of AIDS Treatment: Labor Supply in Western Kenya." *Journal of Human Resources* 43(3): 511–52.

Thomas, D., and J. Strauss. 1997. "Health and Wages: Evidence on Men and Women in Urban Brazil." *Journal of Econometrics* 77(1): 159–86.

Thornton, R. 2005. The Demand for and Impact of Learning HIV Status: Evidence from a Field Experiment. Southern African Regional Poverty Network.

———. 2008. "The Demand for, and Impact of, Learning HIV Status." *American Economic Review* 98(5): 1829–63.

Thurlow, J., J. Gow, and G. George. 2009. "HIV/AIDS, Growth and Poverty in KwaZulu-Natal and South Africa: An Integrated Survey, Demographic and Economy-wide Analysis." *Journal of the International AIDS Society* 12(1): 18.

Tibaijuka, A. K. 1997. "AIDS and Economic Welfare in Peasant Agriculture: Case Studies from Kagabiro Village, Kagera Region, Tanzania." *World Development* 25(6): 963–75.

Timaeus, I. M., and T. Boler. 2007. "Father Figures: The Progress at School of Orphans in South Africa." *AIDS* 21(Suppl. 7): S83–93.

*Times of Zambia.* 2005. "Can Speed Limiters Curb Road Carnage?" Available at: http://www.times.co.zm/news/viewnews.cgi?category=8&id=1169892128

Topouzis, D. 2000. Measuring the Impacts of HIV/AIDS on the Agricultural Sector in Africa. UNAIDS Best Practice collection, Geneva.

Topouzis, D., and J. du Guerny. 1999. Sustainable Agricultural/Rural Development and Vulnerability to the AIDS Epidemic. UNAIDS and Food and Agriculture Organization (FAO), Rome.

Tortora, R. D. 2008. Sub-Saharan Africans Rank the Millennium Development Goals (MDGs). Available at: http://www.gallup.com/poll/116116/sub-saharan-africans-rank-mdgs.aspx

Totin, D., C. Ndugwa, F. Mmiro, R. T. Perry, J. B. Jackson, and R. D Semba. 2002. "Iron Deficiency Anemia Is Highly Prevalent among Human Immunodeficiency Virus–Infected and Uninfected Infants in Uganda." *Journal of Nutrition* 132: 423–9.

Tovanabutra, S., V. Robison, J. Wongtrakul, S. Sennum, V. Suriyanon, D. Kingkeow, S. Kawichai, P. Tanan, A. Duerr, and K. E. Nelson. 2002. "Male Viral Load and Heterosexual Transmission of HIV-1 Subtype E in Northern Thailand." *Journal of Acquired Immune Deficiency Syndromes* 29(3): 275–83.

Townsend, R. M. 1994. "Risk and Insurance in Village India." *Econometrica* 62(3): 539–91.

Transparency International. http://www.transparency.org/

Tsai, A. C., M. Chopra, P. M. Pronyk, and N. A. Martinson. 2009. "Socioeconomic Disparities in Access to HIV/AIDS Treatment Programs in Resource-Limited Settings." *AIDS Care* 21(1): 59–63.

Tuchman, B. 1979. *A Distant Mirror: The Calamitous 14th Century*. Harmondsworth: Penguin.

Tunthanathip, P., R. Lolekha, L. J. Bollen, A. Chaovavanich, U. Siangphoe, C. Nandavisai, O. Suksripanich, P. Sirivongrangson, A. Wiratchai, Y. Inthong, B. Eampokalap, J. Ausavapipit, P. Akarasewi, and K. K. Fox. 2009. "Indicators for Sexual HIV Transmission Risk among People in Thailand Attending HIV Care: The Importance of Positive Prevention." *Sexually Transmitted Infections* 85(1): 36–41.

UN (United Nations). 2001. *Declaration of Commitment on HIV/AIDS*. Available at: http://www.un.org/ga/aids/docs/aress262.pdf

UNAIDS (Joint United Nations Programme on HIV/AIDS). 1998a. AIDS and the Military: UNAIDS Point of View. UNAIDS Best Practice Collection. Available at: http://data.unaids.org/Publications/IRC-pub05/militarypv_en.pdf.

———. 1998b. Report of the Global HIV/AIDS Epidemic. UNAIDS/WHO, Geneva.

———. 1999. A Review of Household and Community Responses to the HIV/AIDS Epidemic in the Rural Areas of Sub-Saharan Africa. Geneva.

———. 2000. Evaluation of the 100% Condom Programme in Thailand: UNAIDS Case Study. Available at: http://data.unaids.org/Publications/IRC-pub01/JC275-100pCondom_en.pdf

———. 2004a. 2004 Report on the Global AIDS Epidemic. Available at: http://www.unaids.org/bangkok2004/GAR2004_pdf/UNAIDSGlobalReport2004_en.pdf

———. 2004b. Policy Statement on HIV Testing. Information note. Available at: http://data.unaids.org/una-docs/hivtestingpolicy_en.pdf

———. 2005a. AIDS Epidemic Update. Geneva, November.

———. 2005b. Evidence for HIV Decline in Zimbabwe: A Comprehensive Review of the Epidemiological Data. Available at: http://data.unaids.org/publications/irc-pub06/zimbabwe_epi_report_nov05_en.pdf

———. 2006a. 2006 Report on the Global AIDS Epidemic. Available at: http://www.unaids.org/en/HIV_data/2006GlobalReport/default.asp

———. 2006b. AIDS Epidemic Update. Geneva, November.

———. 2007a. AIDS Epidemic Update: December 2007. Geneva.

———. 2007b. Global HIV Prevalence Has Levelled Off; AIDS is among the Leading Causes of Death Globally and Remains the Primary Cause of Death in Africa. Geneva.

———. 2008a. 2008 Report on the Global AIDS Epidemic. Geneva: UNAIDS. Available at: http://www.unaids.org/en/KnowledgeCentre/HIVData/GlobalReport/2008/2008_Global_report.asp

———. 2008b. Annual Estimates of HIV Prevalence, People Living with HIV/AIDS, and HIV/AIDS-related Deaths, 1990–2007. (Released in conjunction with UNAIDS (2008a), obtained from UNAIDS website in October 2008). Geneva: UNAIDS.

———. 2008c. Unified Budget and Workplan 2008–09. Available at: http://data.unaids.org:80/pub/BaseDocument/2007/2008_2009_ubw_en.pdf

———. 2009a. AIDS Epidemic Update. UNAIDS, Geneva.

———. 2009b. What Countries Need: Investments Needed for 2010 Targets. Available at: http://data.unaids.org/pub/Report/2009/20090210__investments_needed_2010_en.pdf

UNAIDS (Joint United Nations Programme on HIV/AIDS), UNFPA (United Nations Fund for Population), and UNIFEM (United Nations Development Fund for Women). 2004. *Women and HIV/AIDS: Confronting the Crisis*. Geneva and New York.

UNAIDS (The Joint United Nations Programme on HIV/ AIDS) and WHO (World Health Organization). 1998. AIDS Epidemic Update (December). UNAIDS/WHO, Geneva.

UNDP (United Nations Development Programme). 2008. *Human Development Report 2007/2008*. New York: UNDP.

UNECA (United Nations Economic Commission for Africa), Southern Africa Office. 2003. Land Tenure Systems and Sustainable Development in Southern Africa. Available at: http://www.uneca.org/eca_resources/Publications/srdcs/Land_Tenure_Systems_and _sustainable_Development_in_Southern_Africa.pdf

UNGASS (United Nations General Assembly Special Session). 2008. UNGASS Country Progress Report.

UNICEF (United Nations Children's Fund). 2004. *The State of the World's Children 2005: Childhood Under Threat*. Available at: http://www.unicef.org/sowc05/english/sowc 05.pdf

United Nations Economic and Social Council. 2005. The Flow of Financial Resources for Assisting in the Implementation of the Programmes of Action of the International Conference on Population and Development, Report of the Secretary-General. Commission on Population and Development, 38th Session, April 4–8, 2005. Available at: http://www.resourceflows.org/index.php?module=uploads&func=download&fileI d=89

United Nations Population Division. 2009a. *World Population Prospects: The 2008 Revision – Highlights*. New York: United Nations.

———.2009b. World Population Prospects: The 2008 Revision Population Database. New York: United Nations.

United Nations Security Council. 2000. Resolution 1308 on the Responsibility of the Security Council in the Maintenance of International Peace and Security: HIV/AIDS and International Peacekeeping Operations. S/Res/1308, July 17.

United Nations System in Malawi. 2001. UN Common Country Assessment of Malawi. Lilongwe, Malawi: United Nations System in Malawi. Available at: http://www.undg .org/archive_docs/1676-Malawi_CCA_-_Malawi_2001.pdf

United States Leadership Against HIV/AIDS, Tuberculosis, and Malaria Act of 2003. Public Law 108- 25, 108th Cong., 1st sess.

Urassa, M., J. T. Boerma, R. Isingo, J. Ngalula, J. Ng'weshemi, G. Mwaluko, and B. Zaba. 2001. "The Impact of HIV/AIDS on Mortality and Household Mobility in Rural Tanzania." *AIDS* 15(15): 2017–23.

U.S. Government. 2007. About PEPFAR. Available at: http://www.pepfar.gov/about. 9-28-0007.

USAID (U.S. Agency for International Development). 2002. *"ABCs" of HIV Prevention: Report of a USAID Technical Meeting on Behavior Change Approaches to Primary Prevention of HIV/AIDS*. Washington, DC: USAID.

USAID Bureau for Democracy, Conflict and Humanitarian Assistance, Office of Food for Peace (FFP), and the U.S. President's Emergency Plan for AIDS Relief (PEPFAR). 2007. USAID P.L. 480 Title II Food Aid Programs and the President's Emergency Plan for Aids Relief: HIV and Food Security Conceptual Framework. Washington, DC: USAID.

Usdin, S., E. Scheepers, S. Goldstein, and G. Japhet. 2005. "Achieving Social Change on Gender-Based Violence: A Report on the Impact Evaluation of Soul City's Fourth Series." *Social Science and Medicine* 61(11): 2434–45.

van Dalen, H. P., and M. Reuser. 2008. "Aid and AIDS: A Delicate Cocktail." Available at: http://www.voxeu.org

van der Straten, A., R. King, O. Grinstead, E. Vittinghoff, A. Serufilira, and S. Allen. 1998. "Sexual Coercion, Physical Violence, and HIV Infection among Women in Steady Relationships in Kigali, Rwanda." *AIDS and Behavior* 2(1): 61–73.

Ventelou, B., J. P. Moatti, Y. Videau, and M. Kazatchkine. 2008. "'Time is Costly': Modelling the Macroeconomic Impact of Scaling-up Antiretroviral Treatment in Sub-Saharan Africa." *AIDS* 22(1): 107–13.

Vernazza, P. L., J. R. Dyer, S. A. Fiscus, J. J. Eron, and M. S. Cohen. 1997. "HIV-1 Viral Load in Blood, Semen and Saliva." *AIDS* 11(8): 1058–9.

Vernazza, P. L., B. Hirschel, E. Bernasconi, and M. Flepp. 2008. "HIV Transmission under Highly Active Antiretroviral Therapy." *Lancet* 372(9652): 1806–7; author reply 1807.

Verweel, G., A. M. Van Rossum, N. G. Hartwig, T. F. Wolfs, H. J. Scherpbier, and R. de Groot. 2002. "Treatment with Highly Active Antiretroviral Therapy in Human Immunodeficiency Virus Type 1–infected Children Is Associated with a Sustained Effect on Growth." *Pediatrics* 109(2): e25–31.

Voluntary HIV-1 Counseling and Testing Efficacy Study Group. 2000. "Efficacy of HIV-1 Counselling and Testing in Individuals and Couples in Kenya, Tanzania, and Trinidad: A Randomised Trial." *Lancet* 356(9224): 103–12.

Walensky, R. P., L. L. Wolf, R. Wood, M. O. Fofana, K. A. Freedberg, N. A. Martinson, A. D. Paltiel, X. Anglaret, and M. C. Weinst. 2009. "When to Start Antiretroviral Therapy in Resource-limited Settings." *Annals of Internal Medicine* 151(3): 157–66.

Walker, A. S., V. Mulenga, F. Sinyinza, K. Lishimpi, A. Nunn, C. Chintu, and D. M. Gibb; CHAP Trial Team. 2006. "Determinants of Survival without Antiretroviral Therapy after Infancy in HIV-1-infected Zambian Children in the CHAP Trial." *Journal of Acquired Immune Deficiency Syndromes* 42(5): 637–45.

Wanke, C. A., M. Silva, T. A. Knox, J. Forrester, D. Spiegelman, and S. L. Gorbach. 2000. "Weight Loss and Wasting Remain Common Complications in Individuals Infected with Human Immunodeficiency Virus in the Era of Highly Active Antiretroviral Therapy." *Clinical Infectious Diseases* 31(3): 803–8.

Watkins, S. C. 1993. "If All We Knew About Women Was What We Read in *Demography*, What Would We Know?" *Demography* 30(4): 551–77.

———. 2004. "Navigating the HIV/AIDS Epidemic in Rural Malawi." *Population and Development Review* 30(4): 673–705.

Watkins, S. C., N. Rutenberg, and D. Wilkinson. 1997. Orderly Theories, Disorderly Women. In *The Continuing Demographic Transition*, ed. G. W. Jones, R. M. Douglas, J. C. Caldwell, and R. M. D'Souza, 213–45. Oxford: Clarendon Press.

Watkins, S. C., and A. Swidler. 2009. "Conversations Into Texts: A Method for Studying Public Culture." *Poetics* 37(2): 162–184.

Wawer, M. J., R. Gray, D. Serwadda, Z. Namukwaya, F. Sewankambo, X. Ki, T. Lutalo, F. Nalugoda, and T. Quinn. 2005a. Declines in HIV Prevalence in Uganda: Not as Simple as ABC. Paper presented at the 12th Conference on Retroviruses and Opportunistic Infections, Boston, February 22–25, 2005.

Wawer, M. J., R. H. Gray, N. K. Sewankambo, D. Serwadda, X. Li, O. Laeyendecker, N. Kiwanuka, G. Kigozi, M. Kiddugavu, T. Lutalo, F. Nalugoda, F. Wabwire-Mangen, M. P. Meehan, and T. C. Quinn. 2005b. "Rates of HIV-1 Transmission per Coital Act, by Stage of HIV-1 Infection, in Rakai, Uganda." *Journal of Infectious Diseases* 191(9): 1403–9.

Wawer, M. J., F. Makumbi, G. Kigozi, D. Serwadda, S. Watya, F. Nalugoda, D. Buwembo, V. Ssempijja, N. Kiwanuka, L. H. Moulton, N. K. Sewankambo, S. J. Reynolds, T. C. Quinn, P. Opendi, B. Iga, R. Ridzon, O. Laeyendecker, and R. H. Gray. 2009. "Circumcision in HIV-infected Men and Its Effect on HIV Transmission to Female Partners in Rakai, Uganda: A Randomised Controlled Trial." *Lancet* 374(9685): 229–37.

Wawer, M. J., D. Serwadda, X. Li, T. C. Quinn, N. K. Sewankambo, N. Kiwanuka, G. Kigozi, and R. H. Gray. 2003. HIV-1 Transmission per Coital Act, by Stage of HIV Infection in the HIV+ Index Partner, in Discordant Couples, Rakai, Uganda. 10th Conference on Retroviruses and Opportunistic Infections, Boston, February 10–14, 2003.

Wawer, M. J., N. K. Sewankambo, D. Serwadda, T. C. Quinn, L. A. Paxton, N. Kiwanuka, F. Wabwire-Mangen, C. Li, T. Lutalo, F. Nalugoda, C. A. Gaydos, L. H. Moulton, M. O. Meehan, S. Ahmed, and R. H. Gray. 1999. "Control of Sexually Transmitted Diseases for AIDS Prevention in Uganda: A Randomized Community Trial." *Lancet* 353(9152): 525–35.

Wegbreit, J., S. Bertozzi, L. M. DeMaria, and N. S. Padian. 2006. "Effectiveness of HIV Prevention Strategies in Resource-poor Countries: Tailoring the Intervention to the Context." *AIDS* 20(9): 1217–35.

Weil, D. N. 2004. *Economic Growth*. Boston: Addison-Wesley.

———. 2007. "Accounting for the Effect of Health on Economic Growth." *Quarterly Journal of Economics* 122(3): 1265–306.

Weintrob, A., G. Grandits, B. Agan, A. Ganesan, N. Crum-Cianflone, S. Fraser, S. Patel, G. Wortmann, S. Wegner, and V. Marconi. 2008. Disparate Virologic Response to HAART between Ethnicities. 15th Conference on Retroviruses and Opportunistic Infections, Boston, February 3–6, 2008.

Weir, S. S., C. Morroni, N. Coetzee, J. Spencer, and J. T. Boerma. 2002. "A Pilot Study of a Rapid Assessment Method to Identify Places for AIDS Prevention in Cape Town, South Africa." *Sexually Transmitted Infections* 78(Suppl. 1): i106–13.

Weir, S. S., C. Pailman, X. Mahlalela, N. Coetzee, F. Meidany, and J. T. Boerma . 2003. "From People to Places: Focusing AIDS Prevention Efforts Where It Matters Most." *AIDS* 17(6): 895–903.

Weir, S. S., J. E. Tate, B. Zhusupov, and J. T. Boerma. 2004. "Where the Action Is: Monitoring Local Trends in Sexual Behaviour." *Sexually Transmitted Infections* 80(Suppl. 2): ii63–8.

Weiser, S. D., M. Heisler, K. Leiter, F. Percy-de Korte, S. Tlou, S. DeMonner, N. Phaladze, D. R. Bangsberg, and V. Iacopino. 2006. "Routine HIV Testing in Botswana: A Population-based Study on Attitudes, Practices, and Human Rights Concerns." *PLoS Medicine* 3(7): e261.

Weiss, H. A., D. Halperin, R. C. Bailey, R. J. Hayes, G. Schmid, and C. A. Hankins. 2008. "Male Circumcision for HIV Prevention: From Evidence to Action?" *AIDS* 22(5): 567–74.

Weiss, H. A., M. A. Quigley, and R. J. Hayes. 2000. "Male Circumcision and Risk of HIV Infection in Sub-Saharan Africa: A Systematic Review and Meta-analysis." *AIDS* 14(15): 2361–70.

Were, W., J. Mermin, R. Bunnell, J. P. Ekwaru, and F. Kaharuza. 2003. "Home-based Model for HIV Voluntary Counselling and Testing." *Lancet* 361(9368): 1569.

Westercamp, N., and R. C. Bailey. 2007. "Acceptability of Male Circumcision for Prevention of HIV/AIDS in Sub-Saharan Africa: A Review." *AIDS and Behavior* 11(3): 341–55.

Wheeler, D. A., C. L. Gilbert, C. A. Launer, N. Muurahainen, R. A. Elion, D. I. Abrams, and G. E. Bartsch. 1998. "Weight Loss as a Predictor of Survival and Disease Progression in HIV Infection." *Journal of Acquired Immune Deficiency Syndromes* 18(1): 80–5.

When To Start Consortium, J. A. Sterne, M. May, D. Costagliola, F. de Wolf, A. N. Phillips, R. Harris, M. J. Funk, R. B. Geskus, J. Gill, F. Dabis, J. M. Miró, A. C. Justice, B. Ledergerber, G. Fätkenheuer, R. S. Hogg, A. D. Monforte, M. Saag, C. Smith, S. Staszewski, M. Egger, and S. R. Cole. 2009. "Timing of Initiation of Antiretroviral Therapy in AIDS-free HIV-1-Infected Patients: A Collaborative Analysis of 18 HIV Cohort Studies." *Lancet* 373(9672): 1352–63.

White, P. 2007. Improving Parameter Estimation, Projection Methods, Uncertainty Estimation, and Epidemic Classification: Report of a Meeting of the UNAIDS Reference

Group on Estimates, Modelling and Projections held in Prague, Czech Republic, Nov. 29–Dec. 1, 2006.

Whiteside, A., A. de Waal, and T. Gebretensae. 2006. "AIDS, Security and the Military in Africa: A Sober Appraisal." *African Affairs* 105(419): 201–18.

Whiteside, A., and A. Whalley. 2007. *Reviewing 'Emergencies' for Swaziland: Shifting the Paradigm for a New Era*. Durban: Health Economics and HIV/AIDS Research Division.

WHO (World Health Organization). 1995. Physical Status: The Use and Interpretation of Anthropometry. Report of a WHO Expert Committee. World Health Organization Technical Report Series No. 854: 1–452.

———. 2001. Global Burden of Disease (GBD) 2001 Estimates. Available at: http://www.who.int/healthinfo/global_burden_disease/estimates_regional_2001/en/index.html

———. 2003a. *HIV and Infant Feeding: Framework for Priority Action*. Geneva: WHO.

———. 2003b. *Scaling Up Anti-retroviral Therapy in Resource-limited Settings: Treatment Guidelines for a Public Health Approach*. Geneva, Switzerland: World Health Organization. Available at: http://www.who.int/3by5/publications/documents/arv_guidelines/en/index.html

———. 2004a. Death and DALY Estimates for 2002 by Cause for WHO Member States. Geneva: WHO. Available at: http://www.who.int/healthinfo/global_burden_disease/en/

———. 2004b. *Experiences of 100% Condom Use Programme in Selected Countries of Asia*. Manila, Philippines: WHO, Regional Office for the Western Pacific. Available at: http://www.wpro.who.int/NR/rdonlyres/CDB9792C-3815-44CD-A285-6D28BA88298E/0/100_condom_program_experience.pdf

———. 2004c. *National AIDS Programmes: A Guide to Indicators for Monitoring and Evaluating National HIV/AIDS Prevention Programs for Young People*. Geneva: WHO.

———. 2006a. HIV and Infant Feeding: Update Based on the Technical Consultation Held on Behalf of the Inter-agency Task Team (IATT) on Prevention of HIV Infection in Pregnant Women, Mothers and their Infants. Geneva, October 25–27, 2006. Geneva: WHO.

———. 2006b. *Technical Consultation on the Integration of HIV Interventions into Maternal, Newborn and Child Health Services*. Geneva: WHO.

———. 2007. Scaling Up for Better Health in Cambodia: A Country Case Study for the World Health Organization in Follow-up to the High-Level Forum on the Health Millennium Development Goals. Available at: http://www.who.int/healthsystems/strategy/scaling-up_better_health_Cambodia.pdf

———. 2008a. Effective Aid: Better Health. 3rd High Level Forum on Aid Effectiveness. Accra, Ghana. September 2–4, 2008. Available at: http://www.who.int/hdp/publications/effectiveaid_betterhealth_en.pdf

———. 2008b. *The Global Burden of Disease: 2004 Update*. Geneva: WHO.

———. 2008c. Report on the Expert Global Consultation on Positive Synergies between Health Systems and Global Health Initiatives. Geneva, May 29–30, 2008.

———. 2008d. Task Shifting: Rational Redistribution of Tasks among Health Workforce Teams: Global Recommendations and Guidelines. Available at: http://www.who.int/healthsystems/TTR-TaskShifting.pdf

———. 2008e. World Health Statistics. Available at: http://www.who.int/whosis/whostat/2008/en/index.html

———. 2010. *Guidelines on HIV and Infant Feeding. Principles and recommendations for infant feeding in the context of HIV and a summary of evidence*. Geneva: WHO.

WHO-CHOICE. Choice = Choosing Interventions that are Cost Effective. Available at: http://www.who.int/choice/en/

WHO (World Health Organization), UNAIDS, and UNICEF (United Nations Fund for Children). 2009. Towards Universal Access – Scaling up Priority HIV/AIDS Interventions in the Health Sector – 2009 Progress Report. Geneva: WHO.

WHO (World Health Organization), UNAIDS (The Joint United Nations Programme on HIV/AIDS), UNICEF (United Nations Children's Fund), and UNFPA (United Nations Population Fund). 2008. HIV Transmission through Breastfeeding: A Review of Available Evidence. 2007 Update. Geneva: WHO.

Williams, B. G., D. Taljaard, C. M. Campbell, E. Gouws, L. Ndhlovu, J. Van Dam, M. Caraël, and B. Auvert. 2003. "Changing Patterns of Knowledge, Reported Behaviour and Sexually Transmitted Infections in a South African Gold Mining Community." *AIDS* 17(14): 2099–107.

Wilson, D. 2009. Correspondence on Granich, R. M., et al., "Universal Voluntary HIV Testing with Immediate Antiretroviral Therapy as a Strategy for Elimination of HIV Transmission: A Mathematical Model." *Lancet* 373(9669): 1077–8.

WLSA (Women and Law in Southern Africa). 1997. *The Changing Family in Zambia.* Women and Law in Southern Africa Trust, Lusaka, Zambia.

Wood, R., and S. D. Lawn. 2009. "Should the CD4 Threshold for Starting ART Be Raised?" *Lancet* 373(9672): 1314–6.

Wools-Kaloustian, K., S. Kimaiyo, L. Diero, A. Siika, J. Sidle, C. T. Yiannoutsos, B. Musick, R. Einterz, K. H. Fife, and W. M. Tierney. 2006. "Viability and Effectiveness of Large-scale HIV Treatment Initiatives in Sub-Saharan Africa: Experience from Western Kenya." *AIDS* 20(1): 41–8.

Wools-Kaloustian, K., S. Kimaiyo, B. Musick, J. Sidle, A. Siika, W. Nyandiko, R. Einterz, W. M. Tierney, and C. T. Yiannoutsos . 2009. "The Impact of the President's Emergency Plan for AIDS Relief on Expansion of HIV Care Services for Adult Patients in Western Kenya." *AIDS* 23(2): 195–201.

World Bank. 1999. *Confronting AIDS: Public Priorities in a Global Epidemic,* Rev. Edition. New York: Oxford University Press.

———. 2005. Committing to Results: Improving the Effectiveness of HIV/AIDS Assistance. Operations Evaluation Department. Available at: http://www.worldbank.org/oed/aids/?intcmp=5221495

———. 2006a. Disease Control Priorities Project. The Burden of Disease and Mortality by Condition: Data, Methods, and Results for 2001. Available at: http://www.dcp2.org/pubs/GBD/3/Table/3.B1

———. 2006b. Poverty and Vulnerability Assessment: Investing in Our Future. World Bank Report No. 36546-MW, World Bank, Washington, DC.

———. 2007. *HIV/AIDS, Nutrition, and Food Security: What We Can Do. A Synthesis of International Guidance.* Washington, DC: World Bank.

———. 2008a. World Bank Indicators Database. Washington, DC: World Bank.

———. 2008b. *World Development Indicators 2008.* World Bank, Washington, DC.

Wouters, E., H. Meulemans, H. C. Van Rensburg, J. C. Heunis, and D. Mortelmans. 2007. "Short-term Physical and Emotional Health Outcomes of Public Sector ART in the Free State Province of South Africa." *Quality of Life Research* 16(9): 1461–71.

Xia, Q., F. Molitor, D. H. Osmond, M. Tholandi, L. M. Pollack, J. D. Ruiz, and J. A. Catania. 2006. "Knowledge of Sexual Partner's HIV Serostatus and Serosorting Practices in a California Population-based Sample of Men Who Have Sex with Men." *AIDS* 20(16): 2081–9.

Xiridou, M., R. Geskus, J. de Wit, R. Coutinho, and M. Kretzschmar. 2004. "Primary HIV Infection as Source of HIV Transmission within Steady and Casual Partnerships among Homosexual Men." *AIDS* 18(9): 1311–20.

Yamano, T., and T. S. Jayne. 2004. "Measuring the Impacts of Working-Age Adult Mortality on Small-Scale Farm Households in Kenya." *World Development* 32(1): 91–119.

Yamano, T., and T. S. Jayne. 2005. "Working-Age Adult Mortality and Primary School Attendance in Rural Kenya." *Economic Development and Cultural Change* 53(3): 619–53.

Yamauchi, F., T. Buthelezi, and M. Velia. 2008. "Impacts of Prime-Age Adult Mortality on Labour Supply: Evidence from Adolescents and Women in South Africa." *Oxford Bulletin of Economics and Statistics* 70(3): 375–98.

Yeager, R., C. Hendrix, and S. Kingma. 2000. "International Military Human Immunodeficiency Virus/Acquired Immunodeficiency Syndrome Policies and Programs: Strengths and Limitations in Current Practice." *Military Medicine* 165(2): 87–92.

Youde, J. 2001. All the Voters Will Be Dead: HIV/AIDS and Democratic Legitimacy and Stability in Africa. International Foundation for Election Systems, Washington, DC.

Young, A. 2005. "The Gift of the Dying: The Tragedy of AIDS and the Welfare of Future African Generations." *Quarterly Journal of Economics* 120(2): 423–66.

———. 2007. "In Sorrow to Bring Forth Children: Fertility Amidst the Plague of HIV." *Journal of Economic Growth* 12(4): 283–327.

Yu, J. K., S. C. Chen, K. Y. Wang, C. S. Chang, S. D. Makombe, E. J. Schouten, and A. D. Harries. 2007. "True Outcomes for Patients on Antiretroviral Therapy Who Are 'Lost to Follow-up' in Malawi." *Bulletin of the World Health Organization* 85(7): 550–4.

Zaba, B., E. Pisani, E. Slaymaker, and J. T. Boerma. 2004. "Age at First Sex: Understanding Recent Trends in African Demographic Surveys." *Sexually Transmitted Infections* 80(Suppl. 2): ii28–35.

Zablotska, I. B., G. Prestage, A. E. Grulich, and J. Imrie. 2008. "Differing Trends in Sexual Risk Behaviours in Three Australian States: New South Wales, Victoria and Queensland, 1998–2006." *Sexual Health* 5(2): 125–30.

Zachariah, R., M. Fitzgerald, M. Massaquoi, O. Pasulani, L. Arnould, S. Makombe, and A. D. Harries. 2006. "Risk Factors for High Early Mortality in Patients on Antiretroviral Treatment in a Rural District of Malawi." *AIDS* 20(18): 2355–60.

Zachariah, R., M. P. Spielmann, A. D. Harries, and F. M. Salaniponi. 2002. "Moderate to Severe Malnutrition in Patients with Tuberculosis is a Risk Factor Associated with Early Death." *Transactions of the Royal Society for Tropical Medicine and Hygiene* 96(3): 291–4.

Zimbabwe and Macro International, Inc. Central Statistical Office. 2007. *Zimbabwe Demographic and Health Survey 2005–06.* Calverton, Maryland.

# CONTRIBUTORS

✕✕✕✕✕✕

**Kathleen Beegle** is a senior economist in the Development Research Group at the World Bank. Her research interest includes the measurement of poverty dynamics, socioeconomic dimensions of HIV/AIDS in sub-Saharan Africa, and methods in household survey data collection. Some of her current work includes studies of coping strategies among households in Tanzania using a 19-year longitudinal survey and a study of marriage transitions and HIV in Malawi based on a new panel survey of young adults. As member of the World Bank Living Standards Measurement Study (LSMS) team, she has expertise in the design and implementation of household survey operations and use of household surveys for poverty and policy analysis. She received her Ph.D. in Economics from Michigan State University in 1997 and worked at RAND from 1997–2001 before joining the World Bank.

**Antony Chapoto** is an assistant professor with the Department of Agricultural Economics at Michigan State University and currently associated with the Food Security Research Project in Zambia as the Research Coordinator. He holds a Ph.D. in Agricultural Economics from Michigan State University, a Masters degree in Agricultural Economics from University of Zimbabwe, and a Bachelors degree in Agriculture and Natural Resources from Africa University, Zimbabwe. His current research and professional interests include: grain marketing development in Africa; strategies to reduce the instability of food supply and consumption, involving marketing and regional trade policy; understanding the effects of HIV/AIDS on rural livelihoods and its implications on AIDS mitigation and poverty reduction strategies; and analysis of food system organization and performance in sub-Saharan Africa

**Alex de Waal** is a program director of the Social Science Research Council, a senior fellow of the Harvard Humanitarian Initiative, and a director of Justice Africa in London. He received his D.Phil. in social anthropology from Oxford University in 1988 and has written or edited thirteen books. Among them are, *Famine that Kills: Darfur, Sudan, 1984-1985* (Clarendon Press, 1989); *Facing Genocide: The Nuba of Sudan* (African Rights, 1995); *Famine Crimes: Politics and the Disaster Relief Industry in Africa* (James Currey, 1997); *AIDS and Power: Why There is No Political Crisis—Yet* (Zed, 2006); and with Julie Flint, *Darfur: A New History of a Long War* (revised edition, Zed, 2008). He has served as adviser to the African Union mediation team for the Darfur peace talks (2005—06) and the African Union High-Level Panel on Darfur (2009). He was awarded an OBE in the New Year's Honors List of 2009.

**Damien de Walque** is a senior economist in the Development Research Group (Human Development and Public Services Team) at the World Bank. He received his Ph.D. in Economics from the University of Chicago in 2003. His research interests include health and education and the interactions between them. He is working on evaluating the impact of HIV/AIDS interventions and policies in several African countries. He also develops a research agenda focusing on the analysis of the long-term consequences of mortality crises and on the health and educational outcomes of orphans and vulnerable children.

**Roger England** held senior research positions in health care including medical schools and secondments to the World Health Organization and to the World Bank. He created and directed HLSP (and the HLSP Institute), now one of the world's most experienced private providers of expertise in health systems, public health, aid effectiveness, and sector financing. His first-hand experience in design and implementation of health reform and strengthening covers over 25 countries. HLSP is now incorporated into the global, multidisciplinary Mott MacDonald Group, and Roger has established Health Systems Workshop (HSW), a small non-profit organization providing independent research and comment on issues in international health. HSW also runs http://www.healthstudentnetwork.org, an interactive online meeting and discussion platform for health students and practitioners interested in international health issues.

**Peter Glick** is a senior economist at the RAND Corporation. His research has considered the determinants of HIV-related knowledge and behaviors in Africa, the efficacy of HIV/AIDS prevention interventions, and the impacts of antiretroviral therapy on patient well being and risk behavior in Uganda. He has also undertaken research on the quality of health care and health care demand, on the determinants of child undernutrition and mortality, and on topics such as schooling, gender inequality, and employment and earnings in developing countries. Dr. Glick has consulted on these issues for a range of organizations, including the World Bank, USAID, the Millennium Challenge Corporation, the United Nations Development Programme, and the African Development Bank. He received his Ph.D. in Economics from the American University.

**Markus Goldstein** is a development economist with experience working in sub-Saharan Africa, East Asia, and South Asia. He is currently a senior economist in the Africa Region of the World Bank and in the Poverty and Inequality Group of the Development Economics Research Group, where he works on issues of poverty and gender. His research interests include agriculture, HIV/AIDS, intra-household allocation, risk, poverty measurement, public services, and land tenure. Markus has taught at the London School of Economics, the University of Ghana, Legon, and Georgetown University. He holds a Ph.D. from the University of California, Berkeley.

**Markus Haacker** is a growth and development economist based in London. He holds a Ph.D. in Economics from the London School of Economics. From 1999–2008, he worked at the International Monetary Fund (IMF), mainly at the African Department. Since 2008, he has been an honorary lecturer at the London School of Hygiene and Tropical Medicine, and worked as a consultant to the World Bank. His research focuses on the areas of growth and development, and the intersections of macroeconomics, economic development, and health. Past work includes numerous publications on the macroeconomic and fiscal dimension of HIV/AIDS and HIV/AIDS programs (notably, *The Macroeconomics of HIV/AIDS*, published by the IMF), as well as several publications on the economic role of information and communication technologies in developing countries. For more information, visit http://mh.devgro.com.

**Suneetha Kadiyala** is a postdoctoral fellow in the Poverty, Health and Nutrition Division of the International Food Policy Research Institute (IFPRI). Her research portfolio focuses on HIV and AIDS, and food and nutrition security. She serves as a core member of the team responsible for the development and implementation of research, policy communications, and capacity strengthening activities of the Regional Network on AIDS Livelihoods and Food Security (RENEWAL), an initiative coordinated by IFPRI. She now co-leads the "HIV and Nutrition Security" research theme under RENEWAL. She is the author of several peer-reviewed publications on the subject of HIV/AIDS and food and nutrition security. She is also currently the South Asia focal point for the Agriculture and Health Research Platform, comprising 21 members from involved Consultative Group of International Agricultural Research Centers, WHO, FAO, and other partners. The Platform aims to promote and coordinate research on the linkages between agriculture, nutrition, and health, with the aim of alleviating livelihood and food insecurity through enhanced policy and program effectiveness. Suneetha has a Ph.D. in International Food Policy and Applied Nutrition from the School of Nutrition Science and Policy, Tufts University, Boston.

**Rachel Kline** completed a Master of Education, with a concentration in international education, at Harvard University and a Bachelor of Arts in History at the University of Pennsylvania. She taught high school Spanish at a New York City public school and then taught English in Lesotho, Southern Africa, as a Peace Corps volunteer. Her work as a Peace Corps volunteer included organizing HIV/ AIDS prevention activities for youth throughout the rural area where she lived. She has since worked on various projects related to HIV/AIDS as a consultant for the World Bank. In Lesotho, she worked with the Ministry of Education to set up and assess an orphan assistance program. She has also researched and co-written various reports and academic articles about Africa, on topics such as comparing condom use with different partners, the association between HIV and remarriage, and the response to HIV/AIDS in Lesotho.

**Mead Over** is a Senior Fellow at the Center for Global Development (CGD), where he works on issues related to the economics of efficient, effective, and cost-effective health interventions in developing countries. Prior to CGD, he was lead health economist in the Development Research Group of the World Bank. In addition to his work on the economics of the AIDS epidemic, he has contributed to the economic analysis of malaria and pandemic influenza and to the measurement and explanation of the efficiency of health service delivery in poor countries. His most recent book is entitled, *The Economics of Effective AIDS Treatment: Evaluating Policy Options for Thailand* (2006). He earned his Ph.D. in economics at the University of Wisconsin at Madison and has taught health economics, development economics, applied microeconomics, and econometrics at Williams College and Boston University.

**Elizabeth Pisani** is an independent consultant in infectious disease epidemiology and public health. She has a Ph.D. in epidemiology and has worked in HIV surveillance, prevention program planning, and program monitoring for more than a decade. She was closely involved in developing the WHO/UNAIDS guidelines for Second Generation HIV Surveillance, and has been active in developing methods for behavioral surveillance, population size estimation, data management, and program planning. Most of her work has been in support of Asian governments, including those of Indonesia, China, East Timor, and the Philippines. She is also author of a critically acclaimed book about HIV for non-specialists, entitled, *The Wisdom of Whores: Bureaucrats, Brothels and the Business of AIDS*. Recent research has focused on policies that encourage the sharing of research data and translation of data into policy.

**David E. Sahn** is a professor of economics at Cornell University in the Division of Nutritional Sciences and the Department of Economics. He received his Ph.D. from the Massachusetts Institute of Technology and a Masters of Public Health from the University of Michigan. Prior to coming to Cornell, he was an economist at the World Bank and a research fellow at the International Food Policy Research Institute. He also served as a visiting distinguished scholar at the International

Monetary Fund. Dr. Sahn has published widely on issues of poverty and inequality, and the economics of health and education. Dr. Sahn serves as a consultant to several international organizations and has also been actively engaged in advising various government policymakers, working to translate research findings into practical measures to improve the living standards of the poor.

**Harsha Thirumurthy** is an assistant professor of health economics in the Gillings School of Global Public Health at the University of North Carolina at Chapel Hill and a Faculty Fellow at the Carolina Population Center. He is currently on leave from UNC as an economist at the World Bank. He is also an Affiliate of the Bureau for Research and Economic Analysis of Development. He holds a Ph.D. in economics from Yale University. Dr. Thirumurthy's expertise is in development and health economics, with a focus on the evaluation of policies to combat HIV/AIDS in sub-Saharan Africa and South Asia. His research examines the impacts of health interventions on socioeconomic outcomes and also explores the determinants of health-related behavior; and he has experience in the design and implementation of household surveys in developing countries. In western Kenya, he has conducted an innovative longitudinal survey of HIV-affected households. Using these survey data, his research has documented the social and economic impacts of antiretroviral (ARV) treatment for people living with AIDS. Current research in Kenya, Uganda, and India explores how HIV/AIDS affects individuals' investment behavior and evaluates interventions to improve adherence to ARV treatment.

**Susan Cotts Watkins** received her doctorate in sociology from Princeton University. She has been on the faculty at Yale University and the University of Pennsylvania and is currently a visiting research scientist at the University of California at Los Angeles. With the support of a Guggenheim fellowship (2009–10), she is co-authoring a book with Ann Swidler on the consequences of altruism from afar, the attempts of western countries to stem the tide of the AIDS epidemic. Her work has focused on large-scale demographic and social change, specifically: (1) fertility transitions in historical Europe and the U.S. and in contemporary Africa; (2) the AIDS epidemic in Africa; (3) the role of social networks in these changes. Dr. Watkins and her colleagues have organized two longitudinal survey projects, one in Kenya (http://www.Kenya.pop.upenn.edu), and more recently, a larger project in Malawi, The Malawi Diffusion and Ideational Change Project (MDICP, 1998–present (http://www.malawi.pop.upenn.edu). A collaboration with the College of Medicine, University of Malawi, and Chancellor College, University of Malawi, the study investigates how individuals, couples, and families in rural Malawi are affected by HIV/AIDS, how they respond to the increased HIV/AIDS infection risks in terms of social interactions, sexual relations, and marriage, and how they cope with the consequences of increases in AIDS-related morbidity and mortality.